Great Men, Great Gyms of the Golden Age

By Dave Yarnell

Table of Contents

Introduction — pg 3

Chapter 1	Muscle Beach	pg 9
Chapter 2	More Culver City Secrets	pg 83
Chapter 3	the Dungeon	pg 131
Chapter 4	Gold's Gym	pg 233
Chapter 5	Abe Goldberg's NYC Gym	pg 287
Chapter 6	Bill Pearl's Gym	pg 306
Chapter 7	Vince's Gym	pg 335
Chapter 8	Yarick's Gym	pg 387
Chapter 9	Zuver's Gym	pg 405

Introduction

Most of the gyms we'll focus on here are in Southern California, which has been considered by many to be the "Mecca" of bodybuilding for many decades now. I could well argue that the east coast had a vital role in getting the barbell craze going in the first place, with Alan Calvert's Milo Barbell, Hoffman's York Barbell and Bernarr McFadden's influences in New York city, etc. My last book and some of my other earlier books focused on these aspects, so please don't think I have sold out on my east coast roots. It is just a fact that California has drawn many strength athletes, particularly the bodybuilding crowd for various reasons we will explore in depth here in this book. This Muscle Builder piece makes a nice intro to the book all by itself, I think, so here goes;

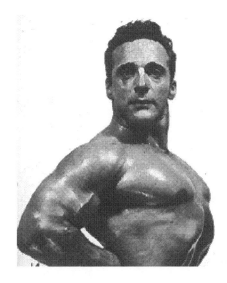

IS IT EASIER TO BUILD A PERFECT BODY IN CALIFORNIA?

Why is it that bodybuilders who leave the East for California make such sensational gains in muscularity and weight, and take top honors in physique contests? Is it the weather, diet, inspiration? What lessons can you learn from the experiences of these stars to use in your own training? Read article for important facts.

Would George Eiferman have become a star if he had stayed in the East? Article supplies answer. —LON.

By BEN WEIDER

TWO years ago he was a tall, well built young man with nothing outstanding about his development. He was big... yes. He had the possibilities... granted. But he was just another bodybuilder. *And then he went to California!* Almost overnight his physique began to take on new form. His shoulders broadened, thickened, became more muscular. His arms swelled into massive size and power. His thighs gained in bulk and muscularity. In 1953, he placed second in the Mr. America contest. In 1954, he won the top American bodybuilding title. Dick Dubois in two years had accomplished a weight-training miracle with the aid of that magic Californian atmosphere.

But is it magic? Is there some unknown, mysterious quality in the air of California and way of living, that makes new bodybuilding champions sprout up out of nowhere... overnight almost? And why are there so many superior examples of physical development in California; why do bodybuilders who move there from the East make such rapid and sensational gains? These are questions *(Continued on page 54)*

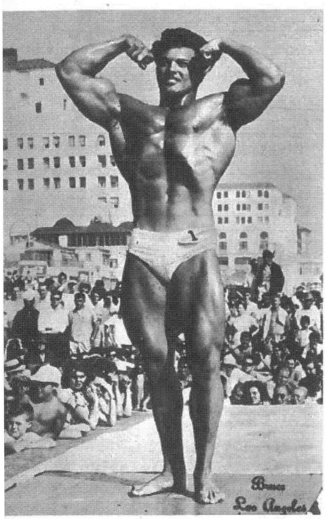

Eastern bodybuilder Dick Dubois was just a local contest winner, then he went to California, in 2 years won Mr. America title. —WARNER.

Within 6 months of going to California, statuesque Lou Degni had made such amazing improvement that he landed stage part with Mae West. —BRUCE.

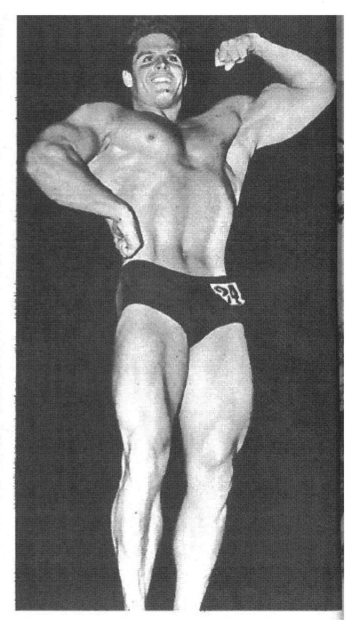

Feature Presentation

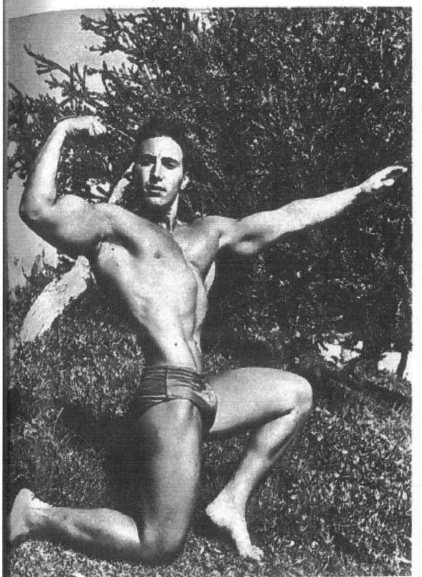

Dom Juliano, formerly of New York, another amazing example of the effects of Californian diet, climate, exercise, on Easterners. —DIXON.

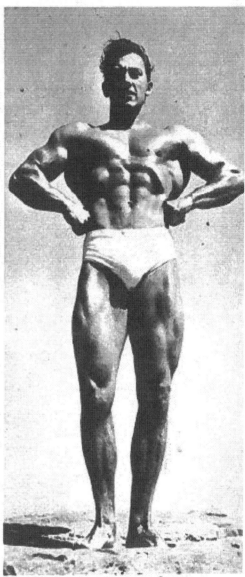

Once he made his home on West Coast, John Farbotnik scored triumph after triumph. SANDTNER.

Build A Perfect Body In California

(Continued from page 15)

which have long puzzled weight trainers all over North America.

First let me make this clear. I sincerely believe that what can be accomplished in California, can be accomplished anywhere else in America. All it amounts to is training as much as possible under conditions similar to those in the Golden Pacific State ... adapting as many of the training practices in use there, to conditions in the East. And yet this does not explain why such men as George Eiferman, Marvin Eder, Dick Dubois, Armand Tanny, John Farbotnik, Ludwig Shusterich, Dominick Juliano, Louis Degni and other stars hit their peak of physical perfection when they moved west.

The greatest asset California has is the climate. In the East the summer is comparatively short with an overwhelming proportion of cold, autumn and winter weather. In California there is a greater proportion of *warm* sunny days, while the temperature in the winter months is mild. Snow is seen once in a generation; a freezing temperature is a rarity. Consequently people in general lead an out-door life, spend more time on the beaches and are *more aware of the importance and attractiveness of a well developed body.*

As a result, there is greater enthusiasm for weight-training, and barbell equipped centers such as Muscle Beach, Venice Beach, and Manhattan Beach are provided for the public, where bodybuilders meet in large numbers, train, give exhibitions, provide instruction for beginners, and take part in contests which are seen not only by those interested in weight training, but by general members of the public. All this helps to promote bodybuilding, create training enthusiasm and provide *inspiration,* a quality without which nothing can be accomplished.

At these out-door training centers, there is a free exchange of bodybuilding ideas. Beginners can watch the Champions work-out, discuss training problems with them, establish friendly relationships with other enthusiasts and become encouraged to train more regularly. The friendships thus formed stimulate the sport even further.

The next greatest Californian bodybuilding asset is *food*. There is a greater variety of the *organic* food substances obtainable in California than in the East. The *sunshine* fruits such as lemons, limes, oranges, and grapefruits grow there in abundance. Sea food with its rich supply of organic phosphorus and mineral iodine is in lavish supply. Honey, dates, figs, raisins, and other energy foods are "dirt cheap." All these huge supplies of fruits are available at moderate prices, are grown in soil full of essential minerals and vitamins, and are literally "eaten-on-the-spot." The effects of such a diet on a bodybuilder need no explanation.

Let's get back to the climate again. In the Eastern and North Eastern States, as we have already pointed out, the proportion of cold months to hot months is in favor of cold temperatures. This means that Nature provides the individual with a sub-skin layer of fat, thus helping to protect him against the cold weather.

And it also indicates that in the East, bodybuilders have a hard time building muscular delineation. And in addition to this, there is a slowing down of activity, a lessening of training enthusiasm. Muscle stimulation is much tougher to produce. There is a greater proportion of sprains and strains, and regular progress is almost non-existent because of the lay-offs due to injuries incurred.

The third most important asset the Bodybuilding Game has in California is the number of gymnasiums. In one section of Hollywood, there are more bodybuilding gyms than there are in the whole of New York City. In the entire Hollywood and Los Angeles area there is a greater number of studios than there is along the entire Atlantic Seaboard.

In some Eastern towns, there are but two or three bodybuilders, who often train alone in a bedroom or garage gymnasium, unaware of the existence of others interested in bodybuilding in their area. This means that an understanding and appreciation of the sport is less, and the spirit of friendly competition totally lacking.

It is a fact that some Eastern States bodybuilders have never seen a Top Star outside the pages of Weider Publications, have never attended a physical excellence contest (one is held practically every week in California) and have yet to meet and discuss bodybuilding with a prominent model of Muscular Might. Is there any wonder that Bodybuilding in the East is not as strong in its organisation, and as productive of Bodybuilding Stars as California?

The fourth Californian Bodybuilding asset is the great variety of training equipment to be found in every studio. Every type of lat machine, wall pulley and floor pulley is accepted as commonplace. A gym would not be fully equipped without a leg press machine, decline bench, squat stands, leg curl and thigh extension bench. What studio in New York City for example, outside of Abe Goldberg's gym at 80 Clinton Street, has these pieces of apparatus? I cannot name at this moment, a single one.

Is there any wonder that the Golden State can turn out new Champions of Muscular form each year? Is there any wonder that Bodybuilding Stars of amazing power and proportion are regularly developed in California? With all the natural advantages, with all the training equipment at their disposal, with all the enthusiasm, friendship and exchange of ideas, it would be a crime, yes a *crime*, if none were produced.

Earlier on in this article I said that what could be done in California could also be accomplished in the East. And I remarked that all it amounted to was training under similar conditions and adapting West Coast training practices to conditions in the East.

First the Eastern weight trainer must stimulate his enthusiasm by making bodybuilding and good health habits part of his daily life. The first step he must take is to subscribe to *Muscle Builder* and *Muscle Power* magazines, so that he can be kept up-to-date on the latest bodybuilding studio equipped with every type of modern apparatus and teaching Weider Methods. If he lives in a suburban area and is unable to join a studio, then he must organise his own little training group among his friends, get others interested in bodybuilding by inviting them to take a work-out with him in his home-gym.

Next he must fully support the local AAU organisation, affiliate his club to that organisation, attend their committee meetings and see to it that more and more contests are run for lifters and bodybuilders. He should support every contest and make sure that as many members of his club enter as possible with the non-competing members lending additional support by attending as spectators in order to encourage those who have entered.

An Eastern bodybuilder should train hardest during the summer, making the most of the warmer temperatures, and working out whenever possible in the fresh-air. Every week end should be spent on the beach in the sun, getting an even coat of tan. Thus definition and proportion will be maintained, or improved, and a reserve fund of energy will be built up for the cold winter months when training enthusiasm is inclined to die down a little.

During the summer months every type of natural food should be eaten. All fresh fruits, salads and vegetables should be part of the daily diet, and at least a quart of milk drunk every 24 hours. During the winter months this diet should be maintained and added to by eating all dried fruits such as raisins, prunes, apricots, apples, pears, and peaches, also honey and such Weider Food Supplements as High Protein tablets, Vitamin-Mineral Food Supplements, and Energy Tablets. During winter training, the bodybuilder should *always* keep himself warm, wearing a track suit when taking a workout, and suitable clothing for normal activity.

In actual workout sessions the Eastern bodybuilder should make use of every conceivable type of equipment. If he doesn't train at a studio, then he should equip his home gym with Double Purpose Exercise Bench, the Multi-Power Exerciser our Multi-Muscle Bars and the Double Tension Krusher in order that he can use the modern training methods of the Californian gyms. If he does not have the ready cash to purchase the extra equipment, then the Weider Organization has a fine Time Payment plan to help him buy all the extra equipment and barbell plates he needs.

Next the Eastern Bodybuilder must follow only a *modern* training course, such as the *Weider Master Championship Course*. Then and then only can he be certain of physical progress and making the most of his potentials, and then only can *we* bring back the Star status of Bodybuilding to the East. And then Weight training will forge ahead and achieve a position that will see a Mr. America from the East crowned year after year. We can do it. Let's start NOW.

Chapter 1   Muscle Beach

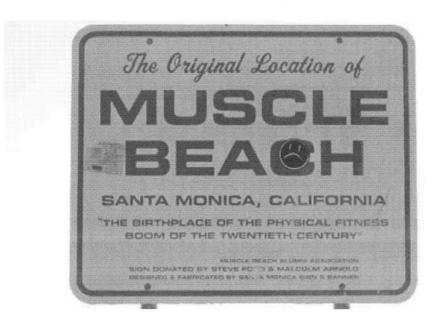

Ok, muscle beach is not exactly a gym, I get that. However, Muscle Beach has been a very important part of the fabric of the iron game in Southern California for so long; it can't possibly be overlooked in a book such as this one. There are so many ties between the various other gyms that we'll discuss here and the folks who trained at them and ran them, etc, that to leave out Muscle Beach would leave a gaping hole in the overall picture of the "golden era" and the times before that. One confusing aspect of the name is that there are really 2 distinct versions of Muscle Beach; the original one, in Santa Monica, and the latter one in Venice. These 2 are often referred to kind of interchangeably, but they were and are 2 separate & distinct locations. The original Muscle Beach was where Abbye "Pudgy" Stockton and her husband Les worked out, along with many other iron game luminaries of the time, having started in the 30s. To get a good overall glimpse of what the place was all about, you might care to read a little book by Marla Matzer Rose, called **"Muscle Beach, where the Best Bodies in the World started a Fitness Revolution"** I read and enjoyed the book and found it to be entertaining as well as informative.

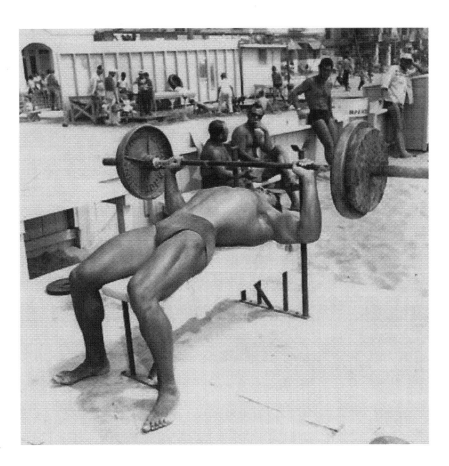

2 shots of the original MB

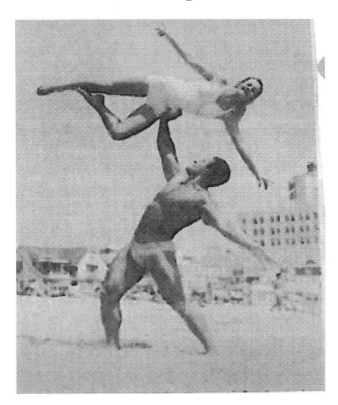

Here is an article from "Muscle Power" when the beach was going strong;

Muscle Power, Vol 7 No 5, Page 30, April 1949

Muscle Beach   by Gordon L'Allemand

Due to the great popularity that the first Muscle Beach article was received by "Your Physique" readers and the many letters asking for more information on Muscle Beach, the editors have decided to release this article to satisfy our reader's requests

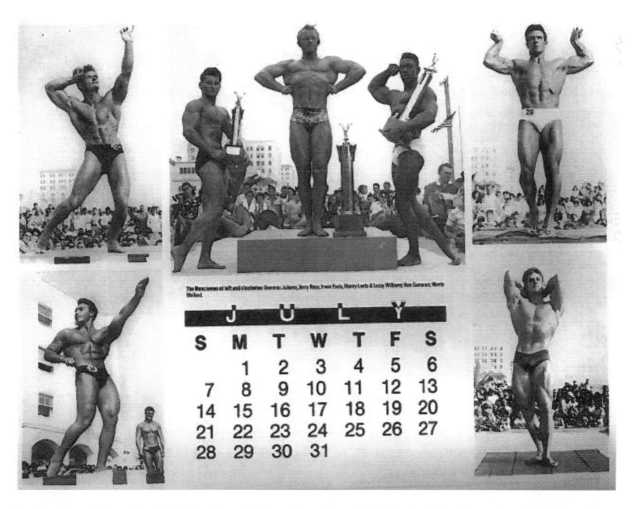

Starting from left, going clockwise; Dom Juliano, Jerry Ross, Irwin Paris, Henry Lentz, Leroy Williams, Ken Cameron & Monty Wolford; are some of the greats of Muscle Beach

MUSCLE BEACH is a national shrine, known around the world, to the body beautiful -- men and gals. . . muscles, muscles, and more muscles and athletic agility and strength. Officially this amazing place is one of the Santa Monica municipal playgrounds basking in the sunshine of this Southern California coastal city. On any sunny day around the calendar the goings on down Muscle Beach way are a composite color motion picture of a one-ring hurdy-gurdy circus, a vaudeville show, a track and field meet, a town-meeting, and a bathing beauty contest -- with laughter, incredible noise, acres of tanned and sunburned skin, swarms of hero-worshipping kids, squadrons of famed and not-so-famed-yet athletes, with ice cream cones and hamburgers thrown in for added color.

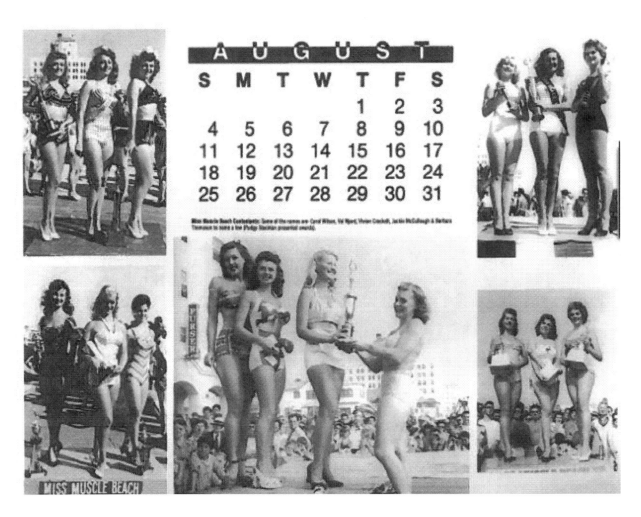

Some of the Bathing Beauties of Muscle Beach

Fourteen years ago a couple of stout lads named Johnny Collins and Barney Frey decided they wanted a place to lift weights, pose with bulging muscles, build human pyramids, work out on the parallel bars, and toss their girl friends around. So they chose this spot on the beach beside Santa Monica pier and near the fishing fleet harbor. The city furnished the apparatus, and health devotees provided the labor to build a small open-air stage alongside the well-known board walk. The adoring public, which loves to sit in the sun and watch someone else work, has well publicized the place by talking. Today Muscle Beach has achieved a deserved world-wide reputation for its weight-lifting, tumbling, adagio teamwork, low and high parallel bars, swinging ring work, and just plain muscle posing. Like Hollywood's Brown Derby, the contestants come here to see and be seen. Muscle Beach will have as many as 2000 contestants and spectators on Saturdays and Sundays. The 15 by 60 foot stage will be a squirming ant-hill of showoff participants from five years to 60: jumping and balancing, building human pyramids four high; tossing each other around the ozone, lifting all sorts of heavy weights -- all to the admiring gaze and occasional bursts of applause of the holidayers massed on the surrounding sands or seated on benches, or standing six deep on the adjacent cement "boardwalk".

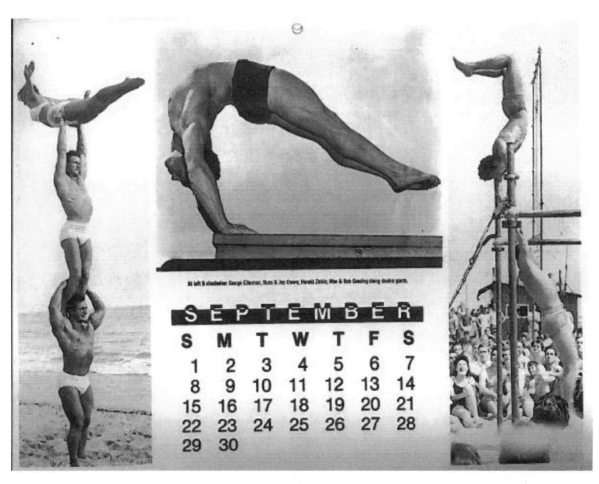

Eiferman, Russ & Joy Crown, Harold Zinkin & Moe (Most) & Bob Gooding

In the little green playground office playground directors Charles McMillan and DeForrest Most (present Pacific Coast light-heavyweight lifting champion) hand out ping pong balls and paddles, iodine, advice, volley balls, and keep a watchful eye on the madcap muscular activities of their enthusiastic brethren and sisters of the padded mats. A burst of applause from the nearby stage attracts you. "That little guy bouncing into the sky from the trampoline," explains Most, "is good. He ought to be. He was a clown with Cole Bros. circus. "Name's Frankie Vincent, from Boston." The crowd likes Frankie's clowning. He hits the canvas bouncing table, then shoots high into the air, running, mugging, posing, or frantically waving. A pretty coffee-brown gal in the office helping McMillan and Most explains the repeated bursts of applause. "We always have special programs on holidays and weekends. This place is really a big laugh from beginning to end. But you can't laugh away the health, the muscles, and the weight-lifting champions."

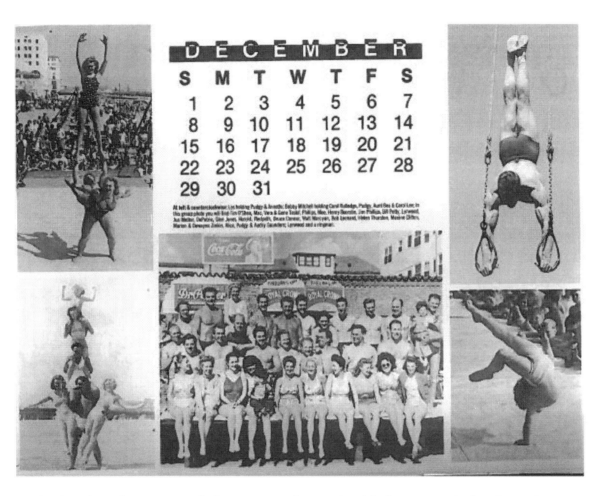

Professionals and amateurs mix here at Muscle Beach with the camaraderie of true devotees of good health. Among the pros on the stage are often famous Hollywood studio stunt men. There is Russ Saunders. These men work out here regularly to keep in shape for their profession as "fall" guys in films. Saunders is one of the world's great all-around acrobats and tumblers. "Oohs!" and "Ahs!" sweep the crowd as he goes through his routine.

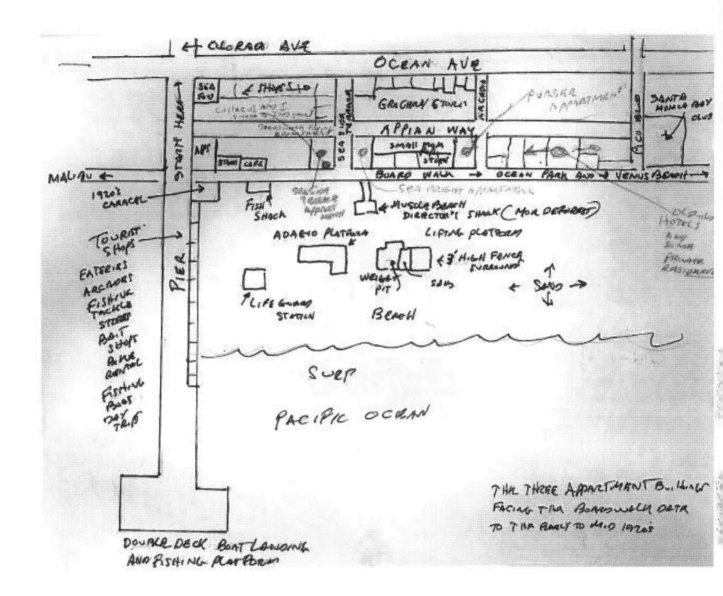

Sam Calhoun provided this hand-drawn map of the original Muscle beach, with his added in notes. Legibility of the notes is not the best, so I'll clarify; the note at top left pointing to the forward-most dot is describing where Sam & Chuck Collras shared an apartment, with the adjacent dot being the Seaside Terrace apartments. Next, working to the right is the dot showing the Sea Bright apartments and on the end of that same block are the higher-end Purser apartments. The last dot shows where some very old apartments and private residences were.

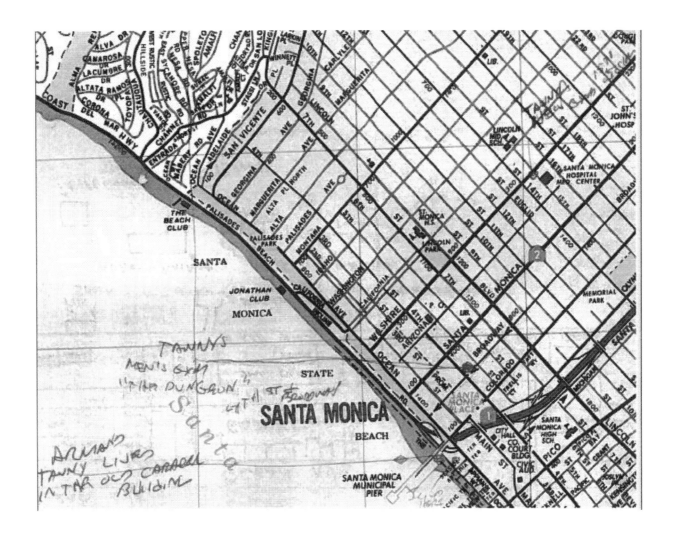

A real map of Santa Monica is shown here, with more notes from Mr. Calhoun. The notes point out where Armand Tanny lived, very close to where Sam lived; as well as the locations of the dungeon on 4th street and Tanny's fancier new gym on 15th st.

A small, dark-headed man takes the center stage, slowly lifts and holds aloft a pair of heavy iron wheels, "That's Tony Terlazzo, two times Olympic champ (1932-36); world champ in 1946; and from 1936 to 1946 U. S. national champ at his weight, 148 pounds." Tony has a body-building studio in Hollywood. Several pairs of men and girls take the stage. Tanned and in perfect health, they engage in adagio: a lifting, leaping, balancing and posing routine. Now and again some impressively handsome couple will be balancing, the girl seven feet up, standing in her partner's hands; then she will lose her balance, wave frantically, and both will tumble to the canvas amid roars of laughter. But it's all in good fun. At times it seems that there are more people on the stage than in the audience, all posing, leaping, and talking at the same time. Several small boys and girls are doing back bends, walking on their hands, being swung around by older acrobats. A slender little Miss of seven whirls over into a half dozen back flips and draws applause. Then a wee lad is lifted in his mother's arms. She points to a tall man lifting the iron wheels. "Watch him, Jimmy. That's Phil Skarin. He's Pacific Coast heavyweight lifting champion." Hollywood big names, famous athletes, and visiting celebrities come and go at Muscle Beach. It doesn't seem very long ago that Jane Russell, now playing with Bob Hope in "The Paleface," was a regular here, playing volley ball. The radio announcer points out celebrities on the stage. "There's Harold Zinkin, Mr. California in 1941 and runner-up to Mr. America in 1945, working out with his adagio partner.... little Dolly Walker. He's one of the greatest tumblers and balancers." The high parallel bars are moved onto the stage and little Frankie Vincent in clown makeup is joined by a lithe blond giant in short pants and clown paint -- Johnny Robinson, a symphony in muscle. Johnny leaps up at the bars and swings up in a circle, whirls over in mid-air and lands on the balls of his feet on the adjoining bar, stares grinning at the roaring crowd. "Johnny Robinson, folks". One of the greatest horizontal bar acrobats in the world. He won the National amateur high bar championship in 1947. "Only missed the Olympics because he doesn't specialize in enough events." Frankie is good on the bars, but he clowns at it while Johnny goes thru a breath-taking routine that would make a monkey nod with approval. The hero-worshipping kids lean on the stage and stare up. "Man, oh man, I wanna be like that Johnny," they say. Johnny Robinson swings around the bars like a greased pendulum, turns loose high in the air, lands neatly on hands or feet with such perfect timing that the crowd thrills. Scores of camera fans with everything from a movie camera to that old family box Brownie or a Speed Graphic are snapping pictures all around the stage. Sea gulls and pelicans float overhead. The roar of nearby waves and the weaving color pattern of humanity make an unforgettable picture. Men outnumber the girls by two to one at Muscle Beach. The way this place grows is that people come to watch, stay to admire, then return to participate. Families bring their kids. Girls and boys from schools and universities come in swarms to see Big Shot athletes do their routines. They can always get the best advice from such stars of the mat as big Armand Tanny and Buford McFatridge (both former heavyweight lifting champs), from Edna Rivers, women's professional "clean and jerk" champ, a rare feat for a woman; from Billy Hamlet and Bob McClellan, two of the best men in the West on the flying rings; and from Jimmy Starkey, one of the few men in the world who can press himself up to a complete handstand with his hands crossed. Muscle Beach grew in fame during the recent war. Many thousands of servicemen visited here during the war, then went abroad on many a lighting front and talked about Muscle Beach, the muscles, the beautiful gals and weightlifters. So hundreds of men have visited this Muscle Beach because of an oft-told tale in Germany or North Africa or Japan. Many hero-worshipping youngsters hitch-hike from across the U. S. to look on or take part in Muscle Beach activities. Some get jobs and stay; others are helped to go home.

On hot summer days hundreds of Southern California school students catch rides the 15 miles to the beach. You never know what names of fame may be working out next to you at Muscle Beach; scientists, engineers, artists, lesser folk among movie players; stunt men, and college athletes. Some of the nation's best volley ball players play here. Jane Russell stopped coming when she became a star. Highlights of the years festive activities are the July Fourth "'Mister Muscle Beach contest for best male physique, and the "Miss Muscle Beach" for prettiest girl, on Labor Day. These events are strictly for amateurs. So Miss "Pudgy" Stockton, the Professional Miss America 1948 $1000 title prize winner in New York can't ever compete. The audience got a bang out of the last July Fourth Mister Muscle Beach men's "beauty contest."' Sixteen men competed, and JIMMY LAWLOR, a Brooklyn boy now majoring in physical education at the University of California, Los Angeles, won the 1948 title. The contestants posed in all the best health and physical culture magazine styles on a small stage. The crowd roared. People come to Muscle Beach to see an exciting free show on a hot day. The men come to build their muscles and show off. The gals are interested in balancing and posing and looking beautiful in the scantiest of suits -- and everybody is interested in seeing and being seen. The poor press photographers have to scramble through a bunch of judges and contestants, admirers, friends of friends of the playground directors. Meanwhile a four-man-high human pyramid is likely to topple from the sky on your neck. The music goes on and on; hamburger stands and soda pop, lost kids and ice cream cones and frantic mamas mill about. Rarely does a contestant or participant get hurt on the stage. They're most likely to fall on someone else or atop a sweating photographer before hitting the deck. But that's Muscle Beach out in Santa Monica, California -- and lots of men and gals hold records with those muscles as well as posing them before the admiring throng.

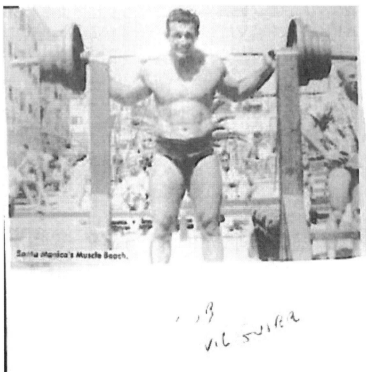

Santa Monica's Muscle Beach.

Bub McQuire

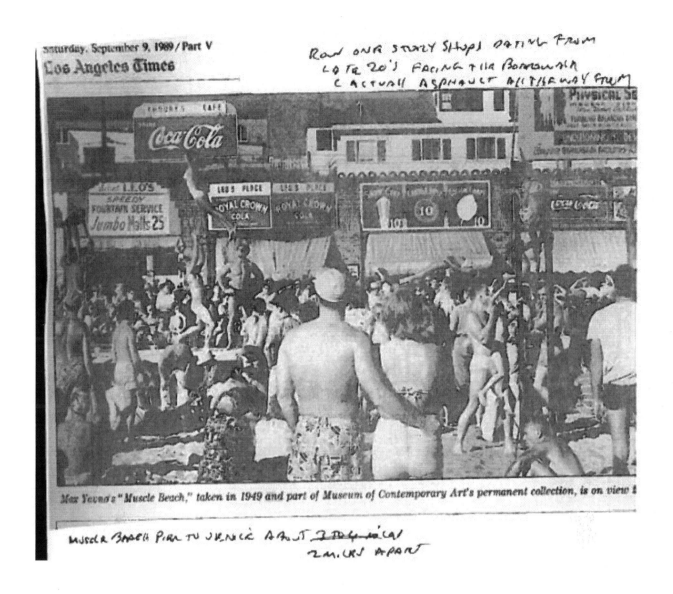

The hand written notes were added by Sam Calhoun, who was kind enough to send the picture taken from an old local paper article

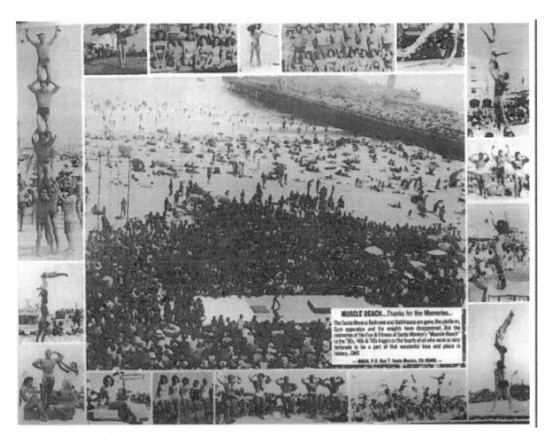

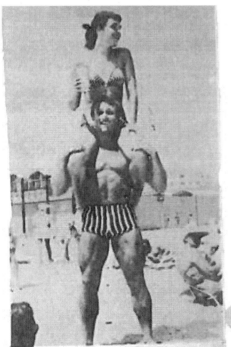

South Africa's gift to Muscle Beach is JOHN ISAACS. No, that's not "manna from heaven" on Johnny's shoulders... just a lovely who descended from outer space. (Zeller) ← GREAT PHOTOGRAPH

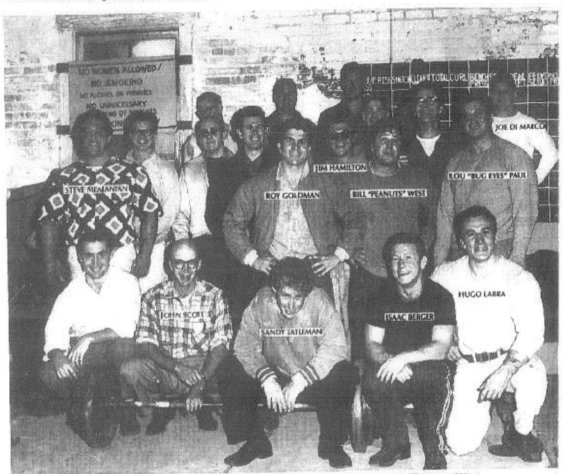

The Muscle Beach Club in 1960 with the Original Westside Barbell Club founders Joe Di Marco and Bill "Peanuts" West

The caption up on top says Westside Barbell club, but the picture depicts the Muscle Beach Club, as you see at the bottom. This is the later version, moved off the beach of Santa Monica's original location.

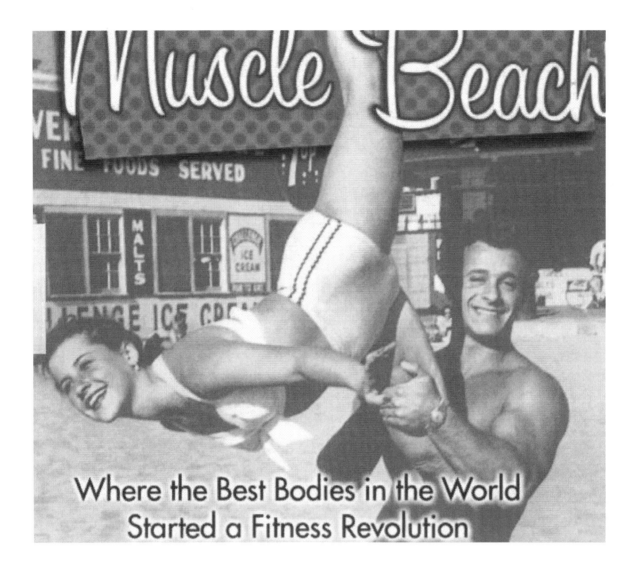

Where the Best Bodies in the World Started a Fitness Revolution

The gentleman on the bottom right is of course none other than **George Eiferman**, a fellow Philadelphian who may have been the nicest and most well liked bodybuilder of all time. Reading an old Strength & Health magazine recently I came across the fact that George's first exposure to the iron was with a teacher in his high school, "Olney High" in Philly, which my older sister attended and where I would also have attended had I not gone to a private school instead. It's a small world, right? I have yet to come across a negative word about the man, and I have read much about him in all my research, so that is saying something. There was a place set up for serious weight training, in addition to what was called an adagio platform, where acrobatics and various forms of dance were done at this original Muscle Beach, but it gradually started to take on a reputation as a hangout for less than savory characters and the local powers eventually shut down the operation and removed the workout platforms and equipment. Some would say it was a trumped up charge that started the beginning of the end, and others would say there were some legitimate concerns for the young residents' moral stature, but whichever side is more correct, the Muscle Beach that many knew & loved for 2 decades or more had basically met its demise. Those die-hards who refused to let a good thing die altogether simply moved the outside workouts to Venice Beach, which ultimately also became known as Muscle Beach.

You will see it referenced throughout the rest of the book, and it was mentioned time and again in the Weider publications with much fondness. The Weider West Coast office was right there in the thick of things, and they fed off of each other's energy.

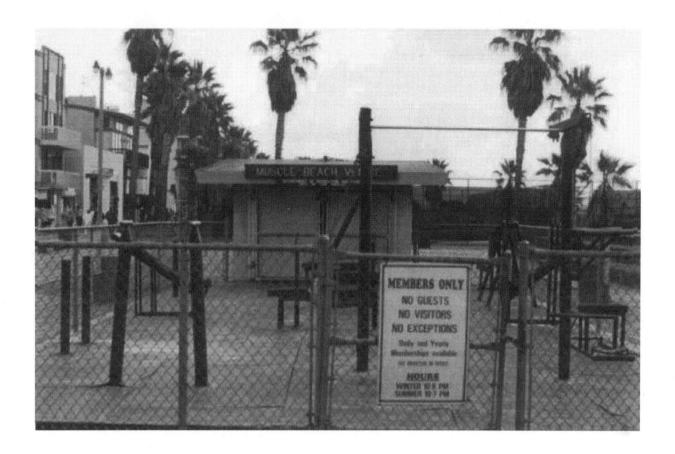

The Venice Muscle Beach

Here is an article I found on the net about Abbye Stockton and her role at Muscle Beach;

In those days it seemed that superheroes were born, created or discovered every other day. Kal-El was shot from his doomed home; Bruce Wayne witnessed his parents murder an Amazonian princess? Life on Paradise Island was interrupted by a crashed plane and a handsome wounded soldier. And in Santa Monica, sometime in the late 1930s, a young woman named Abbye Eville decided she'd put on too much weight in her job as a telephone operator and picked up the dumbbells that her boyfriend had brought her. Then she put them down. Then she picked them up again. The "Foremost Female Physical Culturist." In real life, strength is not a rocket shot or exposure to a wizard or a spider bite: you're not weak one moment and superheroic the next. It's a decision you make daily. Abbye Eville kept lifting the dumbbells. The telephone-company weight dropped away; her childhood nickname, Pudgy, became a fond joke. Her muscles became visible and then impressive. She taught herself to do a headstand, and then a handstand. Her first costume was a two-piece bathing suit jerry-built by her mother: men's swim trunks and a top patterned on an old bra? One-piece bathing suits were too confining for the stunts that she and Les Stockton, the boyfriend with the weights, had started to do with their friends south of the Santa Monica pier, a stretch of sand that picked up the name Muscle Beach. There were plenty of superheroes in the making on Muscle Beach back then: Jack LaLanne, Steve Reeves, and Joe Gold (who would found Gold's Gym). Crowds gathered and gawked. Harold Zinkin, who later invented the Universal Gym, made himself into a belly-up table to support a totem pole of three bodybuilders, feet to shoulders, standing on his stomach. A strongman named George Eiferman? A future Mr. America? Lifted weights with his left hand and played the trumpet with his right. Adagio dancers tossed one another around like javelins; acrobats defied gravity and common sense. In photographs of the Muscle Beach hand-balancers, you can find Pudgy as a top-mounter or under-stander, upside down and right side up, with two women on each arm and a man on her shoulders or alone in a handstand, muscular and pocket-size: 5 foot 1, 115 pounds. Make no mistake: She's not toned or firmed-up or any of those timid terms that even 21st-century women persist in using when they decide to change their bodies through exercise. She's built. Her back is corrugated with muscles as she supports a likewise muscular man. Les Stockton, now her husband, 185 pounds of bodybuilder, upside down over her head. There were strong women before Muscle Beach, pale, leotarded circus and vaudeville performers, and stoic as caryatids as they lifted extraordinary weights. Even their names seem carved from stone: Minerva, Vulcana, Sandwina, and Athleta. But Pudgy Stockton was something brand-new. Every inch and ounce of her body refuted the common wisdom that training with weights turned women manly and muscle-bound. She was splendid as a work of art but undoubtedly, thrillingly, flesh, blood, breath. What does muscle-bound mean, anyhow? It's an insult dreamed up by the underdeveloped. Pudgy Stockton's mission was to show women that muscles could only ever set them free. After the war she ran a gym on Sunset Boulevard called the Salon of Figure Development, and then she and Les opened side-by-side men's and women's gyms in Beverly Hills. Her business card showed her on tiptoes, on the beach, of course, showing off her hamstrings, her biceps, her tiny waist, her impressive bust. Foremost Female Physical Culturist, it read. Writer, authority on feminine figure contouring and cover girl. Women could also read "Barbelles", the column she wrote for Strength and Health magazine. Jan Todd, a friend of Stockton's and co-director of the Todd-McLean Physical Culture Collection at the University of Texas , Austin, and a weight-lifting pioneer herself, says that the columns argued that lifting weights would make you a better athlete. That was a very revolutionary message to be preaching to women. Stockton featured stories of female athletes and ordinary women who trained with weights. This woman over 30 years of age, she wrote of one protégée, with two children, and with no athletic background whatsoever, has brought about, by her persistence, these amazing changes. Her beautiful figure is a living proof of the intelligent application of this system of figure contouring. Pudgy Stockton retired from the gym business in the 1950s to raise her daughter, Laura.

A few years later the Santa Monica workout area was torn down, and Muscle Beach, or a vague idea of it, moved down the coast to Venice. By then, Steve Reeves was Hercules and Jack LaLanne was a TV star. It seems like it was always sunny, Pudgy Stockton said of the first Muscle Beach, her Muscle Beach. In photographs it is. See Pudgy and Les in the brushed-steel black-and-white California sunlight, showing off for the cameras and crowds. You can't see all the work it has taken them to get to this bright beach, both of them looking like sculptures come to joyful life; you can't tell who has kissed whom alive. They have lifted all those weights so they can lift each other. The wind pulls back Pudgy's hair and makes her squint. She stands, blond and lovely, on the palms of her husband's upraised hands while she presses a 100-pound barbell overhead. Then they switch places, and she supports him above her, hand to hand, she smiling up and he smiling down, as satisfactory a portrait of a marriage as ever could be.

Your Physique, Vol 14, No 1, Page 28, October 1950

Mr. U.S.A
Miss. U.S.A
amateur Mr. Western America
Mr. Muscle beach

BY EARLE LIEDERMAN

ON the nights of July 1st, 2nd and 3rd, at the Embassy Theatre, Los Angeles, there were staged three separate events, yet all blended into each other and formed a gala occasion and a treat for all who witnessed this muscle and beauty jamboree. On the first night there was staged the Mr. Western America contest, under the sanction of the AAU. This consisted of the finest amateurs in the West, and it was won by Victor Nicoletti, with Monty Wolford, second, and Pepper Gomez, third. Oddly enough, this is the identical order in which these fellows finished in two previous contests. Nonetheless it was a close affair, for in it were such famous stars as Roy Hilligenn, Malcolm Brenner, Alex Aronis, Joe Sanceri, and numerous others, each worthy of being a prize winner under easier conditions. The second night featured the Miss USA contest in which each of the final eighteen girls was a prize winner, having but recently won a contest staged somewhere in Southern California, in order to be eligible to compete in this gala event. After much judging, the number was weeded down to seven and finally to the best remaining five, and from these was chosen Miss Evelyn Lovequist as Miss USA 1950. Hazel Shaw received second awards, and Lynn Roebuck was third. But the third and final night held the greatest of thrills. It was then that Clarence Ross posed as he never posed before in a special exhibition apart from the USA event which he did not enter. His entire five minute routine kept the audience in constant applause, without let-up, to be followed with shouts and cheers for more and more after Clarence took his final bow. Never before has he received such an ovation! Next came the judging of the seven contestants for the $1,000 cash, large trophy and the title of Mr. USA for 1950. Finally Armand Tanny was proclaimed the winner! He never looked better. His muscles were in great definition and his control over them perfect. His lats and thighs are most unusual and brought most generous applause. Well does he deserve to win, for today; Armand Tanny stands out as one of the finest developed men in the world!

George Eiferman received second honors despite his popularity. He is well liked wherever he goes, for, of all the strongmen, George is about the most congenial and pleasant. He beat our Floyd Page, after a long tie between them, for being the most muscular. Floyd Page who received third honors, showed a most superb body and a greatly improved athlete over previous years. He is a top-flight strongmen and prize winner on his own, and was narrowly beaten by both Eiferman and Tanny according to points. This is about the first time a physique show has been staged for three days in length, and Bert Goodrich, who arranged everything and promoted the affair, deserves credit for the way things went off to everyone's satisfaction. The special vaudeville acts were grand as well as funny, and Jack LaLanne presented his special hand-balancing routine atop uprights which also brought him great applause. John Davis, the champion lifter, was the high spot of the whole contest, for his great lifting was amazing, and at one performance he curled two hands, 205 lbs. without the slightest back bend. Then he did a one-arm military press of 145 lbs., to follow with a 400 lb. jerk. And to top these, he did one squat with 520 lbs. climaxing the previous three days of contests, exhibitions and general physical excitement; on July 4th the annual Mr. Muscle Beach Contest attracted a huge audience. This event is always one of the most popular of the summer season, and each year the winner is selected from a huge group of entrants, for the honor of being Mr. Muscle Beach is a great one and competition is always extra keen. The winner and Mr. Muscle Beach for 1950 is popular PEPPER GOMEZ. Pepper keeps improving with each contest and very shortly will be a serious threat in National competition.

Strength & Health, Page 34, November 1953

Mr. Muscle Beach Contest

By George R Bruce

On July 4, 1953, at famous Muscle Beach in Santa Monica, California, on the shores of the blue Pacific, was held the 7th Annual Jr. and Sr. Mr. Muscle Beach show. Over 3500 people were crowded around the platform on this typical warm and sunny Southern California day. Master of Ceremonies George (Butcherman Bruce started the show at 2:00 P.M. by asking the entire crowd to stand face the flag and pledge allegiance. The great variety show then went on and featured both amateur and professional acts. **DeForrest Most, Playground Director**, featured his juveniles in balancing; Holger and Dolores, adagio; Robinson and Bono, hand balancing and their masterpiece, slow-motion wrestling; Bill and Billy Henry, father and son, Risley and balancing (Bill Henry is a sensational 5-year-old). The Jr. Mr. Muscle Beach contest, held for the first time last year, has already become so popular that next year it will be held as a separate event. There were 24 entries of well-developed young men 17 years of age and under. Lynn Lyman placed 1st (Lynn is 16 years of age, is 5'10", weights 170 lbs., trains at Bob's Gym in Los Angeles, lives in La Habra, California, and has had one year of training); Bert Cedilos placed 2nd and Allen Marshall 3rd. In the Senior Mr. Muscle Beach contest there were 20 entries. **This contest is now open to any man who is not a professional and who has not won a Mr. America contest.** This contest has assumed such national importance that popular demand has caused it to be opened to all comers.

Dominic Juliano placed 1st; Ed Holovchick placed 2nd and Jerry Ross placed 3rd. Dom handles heavy weights at all times during training. He trains three times weekly and his favorite exercise is dips on the parallel bars.

Here is a Strength & Health article from the last days of the original Muscle Beach;

Strength & Health, Page 12, December 1957

Muscle Beach to Remove...or to Improve?

by Thomas Humphrey
pix by Cecil Charles

For more than twenty-five years Santa Monica's Muscle Beach has existed as an unorganized and voluntary enterprise. It has now grown into a phenomenon that is recognized throughout the world by those who practice its particular type of physical activities. Bodybuilding, weightlifting, gymnastics and professional acrobatics are the major forms of athletics at Muscle Beach, while volleyball, table tennis and chess also have their adherents. Each of these groups have some of the nation's best performers, and in some instances, athletes of world-wide reputation. One of the newer sports at Muscle Beach is water skiing. Most of these sports have annual tournaments or a series of summer weekend contests. The Easter, July 4th and Labor Day shows at Muscle Beach are replete with a variety of talent, and attract enormous crowds. Although bodybuilding and weightlifting represent but two of the types of athletes practiced at Muscle Beach, they do constitute the only well organized activities.

The "**Muscle Beach Weightlifting Club**" was formed in 1955 at the insistence of the Santa Monica City Recreation Commission. A panel of officers was elected, a constitution drawn up and by-laws adopted. With part of the funds derived from the annual membership fees an accident insurance policy was set up to protect the members. The Santa Monica City Council was asked to assist with funds in order to improve the beach facilities, and since 1955 the City has allocated approximately $10,000.00 to Muscle Beach. The club membership program proved to be a great success, with almost five hundred dues paying members the first year. With these funds the club has purchased 3800 pounds of YORK Olympic lifting sets and 2300 pounds of dumbbells. Separate bodybuilding and weightlifting platforms, soundly built and covered with 3/4", 3' by 5' "neoprene" rubber sheets were installed, while storage boxes, dumbbell racks, benches and other accessories were also added. The area was then completely enclosed and neatly painted.

In the early summer of 1957 the City officials announced that Muscle Beach was to be moved. Weightlifters, bodybuilders, gymnasts and other enthusiasts descended en masse on the City officials and overwhelmed them with persuasive arguments supporting their desire to keep Muscle Beach at its present location. Some of the following points were brought out:

A. Against re-location

1. Muscle Beach is warmer than other Santa Monica beach areas due to protection from the wind afforded by the nearby pier.
2. Muscle Beach is widely known at its present location.
3. The area proposed for re-location is much too small to allow the present equipment to be safely used.
4. There was no just reason for moving Muscle Beach in the first place.

B. Other suggestions

1. With the $160,000.00 assigned to be used for Muscle Beach re-location, improve the facilities and provide more beach directors.
2. Provide a beach master plan that will include consideration and approval of the Muscle Beach group.

The Muscle Beach group desires complete City administration, for without the City's supervision, in the past, a vicious cycle has been established. Overtaxed facilities became run-down, undesirable elements of society, "beach bums", were attracted and the general public blamed Muscle Beach for conditions that were brought about by a lack of City support. With cooperation from the local press misunderstandings of this type can be eliminated, in time, by public education. Santa Monica is a tennis town, and the City supports this program by helping to send outstanding tennis players to National and World championships. Yet Santa Monica is a beach town too, and they have many more outstanding athletes in weightlifting, gymnastics and volleyball than in tennis. There are also more spectators and participants in these beach sports than in tennis or any other City supported athletics. When the City Recreation Commission was made aware of these facts, they admitted their ignorance of the situation, but with true democratic action they appointed a committee to make a more thorough study of the needs of Muscle Beach. It is difficult for us not to be over-enthusiastic and over-persuasive about the good features of Muscle Beach. What is needed to insure the future of Muscle Beach, however, is an intelligent, diplomatic presentation to the public of the benefits that can be derived from Muscle Beach's particular type of recreation and athletics, and a cooperative attitude to the press. In addition every beach participant is encouraged to present better than average decorum, and to this end the "Muscle Beach Weightlifting Club" excludes members who prove to be a liability. The Muscle Beach weightlifting team has taken one team trophy and placed third as a team at the Jr. Nationals. A member of the MBWC (Dave Ashman) captured the Super-heavyweight title at the national championships this year. Many weightlifting and odd lift contests have been scheduled and the AAU's cooperation and suggestions have been solicited. With Olympic stars and other prominent veterans providing voluntary instruction, encouragement and inspiration to younger, less experienced athletes, the development of an outstanding lifting team seems very probable. The fate of Muscle Beach hangs in balance, but with the expected civic support, improved public understanding and increased participant interest, Muscle Beach will become a real national force in athletics and a symbol of physical fitness and improvement. Keep your eye on the NEW Muscle Beach for you will hear more about it.

The following pages contain snippets from the Muscle Builder magazine's "Let's Gossip" column from the '60s. This will give a little flavor of some of the Muscle Beach happenings from the time.

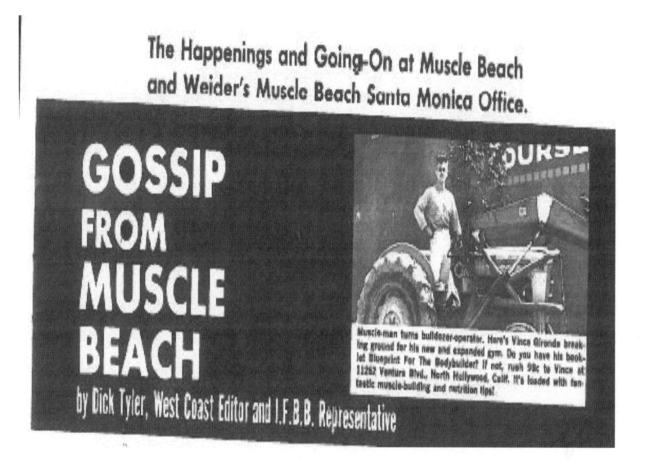

Vince Gironda shown above, clearing room to expand his gym.

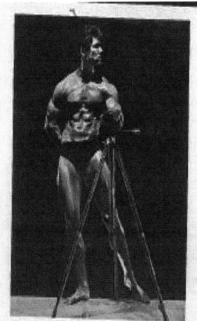

The man with the widest lats in the West (also super-delts, fab-abs, among other muscle stupenda). His physique has an ultra-dramatic look in this exceptional photo.

EVER like to read a good book? How about a good love story? Yeah, yeah, I know. I must have lost my marbles. After all, this is a muscle magazine. Well, sit back and listen will ya! Ya see, there was this guy named Larry Scott, you've heard of him, haven't you? Anyway, not long ago he was in a market when he spies this lovely Japanese girl. (He seems to favor the oriental beauties.) So his muscular heart flexed pretty hard and he realized he was bitten. Only trouble was, she was with this other guy. A few days later he was in the market again. There she was with a different guy. The next time he saw her she was alone. She wore a ring on her finger.

"Are you married?" were his first words to her. She explained that it was just a friendship ring and that she had no desire to tie any knots. No sooner had she said that than she disappeared into the setting sun leaving our hero with his lats spread like a table cloth. To a lesser man that might have meant the end. Larry is not ordinary in any sense of the word. So, in his trusty "batmobile," he hunted for his true love. He prowled around the market until he spotted her walking along the street. Seeing Larry, our little "butterfly" ducked into a doorway to escape. Later Larry spotted her getting into her car. He took the license number

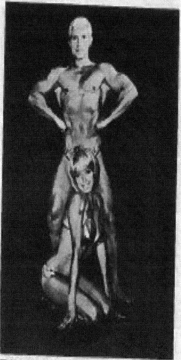

This is famous Mr. Germany and Mr. Europe Junior, Frank Hollfelder in an unusual pose. The gal who has just 'fallen' for him is his beautiful wife, Heidi, who could be Miss Body Beautiful of anywhere!

and traced her address through the police. Honest. Next, he goes to where she lives which happens to be an apartment house and goes from door to door asking for a lovely Japanese girl. With no luck he starts to drive away when guess who drives up. He blocks her way. She threatens to call the police.

"No!" he cries, and they decided to talk. And talk he does (You guys who wonder about the secrets of some of the champs like Scott just remember that Larry tackles his workouts like he does his romantic life. He WORKS for what he wants.) The ending? Larry and Rachel were recently married!

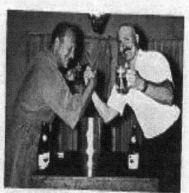

No, no! If you think the guy with the handle-bar moustache is a thin Mac Batchelor, you're wrong. He's famed lifter-physique star Bert Elliot. Mac and Bert are the best of friends, and Bert is now interested in duplicating many of Mac's fabulous feats of strength... like wrist wrestling.

Have you heard about the near-fatal accident Don Howorth was involved in? It was just a short time before the MR. AMERICA when he and a friend were taking a ride in a little sports car. Speed and the wrong moves caused the car to spin out and roll. Don's friend went sailing out of the car and sustained very serious injuries. Don? Hardly a scratch.

From my "Who Cares about that Guy" file comes this gem. I've noticed that I have directed some of my disparaging remarks about the sorry shape I'm in at me. It was getting so that the *(Continued on page 52)*

Don Howorth, Larry Scott & Bert Elliot seen in the page above, we'll see more of Bert in the Zuver's chapter.

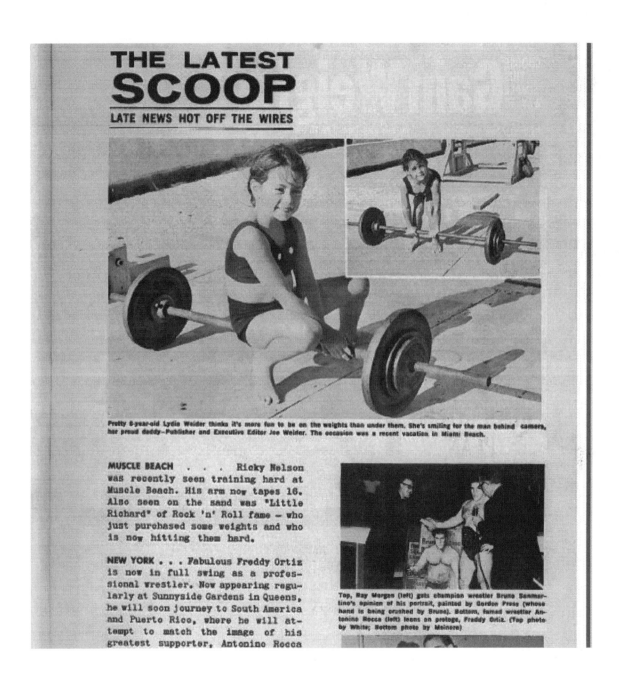

Above you see Lydia Weider in the picture, and a little clip about Ricky Nelson training at Muscle Beach. On the Bottom right, you see something about Bruno Samartino.

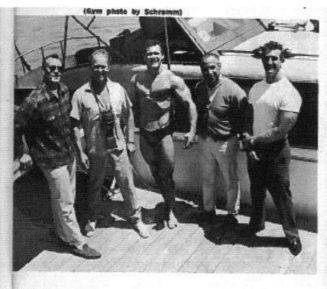
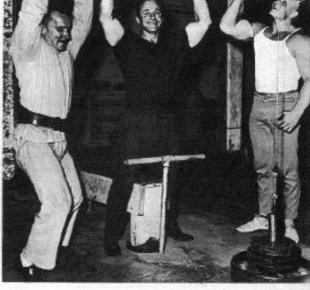

LET'S GOSSIP

HOT NEWS ON THE IRON FRONT

MORE WEST COAST GOSSIP by ARLEY VEST

Results of the West Coast's big show of the year, the Pacific Coast Championships . . . the show was dedicated to the late President John F. Kennedy. Even before emcee Gene Mozee could wind-up the announcement of dedication, the audience rose to its feet in a standing ovation to the memory of a great man — a great American — a great President — a man who was also an enthusiastic booster of physical fitness.

The power lift portion of the meet afforded plenty of thrills. Thirteen record attempts were made. Champ Ralph McCoy at 165 pounds nearly succeeded with a 515-pound Squat. He should make it on a "good" night. Heavyweight Lee Phillips didn't try for a new Squat record because of a bout with the flu . . . he settled for 650 on this occasion. Outstanding lifter was Herculean Harold Love. Lifting in the 198-pound class, Harold made a Strict Bench Press with 425 and a Squat with 605!

Then came the physique men . . . each looking like a young God under the unusual lighting. Don Howorth won the title of Mr. West Coast, (Continued on page 70)

Labra, Eifferman & Draper above right, and some other well known guys on the left;

Clarence Ross, Weider photographer, Russ Warner, Ken McCord, Abdu Allen & Bob Mendelsohn

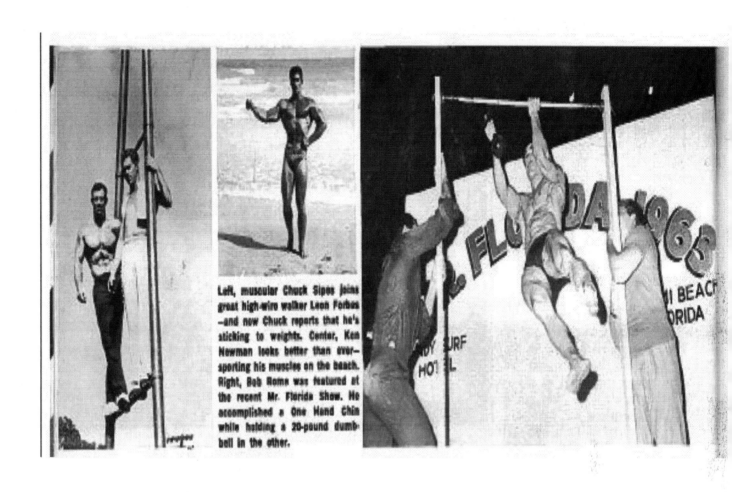

Chuck Sipes tries the high wire, probably both the first and the last time.

special training routine, working harder than ever at his gym. Can he top his already super shape? As you know, Vince boasts such gym members as Larry Scott, John Tristram, Clint Walker ("Rawhide") and James Drury ("The Virginian").

NEW YORK . . . Congratulations to Fred Randall and Renee Lee on their recent marriage. Fred and partner Jerry Howard are professional handbalancers. They have to their credit numerous television, stage, nightclub and movie appearances—and have performed in several big IFBB shows. And many IFBB fans will recall the beautiful Renee, who sang at the 1962 IFBB MR. UNIVERSE-MR. AMERICA SHOW. At present, Fred and Jerry are appearing in high-school physical fitness shows—and Renee is singing her way through Broadway in a new musical, "High Spirits."

Did you see Jerry Winick on television recently? He appeared as a quiz contestant on the popular program, "Who Do You Trust?"—and emcee Woody Woodbury had Jerry go through a few poses for the fans and then arm-wrestled him. Woody won the match . . . with a bit o' help from his opponent, of course.

MIAMI BEACH . . . Ken Newman is really climbing the muscle ladder of success. Shortly after winning the recent IFBB MR. FLORIDA CONTEST he won the MR. FOUNTAINBLEU HOTEL CONTEST. The prize? Why, a week's free stay at the famed hotel, of course. Brooklyn's Nick Perrotti placed 2nd, by the way. Kenny's present statistics are: 180 pounds; 47 chest; 17½ arms; and 23 thighs. He hopes to weigh 200 by mid-summer.

Popular television show "Surfside 6" recently sported a scene involving one of its stars performing a Barbell Bench Press and Dumbbell Curls. Just goes to show that everyone is becoming more and more conscious of weights these days —and of training benefits.

SANTA MONICA . . . Famed physique photographer Russ Warner is now Manager of WEIDER WEST COAST at 1220 Fifth Street, just off Muscle Beach. He moved in to replace George Eiferman, who is now in Hawaii. Big Dave Draper is still in charge of shipping, and the office is staffed with many West Coast stars—frequently seen in MUSCLE BUILDER and MR. AMERICA. Drop by for a visit next trip out Santa Monica way!

Ed Jubinville writes that U.S. Air Force Sergeant Emmet Jones (1963 IFBB MR. NEW ENGLAND) is now stationed in Pakistan. Happy stay, Emmet, and here's hoping for your frequent appearance as an IFBB contestant in 1964!

CANOGA PARK . . . Bert Goodrich is now Athletic Director at Rocketdyne— a branch of North American Aviation. Stationed in Canoga Park, California, Bert trains the top brass there.

NEW YORK . . . Pioneer physique photographer Lon is now capitalizing on his musical talents. He is now demonstrating for Hammond Organs. Even when Lon was one of the world's leading physique photographers he was an accomplished musician—and now that he has put his camera aside, he is devoting all his time to music.

Some very kooky bodybuilders we know have taken to "mooning"—a shocking exposure of the gluteus maximus in public. Some odd-balls will do anything for a laugh, and this college craze is a "natural" for those way-out musclemen who love to show-off. MUSCLE BUILDER does not encourage this asinine behavior.

STATEN ISLAND . . . IFBB champ Larry Powers has put together a Rock 'n' Roll combo. The troupe is packed with good music and pretty gals. Larry sings, dances, jokes and poses—and the group performs free for all worthwhile organizations.

NEW YORK . . . Stanley Nudelman is now in heavy training at Tom Minichello's Mid-City Health Club—after a long absence from the barbell scene. Stan belongs to the era of Abe Goldberg's old Clinton Street gym—when fellows like Al Berman, Marvin Eder and Artie Zeller were in prime condition. The Mid-City is training grounds for top Weider bodybuilders and wrestlers in New York. It is located at 883 Sixth Avenue.

Latest gym fad in the New York area is training in over-sized pajamas . . . they're warm, comfortable and hide the muscles for that surprise appearance come IFBB contest day.

WAIKIKI BEACH . . . George Eiferman reports that Dr. Richard You's new physical fitness center—a huge building in downtown Honolulu—will be completed shortly. It will serve all of Hawaii —and will house a Weider distribution center. George and Dr. You will be at the helm. Until then and later in conjunction with the new center, the Hilton Hawaiian Village on Waikiki Beach will serve all bodybuilders and health enthusiasts. George and Dr. You are in charge —and the Village boasts physical mathematics (weight-gaining and weight-reduction), a huge pool, a solarium, massages, grooming consultation and other services for men and women. All this—the sun and the palm trees and the balmy breezes and the cool water a paradise!

NORTH HIGHLANDS . . . The newest addition to the Chuck Sipes household is little Patricia—really sproutin' up. That makes three girls. And in addition to home life, Chuck keeps busy making special posing appearances, writes a physical fitness column for a newspaper, skin-dives and enjoys mountain-climbing. He recently did a show

Check out the Santa Monica piece above

Let's Gossip

(Continued from page 24)

drums or tom-toms, and which he mixed with broad smiles. Anyway, it was something different and well liked.

STEVE REEVES is back again after spending about a year in Italy and on the island of Majorca in the Mediterranean where he told me that he had a glorious time. Steve has bought a ranch near San Diego and plans to live on it beginning next July. He said he will raise horses and avocados. Maybe my ears heard wrongly and perhaps he said "horses and flies" as these usually go together. Steve, by the way, is in grand shape at 205 lbs.

PAUL ANDERSON also returned to Hollywood after spending some time at his home in Georgia. He is awaiting call, y' know, from a motion picture studio so as to start his second feature film. His first one, "Once upon a horse," will have been released before this hits print. You gotta see it — a *must*.

MILLARD WILLIAMSON the fellow with the huge musculature and who always gave spectacular posing exhibitions at physique contests wherein he displayed his immense chest expansion, informs me that he has quit all bodybuilding and, as of now, only exercises for health's sake. He says he prefers to educate his mind rather than enlarge his muscles. Maybe he's smart at that.

DON SCOTT expects that stork to drop a bundle upon his abode in June. Yeah, I'm betting him that it'll be a gal. Don, as you may know, has a superb physique, all barbell trained.

ART ZELLER who deserted New York for Muscle Beach has turned into a super enthusiast for photography. He can be seen almost daily at Muscle Beach where he shoots candid shots of *who's who* along the sands. Art is cooperating with me, too, and has promised to keep me supplied with lots of photos. So if this comes true, look for them in this magazine very soon—O, sooner than that! O yes, Art Zeller is also a chess nut. I mean he is also super enthusiastic at playing chess. He is just about the best player at Muscle Beach and points South (which is the ocean). Well, he can beat me at the game most of the time. In fact, nearly all of the time, I admit with reluctance.

Guess what! When Paul Anderson first returned to Hollywood after being away for so long, what do you suppose he did? He immediately went fishing with Howard Cantonwine, his manager, that's what. But Paul as a fisherman had better stick to his weights for he caught nothing — not even a bite.

ALAN STEPHAN came to Hollywood for a brief visit to the AHS studios and had just time enough to shake hands with me and say "Hello." We meet and part and meet again; and such is life.

Mr Death Valley sez . . . The only danged exercise Ah gits these here days, podner, consists of jumpin' at conclusions, stretchin' the truth, an' runnin' up bills. An' Ah used t' bend over backwards in a-helping' folks, but Ah cut this out lately. 'Twas too danged strenuous.

Muscle Beach in early January . . . It was like a summer day and with a summer crowd when I, too, mingled with the gang under the warm sun streaming through the fresh air without a whisp of a breeze. The blue Pacific ocean sent its foaming waves creaming and crashing along the shore and hundreds of the regular fellows together with new faces enjoyed it all. And so did I. I reluctantly left just as the flaming sun was about to dip beyond the horizon. Thought you'd like to know how it is out this way.

FRANK STRANAHAN, the heavy muscled barbell enthusiast, and who was the world's leading amateur golfer throughout the years, and who turned professional a year or two ago, is beating the best of the top players. Frank recently won the *Los Angeles open* tournament by defeating the world's

July of '52 Muscle Builder gossip column excerpt marking the start of Art Zeller's photography career with Weider, some other interesting tidbits from the time.

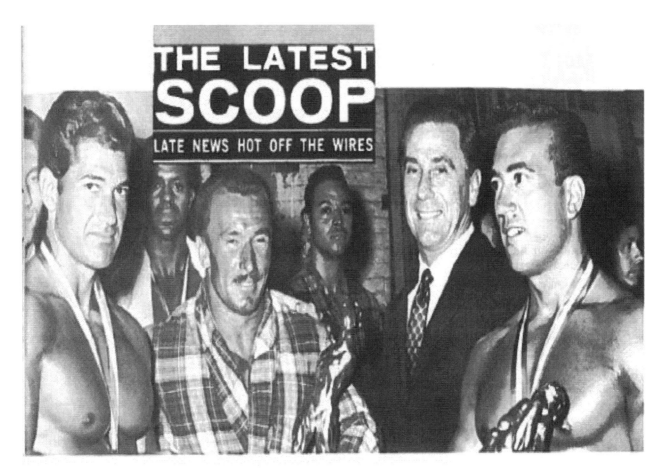

MUSCLE BEACH... The incredible Larry Scott, recently voted the #1 bodybuilder of the year in an international "Top 10" Poll conducted by MR. AMERICA magazine, has been besieged by offers to exhibit his phenomenal physique all over the world. He has received pleas from Yugoslavia, Mexico, Hawaii, and South Africa — among many others. Following his appearance at the Brooklyn Academy of Music on September 17th, when he will defend his MR. OLYMPIA title, he is expected to tour Western Europe. This all goes to show the great power of the IFBB and MUSCLE BUILDER and MR. AMERICA magazines — what they can do in promoting a deserving bodybuilder to the point of international fame and fortune. Larry Scott has certainly taken his place among the bodybuilding greats of all-time. He's earned it — and deserves it. History may prove him to be the greatest of all greats.

HOLLYWOOD... Where does big Dave Draper find the time to do it all? He manages the Weider office at Muscle Beach, writes feature articles for MUSCLE BUILDER and MR. AMERICA magazines, occasionally acts in the movies, performs on television, recently performed with Jayne Mansfield in promoting one of her movies, is now in heavy training for this year's IFBB MR. UNIVERSE, MR. WORLD and, possibly, MR. OLYMPIA contests — and just completed an ad for Drake's Cakes. (This last item causes the "blond bomber" to chuckle. In the television commercial he portrays a circus strongman, and gobbles up the cake — loaded with bleached flour, refined sugar, preservatives, corn starch and additives. In fact, eating this breaks every nutrition rule he normally follows. Anyway — Dave dissolves it with liquid Crash Cut and heavy training. So — he eats the cake, chuckles and trains
(Continued on page 54)

This picture has Hugo Labra in the foreground, Weider standing behind, and the text is about Larry Scott & Dave Draper

The first article back in the introduction mentioned some East Coast transplants that flourished in Southern California

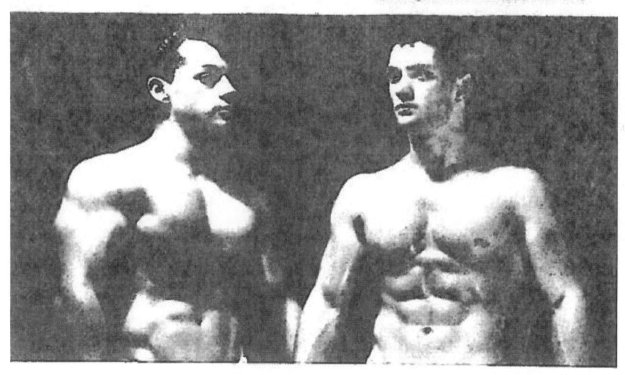

These magnificent bodies, possessed by Marvin Eder and Arthur Zeller, were developed by following Advanced Principles of Training.

Here are a couple of transports from the east that became Weider west coast men.

Artie Zeller became a great photographer for the Weider organization, and in fact many of the photos you'll see in the book, especially in the Zuver's gym section, were taken by Art. The following letter provided by Sam Calhoun, who actually was a close friend of art's, shows his sense of humor;

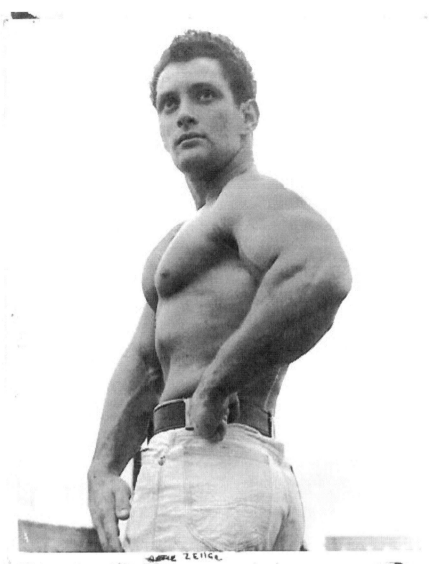

THA ONR's ONLY ARTIR ZELLER ANOTHER FRIEND
SEE LETTER ATTACHED

Dec. 6, 1958

Dear Cosmo,

Terrifying news ! The "heat" swooped down on the Seaside Terrace last night, surrounded the place and proceeded to make several arrests. It was about 2 a.m., I was sleeping at Isaacs pad, (he was out), and Bob Baker was sleeping in the bedroom. Suddenly a pounding on the door.. " Who the hell is it ?" I ask in my irritated half sleep. " The police !" A typical reply at the Seaside, what with all the constant buggery. So I answer, " C'mon, cut the shit.. I'm sleeping." The next knock almost breaks the door down. I realize it's no gag. By this time my heart is pounding and I open the door... four flashlights right in my eyes held in four hands owned by four 8 foot police plainclothesmen. They come in and with them is Dave Sheppard, handcuffed with hands behind his back and George Sheffield handcuffed to a M.B. newcomer from Vancouver. " Where's Isaac Berger ?" " I don't know." And I didn't. More questions, heavy searching action and finally they all leave. They come back 3 more times that night looking for Ike.

It's all to do with the 2 little girls scene, or so hearsay has it. Except this time there's a ring of authenticity to the rumors. John Carper is being charged with Statutory rape, contributing to delinquency of a minor, and sex perversion. I think they are going to charge the rest of them with the same. And they're looking for Isaac on the same charge! I can see the headlines now.. OLYMPIC CHAMPIONS ETC. If they get a hold of simple Isaac he will confess to every crime that has remained unsolved around here for the past 10 years. Great heavens. Of all nights to be at his pad, now I'm needlessly involved. And you know the way their minds work.. guilt by association. Well, of course I'm innocent of having anything to do with the entire affair.. but since when has that ever saved anyone. I'm exaggerating.. probably nothing at all will happen to me.

I would probably have more to say but we're all so overwhelmed by this that I will end this alarming note here. Anything else would be anticlimactic.

I'll write more later.

Love,
H

Here is another item from friend Sam Calhoun's archives I doubt you'll find elsewhere;

THE MUSCLE BEACH BUGLE

(The Muscle Beach Bugle is a comprehensive, all inclusive article and analysis of the latest trends, news and dirt at Muscle Beach.)

John Burns, the Albert Schweitzer of Muscle Beach, was awarded the Hymie Schwartz Peace Prize for his unexcelled work in organizing this years Brotherhood week at M.B. The Sheffield Brothers ran a close second in their efforts at easing racial tension.

Welcomed back after a Hawaiian Soul Saving Campaign was former Mr. America and Mr. U.S.A. Dick DuBois. He is quickly gaining recognition as the most influential spiritual leader ever to hit Ocean Parks skid row. DuBois right hand man is recently saved Bert West, a graduate of the eccleciastic department at Camarillo.

Scheduled to dance the male lead in Swan Lake at Santa Monicas new civic center is Adam Blatman. He will dance opposite Maria Tallchief. Adam is the cultural leader of the Truck Drivers Union.

Latest devotee of Muscle Beach is Gene Bohaty who's numerous physique awards are known to all. Gene is a mathematician who specializes in integral calculus and is famous for his world renowned contributions in atomic research. We last saw Gene at the unemployment office, standing in line behind Chuck Cholras.

The Muscle Beach Weightlifting Club extends congratulations to newlyweds Mr. and Mrs. Chuck Cholras. As a wedding gift the club bought them a shotgun, and a copy of Dr. Isaac Berger's best selling book on birth control, entitled, " Eat More-Worry Less ".

Mr. Muscle Beach of 1957, Sam Martin, has recently published a tune which will soon be distributed in the juke boxes of America. It is entitled, " I'm sittin' on top of the Earl ".

Tom Humphry has been suspended from the club indefinitely pending further investigations of the reports that he and Edna were caught in a compromising position under the pier.

Don Blast wins in neck in neck race with mountain goat for best dressed male in Topanga Canyon. Blast is rumored to be nominated for treasurer of the West Coast Bank of America.

After 2 months of intensive research, experts in the field of physical culture and development have announced that Paul Nutter can go no further... He has reached the pinnacle of muscularity.

Charlie Finklestein wins Mr. Tijuana !! , claims Mr. Jr. Nicaragua is his next step on the ladder to fame. Mr. Ocean Park Blvd. his ultimate goal.

After secretive investigation by the P.B.I. Deforrest Most has been cleared as a security risk, it was announced today by Bob Baker; Local head of Un-American Activities Committee.

Art Fields arrested for vagrancy. " I guess I'm just a bum !", he said dejectedly. He was bailed out by the M'aitre De of Zucky's who brought Field's Chef-Salad dinner along.. with roquefort on the side. " Tonite it's <u>unusual!</u>", said Fields.

Flash!! Esther, wife of Muscle Beach's grocer Norman, was seen riding down the Promenade at 2 a.m. on a unicycle. " She was apparently on her way to a love tryst ", decided Abie Feinstein, expert in such matters.

HYMIE SCHWARTZ BEATS CITY HALL !!! Hymie Schwartz was arrested today when he was caught behind the city hall beating on the building with a broken dumbell handle. " I guess you can't beat city hall ", Hymie said.

Emil Obando noted top salesman for Slenderella int.

LETTER TO COSMO MCMOON N/R   ARTIE ZELLER

While the old workout area of the original Muscle Beach was shut down in '59, Muscle Beach lived; it just moved down the road a bit to Venice Beach. This movie was released in 1964, and the article here is from June of that year.

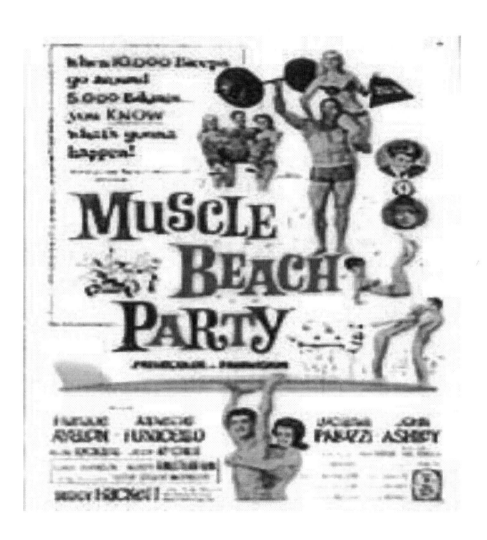

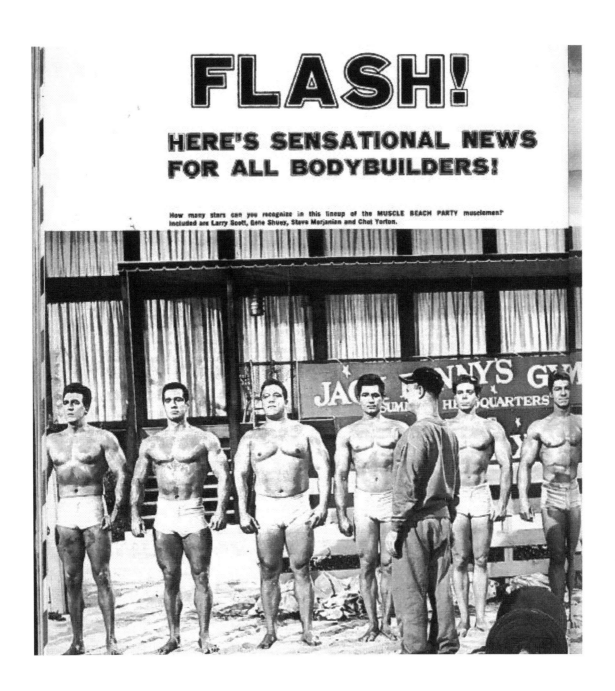

There is some serious beef in this lineup!

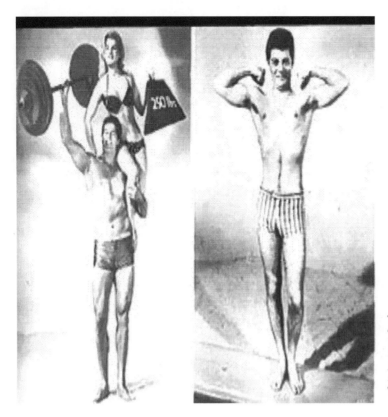

The massive muscleman lifting the barbell (and barbelle!) is Pete Lupis, another Weider star who is the muscle lead in MUSCLE BEACH PARTY. Right, star Frankie Avalon flexes his budding muscles! He was so inspired by movie that he will take up Weider training shortly.

Recognize Pete Lupis at top left? He had a long term role in the hit show "Mission Impossible" Of course; the other guy was pretty popular at the time also, though not for his great musculature.

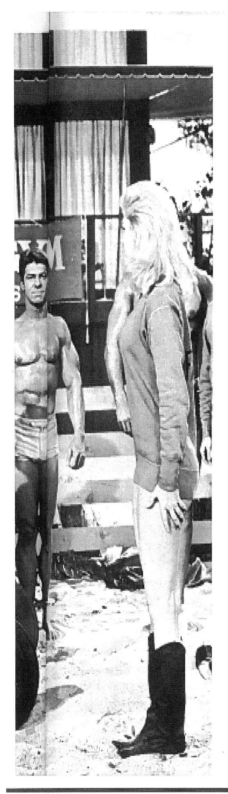

★ MUSCLE BEACH PARTY, that hot new muscle movie direct from American-International Studios, is at your theater now . . . don't miss it! This is a movie all muscle builders should see, for not only will you see your IFBB champs in featured roles but such great favorites as Annette, Frankie Avalon, Buddy Hackett and Dick Dale make this a really enjoyable picture.

This month's issue of **Muscle Builder** is devoted to getting in shape by summer, and **Muscle Beach Party** is perfect summer entertainment. You'll see on the beach such top Weider stars as Steve Merjanian, World Record strength star; Gene Shuey, **IFBB 1961 Mr. America;** incomparable **IFBB 1962 Mr. America Larry Scott** in a featured role; and top Weider champ Pete Lupis (on the screen he's "Rock Stevens") as the muscle lead. In case you don't remember Pete, check back in your recent **Muscle Builder** issues and you'll see a feature article on him by Reg Lewis.

And, all your entertainment stars such as beautiful Annette, singer Frankie Avalon (who now trains with Weider weights! . . . watch for an exclusive feature on Frankie in the July Mr. America) and top comedians Buddy Hackett, Morey Amsterdam and Don Rickles (he plays "Jack Fanny" top gym instructor!) make this a really wild, swinging picture! Add to this the music of Lex Baxter, the surfing sounds of Dick Dale and top rock-n-roller, Little Stevie Wonder, and you've got an entertainment package that

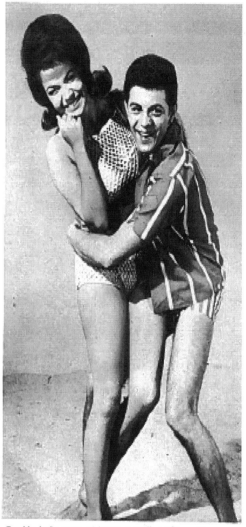

Frankie looks more at home grappling with pretty Annette, his co-star in MUSCLE BEACH PARTY. Their refreshing antics are the focal point of the movie.

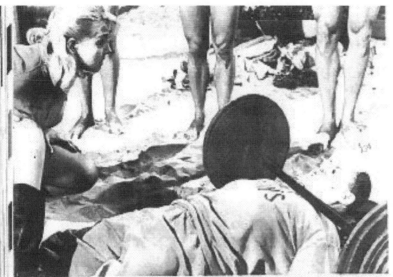

Wha' happen! It seems Jack Fanny (laughingly played by Don Rickles) can't quite practice what he preaches. Below, Larry Scott shows why he won the IFBB Mr. America title . . . he certainly looks more massive and cutup than ever in the movie.

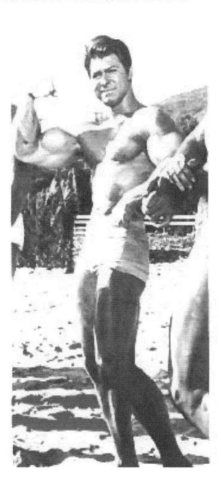

What's everyone looking at?

spells dynamite to all young and fun-loving movie goers.

And, muscle building fans, here's the best news of all! Features Editor Jon Twichell states that American International, producers of the picture, and the Weider Barbell Company will co-promote the movie throughout this country and abroad. Every state in this country will have muscle contests in connection with the picture, with first prize being a Weider Championship Barbell-Dumbbell set! Second prizes will be the incomparable Weider Cable Sets and many other food supplement and equipment prizes will be given. All the theaters showing the picture will have **Muscle Builder** and **Mr. America** magazines available to

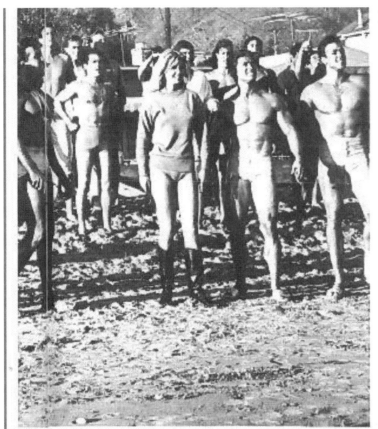
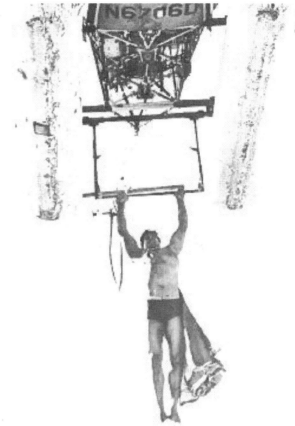

Why, it's Flex Martian (played by Pete Lupus) coming in for a landing in another spectacular scene from MUSCLE BEACH PARTY.

them, and if your theater doesn't have them, ask them why!

Why is the Weider Company doing this, donating this equipment? We believe this movie, the first American "muscle" movie in ten full years is great for bodybuilding, is a really good movie and top entertainment for all. And, whatever we feel is good for bodybuilding, we will support to our fullest extent . . . unlike other barbell companies, we back our words with deeds!

We strongly urge all our readers to see this movie. In it are IFBB champs posing . . . beautiful girls . . . top singers . . . a top entertainment package for all! See it today!

Yet another high point of the movie is its great music; here Dick Dale and his Surfer group perform. (All photos courtesy American International Pictures)

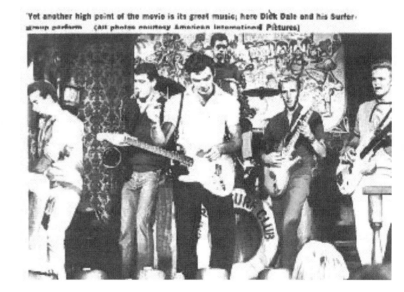

So I'm sure you noticed **Don Rickles** playing the role of "**Jack Fanney**" in this fun flick. Can you guess who they are poking fun at with this one? That's right… the one and only **Vic Tanny**, who we'll discuss further on in more detail. Also having a prominent role in the picture was big **Steve Merjanian**, who trained with my friend **Joe DiMarco, Bill West** & the rest of the guys known as the original **Westside Barbell club.** Steve and Bill both got quite a bit of television and movie work as was discussed in my "**Forgotten Secrets of the Culver City Westside Barbell club revealed**" DiMarco opted for the security of a regular nine to five job of a more mundane nature, and perhaps this was one reason he never got as much recognition as some of the other crew members, though he was an integral part of the core group. For a very in-depth and detailed look at the club, I suggest you grab a copy of my book, but since I wrote that one, I have found some additional stuff on the guys that I thought would make a nice addition to this new one. You'll get to that chapter soon enough.

This interesting 2 part interview with **Ellington Darden** starts in part one with Darden reminiscing about his early days starting out with the weights, in Texas, his encounters with Arnold, Arthur Jones, Casey Viator and others. He gives his ideas on high intensity full body training vs. split routine, higher volume training. It is from the T-Nation website;

http://www.t-nation.com/free_online_article/sports_body_training_performance_interviews/a_return_to_the_golden_age_ii

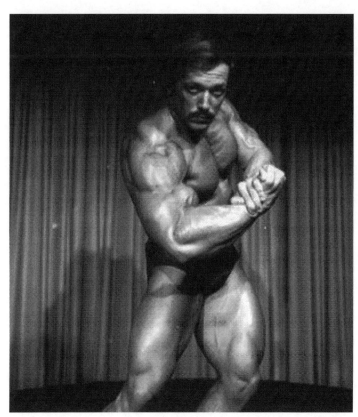

Casey Viator

Darden trained at Muscle Beach and the Dungeon in the early '60s, which many of you may not be aware of.

One particularly interesting story he tells about is when he and Arnold both spoke at a new nautilus facility opening ceremony that took place in Bethlehem, Pa, which is minutes from where I currently abide. Here is an excerpt from part one describing that;

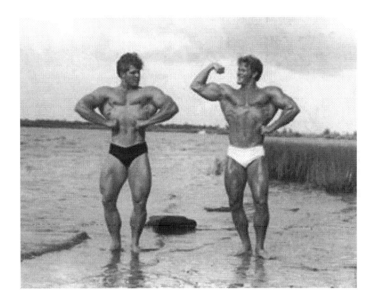

Darden with Jim Haislop

> phia. Haislop's outstanding legs and broad shoulders are somewhat reminiscent of Steve Reeves, but he possesses a much deeper chest than Reeves. Third place went to Captain Craig Whitehead of the U.S. Air Force Medical Corps. Dr. Whitehead's showing was a notable improvement over his ninth place finish in the 1967 Mr. America event.

Above is a piece from a lifting report out of Muscle Builder, mentioning Haislop in a positive way

My first quality meeting with Schwarzenegger was in 1977. I was director of research for Nautilus Sports/Medical Industries and a new Nautilus Fitness Center was having a grand opening in Bethlehem, Pennsylvania. The owner invited Arnold and me to speak at the local high school. He met both of us at the airport in Philadelphia and drove us to **Bethlehem**, which was north about 50 miles. So we had more than an hour to talk. Arnold hadn't yet made it in the movies, but he'd won five consecutive Mr. Olympia titles. The more we talked (it was mostly Arnold talking and me listening), the more I was reminded of a book, *Your Erroneous Zones*, by Dr. Wayne Dyer. I soon realized that Arnold had learned little from his success. Dyer, in one chapter of his book, noted that "success often keeps you applying the same old misinformation and faulty beliefs." When I could finally squeeze a couple of words into Arnold's discourse, I boldly said, "Nothing fails like success," and I proceeded to share with him what I'd read in Dyer's manual. That got his attention and he sincerely asked me to tell him more. "Just about the only thing we can learn from is *failure*," I continued. "But to do so, we must recognize what we're doing as a *mistake*. Then we must correct that mistake." In the same vein, Arthur Jones once told me, "Good judgment comes from experience. Experience comes from bad judgment." It's unfortunate that we have to make mistakes to learn. But apparently we do. Success can often lead us on a path of self-destruction. We must constantly evaluate and reevaluate both our successes *and* failures. Arnold listened intently for a few minutes and he changed the subject to something less thought provoking. Later, in his speech that night, he challenged the young bodybuilders in the audience who wanted to look like him to apply his training advice.

His training advice is well documented in his books, which have been published by Simon & Schuster. For best results in building your body, **Arnold recommended the following:**

• Perform at least 20 sets for most body parts.

• Do high-repetition sets for definition and low-repetition sets for mass.

• Adhere to a split routine by concentrating on different parts of your body on different days.

My advice to the audience that night was quite different from Arnold's, and I might add, I delivered it before Arnold spoke. For best bodybuilding results, I noted that you should:

• Perform only one or two sets per body part.

• Do 8 to 12 repetitions per set for most body parts. Definition is almost entirely related to following a diet to reduce the percentage of subcutaneous fat.

• Train the whole body in each workout and rest the whole body the following day. Do not split the routine.

Arnold was a believer in **high-volume, four-hours-per-day, six-days-per-week, high-volume training (HVT).** My bodybuilding philosophy was dissimilar: **brief, high-intensity, 30-minute routines that are repeated three times per week (HIT)**. Naturally, Arnold, with his impressive size, titles, and ability to work an audience, had the upper hand. "Who are you going to believe," Arnold said to the audience near the end of his speech, "him?" as he pointed my way and laughed, "or me?" as he flexed his Mr. Olympia arms in a double-biceps pose.

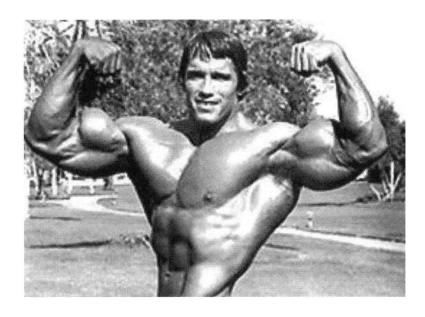

I was no match for Arnold that night and I knew it. Political researchers have known for years that most voters respond to how a candidate looks more than they do to what he says. Arnold, with his massively developed physique and high-peaked biceps, would be able to sway almost any group of exercise enthusiasts his way. And he did.

In another part of this interview, **Darden talks about Vic Tanny, Joe Weider, etc;**

T-Nation: When you first started competing, how did you and most bodybuilders train?

Dr. Darden: **All of my early training, from 1958 to 1963, was based on three times per week, whole-body routines.** My first barbell set was from **Healthways**, and the enclosed booklet pushed that type of training.

The booklets shown on the following pages are from other companies, but are likely very similar in the advice given in the Healthways manual that came with their barbell set;

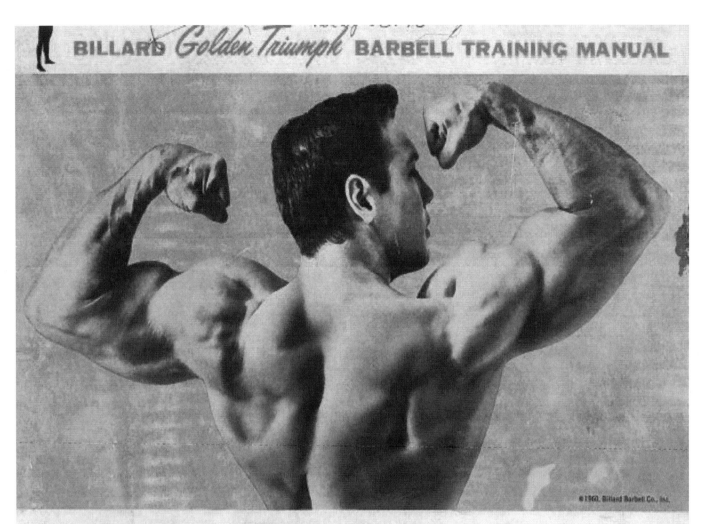

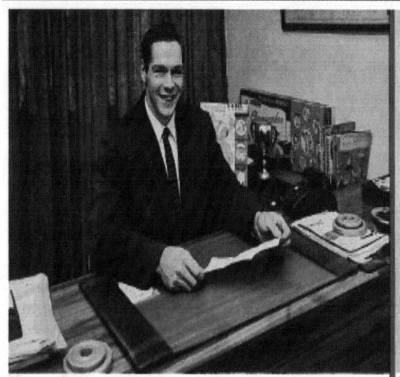
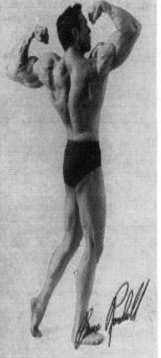
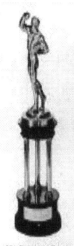

Mr. Universe Trophy Awarded to Bruce Randall, Mr. Universe 1960, for having attained the highest standard of body development. His prize-winning measurements achieved with barbell training: arms 19½", chest 55", waist 31", thighs 27", calf 18½", neck 18". Wt. 225 lbs.

A message from BRUCE RANDALL
Mr. Universe 1960

Congratulations! You now own a Billard precision-made Barbell Set, equipped with exclusive, patented "Loc-Fast" Collars. It's the finest barbell set made today, and the choice of outstanding athletes and weight lifters as well as leading health gymnasiums, schools and hospitals throughout the country. ■ And with your set you get this expert barbell "trainer" – the "Billard Golden Triumph Barbell Training Course." Professional athletes and trainers have collaborated in this book and, of course, I have drawn on my own experiences demonstrating correct barbell procedure in schools and health clubs throughout the country, and while training for the Mr. Universe Contests. Most of the exercises are illustrated by Abe Goldberg, owner of one of the finest health studios in New York. I think you'll enjoy working with this book that also includes informative facts on barbell training and records. ■ Did you know that barbell training is the only proven scientific method of developing a powerful and balanced body? With barbells you can build robust health and increase strength and stamina. This is not a super-human goal attainable by "some other fellow." It's a goal you can easily achieve. Beginners find this difficult

(continued Page 6)

GENERAL TRAINING INFORMATION

From beginner to advanced exercises, follow these suggestions for best results: Monday, Wednesday and Friday are perfect days for a workout schedule. Ideally, barbell training should be done 3 times a week, with not less than 30-minute workouts. This amount of exercise is enjoyable and necessary for muscular development. Give yourself a day's rest between each workout and a complete weekend of relaxation after the Friday workout. Remember, rest periods are important for muscle recuperation and build-up. ■ Begin training periods before the evening meal, leaving a half hour for rest before eating. Breathe in as you start each exercise movement, exhale on completion. To be successful in barbell training, you must exercise regularly, maintain a proper diet, and always get enough sleep. ■ Now read the Introduction to Beginner Exercises on page 2.

The inside-cover from the manual shown on previous page

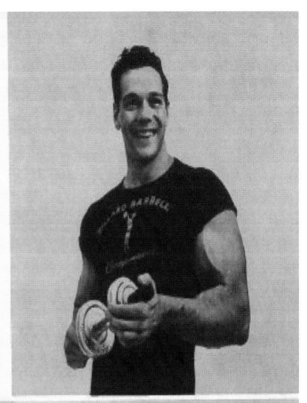

INTRODUCTION TO INTERMEDIATE EXERCISES

3 months with Billard Barbells and Dumbbells

Now that you've developed good form doing complete movements in each exercise, you're ready to select the number of plates and proper weights from the exercises that follow. But if you haven't kept pace, find out why. Did you skip a workout occasionally? Or do you just need more time on the same exercises? If so, take another week or two and repeat the beginner exercises. Remember your aim is to train, not to strain.

GOOD EATING HABITS

... are a must in successful barbell training. You need plenty of energy to get first-rate results. And energy depends on the food you eat. Good eating habits are easy to follow. Be sure you get your daily minimum requirements of vitamins, calcium, minerals—and nature's very important life-giving substance, protein. Remember, protein is as important as the air you breathe. And, like air, protein can't be stored by the body. You need a new supply of protein daily to keep building muscle and tissue. Meat, fish, eggs and cheese are among the high protein foods. Even for people who don't get much exercise, three hearty meals a day often do not provide the daily protein requirement.

The person who exercises with barbells to lose weight needs protein just as much as the one who exercises to gain weight. Based on the scientific principle of balanced exercising, barbell exercises develop a powerful and balanced body. This means your natural needs are fulfilled for either a weight gain or loss.

To be sure of sufficient protein, most successful athletes now supplement their daily diet with high protein tablets. Sufficient protein gives you the energy for effective exercising that helps break down unwanted fat deposits in the body and builds muscle.

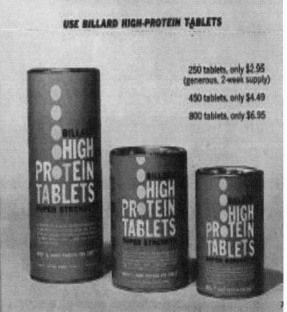

USE BILLARD HIGH-PROTEIN TABLETS

250 tablets, only $2.95
(generous, 2-week supply)

450 tablets, only $4.49

800 tablets, only $6.95

The inevitable supplement pitch on the back cover

Here is one of the exercise illustration pages featuring Mr. Universe, Bruce Randall;

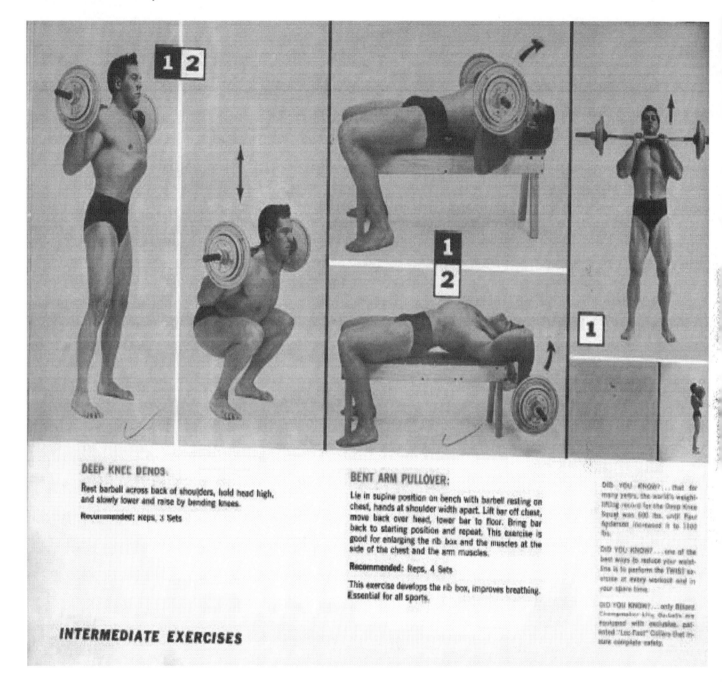

On the back panel of the booklet, we see Bruce demonstrating Olympic lifts…. Bruce was very versatile!

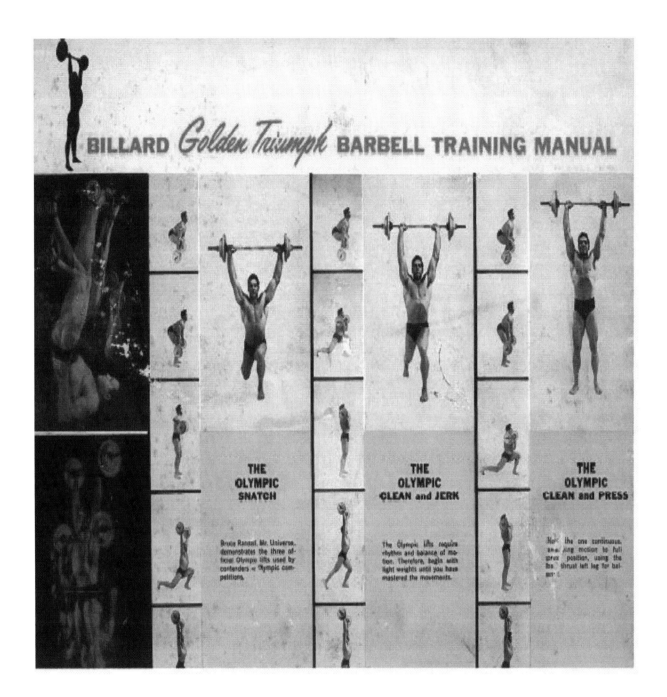

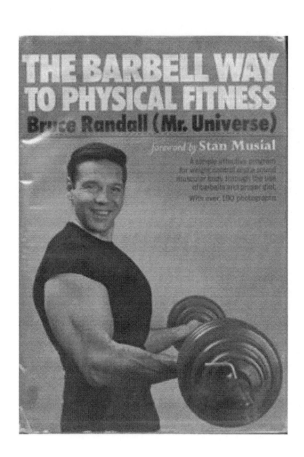

This booklet from the same era would have offered similar advice:

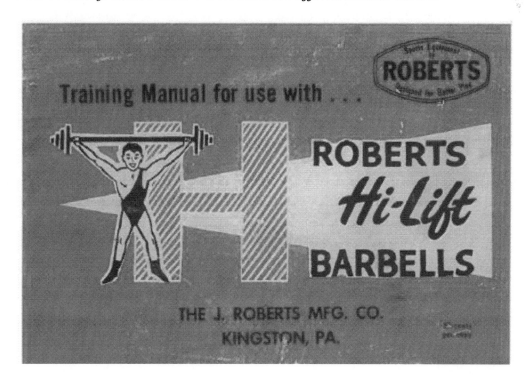

IT'S FUN TO BUILD A STRONG, HEALTHY BODY

Follow the instructions in this manual carefully and you will receive the full benefits of this wonderful means of building a strong, healthy body. Try to establish a routine which you can faithfully follow. The exercises should be completed at least a half hour before a meal. Spend at least 30 minutes exercising each time.

Most athletes prefer to train 3 times a week with a full day's rest in between workouts. Some train Mondays, Wednesdays and Fridays, giving themselves an extra day's relaxation over the weekend. After you have been in training for a while, you can decide what schedule is best for you.

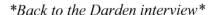

Back to the Darden interview

And I carefully studied **Bob Hoffman's *Strength & Health* magazine,** which was the main training journal of that day. Hoffman was big on the basics and **three-days-per-week, whole-body workouts.** I built the majority of my muscular size and strength (from 138 pounds to 202 pounds) using these methods. In 1984, **Vic Tanny**, who had one of the first bodybuilding gyms on the West Coast and knew all the contest winners, shared the following about whole-body and split-routine training: Tanny realized in the early 1940s that to make gyms profitable, he had to get women involved. **He did this by adding carpet, chrome, mirrors, and one other thing: He discovered that women didn't like to exercise around men.** Instead of having a facility for men and a separate one for women, however, he simply used the same location and went to a **Monday-Wednesday-Friday schedule for men, followed by a Tuesday-Thursday-Saturday schedule for women**. This every-other-day schedule made every-other-day training the norm, and it remained that way from 1950 to well into the 1960s. It wasn't until the mid-1960s, Tanny remembered, that he had enough clubs throughout the United States (and enough revenue) to create separate clubs for men and women. After that, an enthusiastic man or woman could exercise four, five, or even six days a week – and many of the bodybuilders started training in a "more-is-better" way. Tanny had a keen sense of making money, but he also understood which training produced the best results. **He was a die-hard believer in three-days-per-week training.**

Author's notes

You will see an article later on in the section about Tanny & his gyms that at least somewhat contradicts Darden's assertion above about Vic being a die-hard believer in 3 days per week training. Perhaps Vic pushed the concept hard during his early days with his gym members out of financial considerations.

Speaking of Strength & Health & the whole brevity of workout issue, here is a cool little snippet from a 1948 Strength & Health issue that sheds a little humor on the subject, from a guy who was a bit more in tune with the rationale of the Darden philosophy. Scan down the second column to near the bottom for the piece that starts with "how long should a workout last?"

The S&H article will digress momentarily from the Darden interview, but then we'll jump right back into it again without skipping a beat

The article on the following 2 pages was originally laid out on one page. Please read down column 1, both pages, then column 2 both pages, etc.

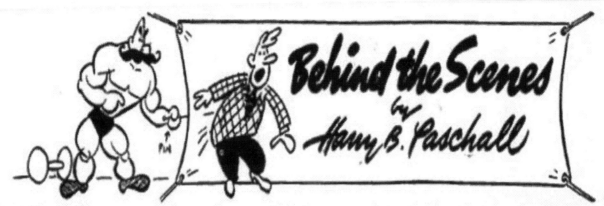

Behind the Scenes by Harry B. Paschall

ON this month's cover we proudly present the picture of one of our native sons, Fraysher Ferguson, of the Apollo Health Studio, Columbus, Ohio. Since Fraysher is one of our particular pals, perhaps we may be allowed to gloat for a couple of paragraphs. An old-timer of the open road once told us that the way to get to really know a man was to go fishing or hunting with him. Since we would rather lift weights than go fishing, we have come to the conclusion that one of the best ways to know a man is to train along with him. We have worked out many, many times with Fergy, and we have gone on trips with him to Cincinnati, to Cleveland, to Akron, to Chicago, to Philadelphia, and we have enjoyed these friendly outings so much that we can truly say, as the Texas cowboys used to put it, "He's a man to ride the river with."

Fraysher is just a shade under six feet, and weighs a natural 181, and he has just about the finest muscular definition these old eyes have ever seen. He started barbell work to correct a very fragile frame back in his Ozark home a bit over a decade ago, made a great deal of progress until a service injury put him in the hospital for nearly two years, and robbed him of all the physical gains he had made. His comeback since that time has constituted one of the greatest health and strength barbell miracles. He became well known several years ago as a repetition bent presser (we have seen him do 8 repetitions with 200 pounds), and also won the Ohio 181 pound lifting title, as well as the 1945 Mr. Ohio contest.

Lately Fraysher has been doing some real lifting training, and as we are writing this a week before the Junior Nationals, we are going to venture the assertion that he will fly down to Louisiana next week and not only win the lightheavyweight lifting title, but also the Jr. Mr. America crown. He has done 255, 255, 315 for an 825 total in training on a tiny and very delicate lifting platform. He should do even better in the Juniors in competition, and we figure anything over 825 should win handily, as this figure in itself would break all previous junior records. Ferguson is an athlete who combines great strength for three or four hours. As we recall, one expert some years ago ran an experiment in his gym to see how fast a man could take a complete workout, which included all of the standard exercises; curls, presses, rowing, bendovers, squats, side-bends, sit-ups, leg-raises, and several dumbell routines. One man did the whole layout in eight minutes, and was not too fagged.

We have a feeling that some of the boys are overdoing this workout business by training daily for hours on end, and by using the multiple series system ad nauseam. That is, exceeding the point where exercise is beneficial and becomes a tearing down process rather than a building program. We will go along with the series idea for specialization up to three sets, but over that it becomes muscle-spinning. However, to get back to the length of a work-out, we can recall the cunning use made of this streamlined program by one gym owner of our acquaintance. He had a habit of closing his place at nine o'clock in the evening, and was pretty anxious to get through and get home, but he had, as so many gym operain his Ozark home a bit over a decade ago, then went to Springfield College to become a physical director, and while there he was instrumental in having the York boys give an exhibition at this most famous of all physical education schools. He had is an athlete who combines great strength with flashing speed, and has the capacity to do 260, 275, 350 by the time the Olympic games roll around in August, if he were able to train a few weeks with the "derned demons" in York. We particularly love the way he thrusts out his arms to a terrific solid lock on both snatches and jerks. Once the weight has passed the top of his head on either lift, there is no longer any question about it.

You can check the results of the Junior meet in this same issue (I hope), and see how well I make out on this prediction. But win or lose, Fraysher is the sort of fine athlete we are proud of attracting to the iron game.

* * *

Ever since our charming co-worker, Abbye ("Pudgy") Stockton has set up housekeeping in the next apartment, (just turn the page) we have been having difficulty in keeping our model Bosco under proper control. As you can see, he got away from us this month. Our slot in the makeup of Strength and Health has kinda put us in the middle. You might say we are between Beauty and the Beast.

* * *

How long should a workout be? We have run into some heated arguments concerning this simple subject in our years of hobnobbing with barbell fans. Some say thirty minutes is enough, others hold out

home, but he had, as so many gym operators have found out to their sorrow, one of those three-hour work-out boys who made a habit of getting into the place just under

(Continued on Page 28)

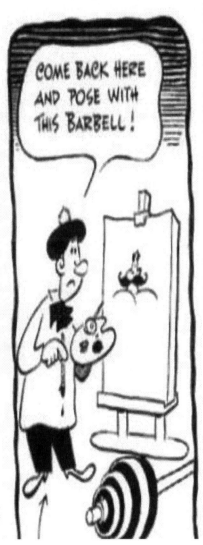

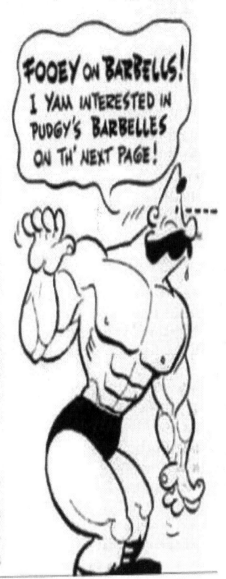

Behind the Scenes

(Continued from Page 21)

the wire at 8 P. M. and then proceeding to take his leisurely time over a thousand exercises. Naturally everybody around the gym coined the name "Bottleneck" for this character; and I have seen the gym director so boiling mad as hour succeeded hour, and his dinner grew cold, and Bottleneck sauntered from rack to rack without heed to hints to hit the shower, that apoplexy was actually imminent.

However the Bottleneck problem was solved in a very clever way. The Professor told him that he had a great new idea that would build muscle so fast you wouldn't believe it. "What is it?" screamed Bottleneck, who was really interested in muscles. The wily professional then unfolded his brainwave, "The way to build big muscles fast is to get all the blood into the muscles, and then don't let it get out. You do fifteen curls and your biceps swells up; it's full of blood, see? Now let's keep that blood right there. How? Do every exercise with lightning speed . . . fast . . . *fast* . . . FASTER! Don't pause and let the blood run out; jump right from curls to presses, to squats, to pullovers, to rowing, to side-bends, to sit-ups and then run to the showers!

You should have seen Bottleneck go through this work-out! It took him all of seven minutes, with the instructor standing right behind him prodding him on; grabbing his arm and hustling him to the shower, and then handing him his towel and telling him to get a brisk, FAST rubdown.

I don't know whether Bottleneck ever got wise that the new muscle building system was especially tailored to his particular needs, as I lost sight of him not long afterward. However, if he is in our audience right now he will recognize the name "Bottleneck" and know whereof we speak.

returning to the Darden interview

Joe Weider's *Mr. America* **and** *Muscle Builder* **magazines**, which were **predecessors to** *Muscle & Fitness*, were around during the 1960s but difficult to find consistently on the newsstands. Its true Weider pushed split routines and high-volume training, but most bodybuilders at that time didn't take his magazines seriously. **Weider wasn't taken seriously until he brought Arnold Schwarzenegger to the United States, made him into the 1970 Mr. Olympia, and began writing about him in his magazines.** You could say that *Arnold really popularized Joe* and that *Joe really popularized Arnold*. They both needed each other. Together, Arnold and Joe – along with the writers at Joe's magazines – promoted **split routines, double splits, bombing, blitzing, and many other razzle-dazzle techniques** to keep guys exercising longer and more often. Of course, Weider knew exactly what he was doing, because in almost every article he published, he peppered the writing with his food supplements and the fact that, if you really want to make progress (like the champions do), you *must* consume Weider supplements.

In the second part of this T-Nation interview, Darden talks more about Muscle Beach & the "Golden Age"

Uncovering Muscle Beach

When many of us think of perfect physiques, we think of those belonging to **Golden Age bodybuilders.** These champions of the past were muscular, strong, healthy, and athletic. It's cliché but it's true: women wanted them; men wanted to be them. But how did these Golden Agers train? How did they eat? What was the vibe like back in the glory days of bodybuilding? How did it all begin? One person who knows is Dr. Ellington Darden. Dr. Darden knows because he was there through much of the Golden Age. **He won his first contest in 1964, which of all things was called Mr. Muscle Beach.** The contest was held in conjunction with the grand opening of a movie called *Muscle Beach Party*. This beach parody starred Annette Funicello and Frankie Avalon, and featured bodybuilders **Larry Scott, Peter Lupus, and Chet Yorton, among others.**

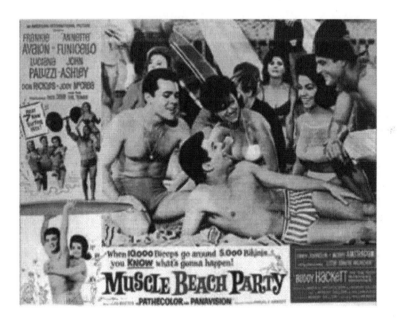

In Part I of the interview, Dr. Darden talked about full-body training and bodybuilding in the 1960s and 70s. In this installment, he talks about **what can be done to save modern bodybuilding,** and he delves further into the past, into what many consider to be the beginning of American physical culture: the real Muscle Beach.

T-Nation: Most people have heard of Muscle Beach, but few know much about it. Where was Muscle Beach and exactly what went on there?

Dr. Darden: The original Muscle Beach, California, was located on 200-square yards of sand, just to the south of the main pier in Santa Monica. **From 1940 to 1958, Muscle Beach was the most famous playground in the world for bodybuilding, weightlifting, and gymnastics.** The long pier shielded the nearby beach from prevailing winds and allowed fitness activities to be practiced year-round. At the center of the beach activities was an L-shaped platform/pen, with an enclosed shed at one end. The shed was designed to house a selection of barbells, dumbbells, benches, and racks. The equipment was stored in the shed each night and organized outdoors for use each morning. The open-air gym buzzed with participation and fan appeal. Eventually, the pen was surrounded by a short fence and became officially known as the "**Muscle Beach Weightlifting Club.**" Approximately 50-yards east of the club area was a 12-foot by 60-foot, raised wooden platform, which extended north to south. Acrobats, gymnasts, hand-balancing teams, and adagio acts trained and performed on this improvised stage. In between both platforms were various high bars, parallel bars, flying rings, and volleyball nets.

Perhaps most important, the entire beach-training atmosphere was enveloped by the renowned California sun and surf, with a dash of Hollywood mystique thrown in for amusement. Athletes came from all over to display their acrobatic, gymnastic, weightlifting, and bodybuilding skills. As the years went by and the popularity increased, portable bleachers were brought in to appease the spectators. From 1947 to 1958 – when strength and physique contests were scheduled on holiday weekends – the audience might number more than 5,000.

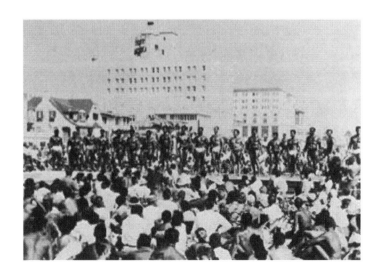

T-Nation: Interesting. So, everything we've heard about Muscle Beach and the training that originated there, actually took place outdoors on the beach?

Dr. Darden: Some of it did, especially on the weekends. But a lot of the so-called Muscle Beach training took place five blocks away in **Vic Tanny's Gym.** Shortly after World War II, Tanny converted a 7,000-square-foot USO center, which was **located in a basement on 4th Street**, into the best-equipped gym in the United States. To serious trainees, this beloved gym became known as **the Dungeon.**

The Dungeon was where a long list of famous bodybuilders trained, men such as **Steve Reeves (1947 Mr. America), George Eiferman (1948 Mr. America), Armand Tanny (Vic's brother and 1950 Mr. USA), and Joe Gold (original owner of Gold's Gym)**, just to name a few.

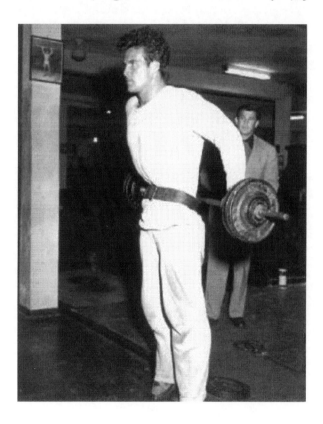

Steve Reeves performs a hack squat at the Dungeon in 1947. That's Vic Tanny in the background.

T-Nation: Did you ever visit Muscle Beach?

Dr. Darden: No, not the original Muscle Beach. I was too young in the 1950s and really didn't develop an interest in training until the 1960s. Muscle Beach, from my research, was forced to close in late 1958.

The politics surrounding certain problems caused the Santa Monica city council to mandate that the weightlifting and bodybuilding equipment be removed, athletic contests be suspended, and the name "Muscle Beach" be discontinued. According to several people I've talked to about this, the decisions and equipment removal happened literally overnight. **Afterward, the beach regulars united and moved their training a mile south to Venice Beach. In 1959, Venice Beach, with newer and better outdoor facilities, became the new hangout for the muscle crowd.** When I became interested in bodybuilding, there was a guy in our town who was into karate. He wasn't very big – about 5 foot 3 inches tall – but he had some big arms for his height. Anyway, this guy had a large collection of muscle magazines from the 1950s that he let me borrow. They were mostly **Weider's *Muscle Builder* magazines** and each one had a column about Muscle Beach gossip. (**Just like the clips shown earlier)* Over several weeks, I eagerly read over a hundred of these magazines. I became well versed in what was going on at Muscle Beach, even though I was always from three to ten years behind the actual happenings. And, of course, **Weider's magazines from the 1960s reported on activities at Venice Beach**.

But I had never talked to anyone who'd actually been to the original Muscle Beach or Venice Beach until I met **Dan Ilse** in Waco in 1963. I mentioned Dan in the first interview, as he had won 1962 Mr. Texas. Ilse had actually hung out there for a while and he was always talking about the guys and the atmosphere. Ilse told me that if I ever decided to drive out to California, he'd go with me. In the summer of 1963, I made up my mind to go, but Ilse backed out, and I went alone. I checked into a cheap hotel, two blocks from the Venice Beach outdoor weight pin, and my adventure began.

T-Nation: Okay, so it's the summer of 1963 and you're in California training at **Venice Beach**. What was that like?

Dr. Darden: There was always something interesting going on at the beach. And I met a lot of guys I'd read about. For example, I talked with **Reg Lewis**, who won the IFBB Mr. America later that year, as well as his wife Shari. Shari was the first woman I'd ever seen who could do chins and dips. They were both tan, lean, and in great shape.

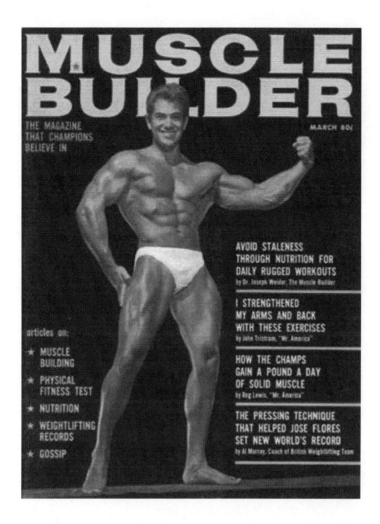

An athletic-looking Reg Lewis lights up the cover of the
March 1964 issue of *Muscle Builder* magazine.

I got a chance to workout with **Hugo Labra, Chuck Collras, and Bernie Ernst**. Ernst was winning most of the California contests at that time, and he was particularly helpful to me.

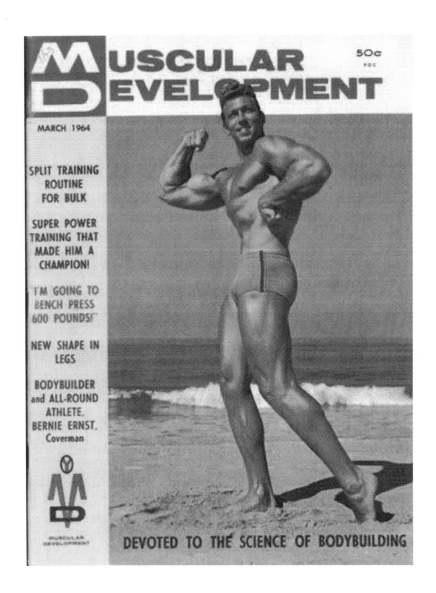

Bernie Ernst as cover man for Hoffman's Muscular Development

The guys who impressed me the most, however, were a couple of powerlifters: Steve Merjanian and Billy "Peanuts" West. Merjanian was 6-feet tall, weighed 285 pounds,* *author's note: 290 according to Joe DiMarco who trained regularly with Steve for a while, in fact that was his nick-name-290)* and was incredibly thick through the chest and shoulders, so thick that the only thing that he could wear over his upper body was a blanket with a hole in the middle for his head.

Many mornings he'd come striding down the beach wearing beige shorts and this colorful blanket over his upper body, with a shaved head sticking out. He was a friendly guy and he always sported a big grin. Slightly behind him was West, who was smaller and who couldn't match Marjanian's long stride. West carried their training logs and he was more talkative and always seemed to be charting their progress. Marjanian's specialty was the incline press and I remember seeing him do 480 pounds, which at that time was probably close to a world record.

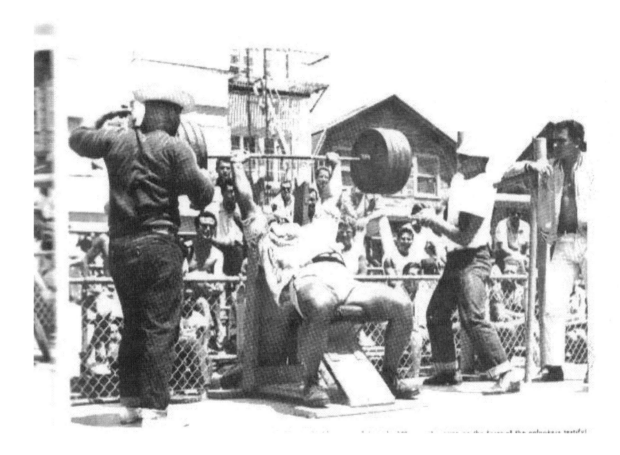

Steve Merjanian had the thickest upper chest development that I've ever seen, before or since. **Someone told me that Merjanian and West did their squats and deadlifts down the road in a basement training area called the Dungeon. Several days later, I visited the Dungeon.**

It was dark, dank, and filled to the brim with bars, benches, and weights. I didn't make the connection at that time, but **that was the original location of Tanny's gym, which had changed hands several times since the late 1950s.** All in all, my six weeks in California were meaningful. I came back to Texas with more enthusiasm than ever for bodybuilding.

On another note, when I entered the 1970 AAU Mr. America, which was held in Los Angeles, I visited Venice Beach and had a look at the outdoor area where I'd trained in 1963. The scene, however, had changed. It wasn't the friendly "come on in and join us" atmosphere that it had been seven years earlier. And in Santa Monica, the Dungeon had been uprooted and the entire building turned into a parking lot.

T-Nation: You've mentioned **Vic Tanny** several times. How did you meet him?

Dr. Darden: Vic showed up one day at the Nautilus headquarters in Lake Helen, Florida, in 1980 to visit Arthur Jones. **Jones had trained for a couple of months at Tanny's Gym in 1947 and Vic remembered him.** Let me tell you, Arthur Jones had a lot of stories, but Vic Tanny had just as many – and he loved to share them. Tanny, perhaps more than any single individual, helped bring modern weight training to the masses. During the 1950s and 1960s, he owned and operated more than 100 Vic Tanny Health Centers throughout the United States. Furthermore, while he had his landmark club, the Dungeon, he wrote a popular column for *Strength & Health* magazine called the "**West Coast Scene.**" As much as anyone, **Vic helped make Muscle Beach into the Mecca for bodybuilding that it became famous for.**

T-Nation: Didn't Tanny sponsor the Mr. USA contest in the late 1940s that featured the famous John Grimek/Steve Reeves confrontation?

Dr. Darden: Yes, Vic told me all about that event. It was the **1949 Mr. USA, which was perhaps the best-promoted and best-attended physique show ever.** This was the contest that brought **John Grimek out of retirement to face Steve Reeves, George Eiferman, and Clancy Ross,** all of whom had previously won the AAU Mr. America. It was held at the Shrine Auditorium and 4,500 people attended.

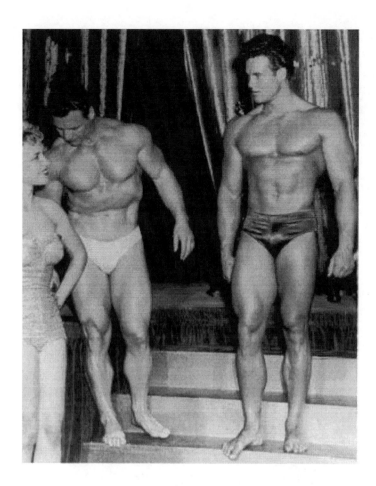

John Grimek (left) and Steve Reeves battled for the
1949 Mr. USA. Grimek was the eventual winner.

In those days, John Grimek – who'd been in the 1936 Olympic Games in weightlifting and who'd won the Mr. America in 1940 and 1941 – was a living legend. His posing routine included acrobatics, muscle control, and flexibility feats. In some 15 years of competing, John Grimek had never lost a physique contest. "Because of who he was," Tanny remembered, "Grimek could have won the contest wearing his street clothes. Was he the best-built man there? No, that belonged to Steve Reeves. But I couldn't say that then, and I even have difficulty admitting it now. That's how much we all admired Grimek." The final outcome of the 1949 Mr. USA was 1) John Grimek, 2) Clancy Ross, 3) Steve Reeves, 4) George Eiferman, and 5) Armand Tanny. Vic went on to say that he supervised Reeves training for the better part of a year, and that Steve Reeves – more than anyone else he'd ever seen – had the complete physique. Here was Tanny's revealing, off-the-record sidebar: He said that if the situation had been reversed: if Reeves had been older than Grimek, and if Reeves had starred in his Hercules movies first (similar to Grimek going to the Olympics and winning the first two Mr. Americas), then Reeves' presence would have had similarly invoked the enigmatic star-quality expectation that seemed to have produced such a profound psychological effect on the pro-Grimek judging panels of the day.

Had this been the case, then in Tanny's assessment, no one would have ever defeated Steve Reeves in a bodybuilding contest. In fact, no one would have even entered against him.

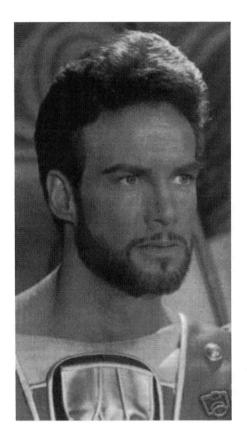

Steve Reeves not only had the ideal body to play Hercules – but his face was also heroic, especially with his beard.

T-Nation: I've often wondered if the early contests had some of the same political overtures that exist in today's professional contests. Did you ever talk to Steve Reeves in person?

Dr. Darden: I sure did. Reeves had a chronic shoulder problem and visited the Nautilus headquarters in 1978 to consult with our sports-medicine physician. When we asked him how he injured his shoulder, his response was anything but typical:

"I was racing in a chariot," Reeves said calmly. "The thing got out of control and slammed into a tree, and I jammed my right arm. The next morning, chased by a crocodile, I had to swim 50 yards under water while oil burned on the river's surface. With every stroke I could feel my right shoulder tear a little more. But there was no turning back."

The picture Reeves painted caught everybody by surprise. No one smiled since Reeves was very serious. Finally, Arthur Jones said, "Damn, Steve, that last bit of action would make a dramatic scene for Tarzan. Have you ever thought about getting into the movies?" That cracked everybody up and we all had a good laugh. Unfortunately, there was little we could recommend for Steve's shoulder (except specific strength-training exercises, which he was already doing, and surgery, which he didn't want to go through). Later that afternoon, Reeves told me that he was thoroughly burned out on the bodybuilding scene, that he wanted nothing to do with it. Casey Viator and I both could tell by looking into his eyes that he'd been disappointed numerous times by disingenuous people and probably taken advantage of too many times to remember. But Reeves continued to hang around the Nautilus gym, which was just off my office. He interacted with some of the regular trainees who dropped by to workout that day. And he continued to chat with Viator and me. Slowly he began to open up – **especially when I brought up the topic of Muscle Beach and his training time at Tanny's**. Then he alluded to something that I won't forget. He said **he missed those hard training sessions at Tanny's and he remembered how quickly his body had responded. But most of all, he said that he missed those innocent times when the older bodybuilders at Tanny's offered help, sincere help, to the younger guys who had just joined. He used the word "mentoring" several times and noted that he seldom saw such behavior in the gyms he visited today**. He graciously thanked Viator and me and said the workout area we had at Nautilus reminded him, at least the atmosphere, of what went on inside of Tanny's. As he was leaving, we asked him to show us his calf. Steve slowly rolled up his left pant leg and contracted a mound of muscle that must have easily been 17-1/2 inches in circumference – and he said he hadn't performed a calf raise in years. Oh, to have such genetics!

T-Nation: The lack of mentoring appears to be even more common in 2006. In most gyms, to get any kind of help at all, you have to hire a personal trainer at $50 to $100 an hour – and this personal trainer probably doesn't know, or care to know, the difference between Steve Reeves and Steve Martin or between a regular curl and a reverse curl.

Dr. Darden: So true. This reminds me; last year I spent four hours with the manager at Tanny's Gym from 1947 to 1949. **Ben Sorenson** is his name. Sorenson was well versed in what went on in what he called not only the world's best, but also the world's "friendliest" gym. "The bodybuilders at Tanny's," Sorenson recalled, "made the place special. Need a spot? No problem, George Eiferman would hand you a heavy barbell and stand by. Need a new chest routine? Steve Reeves would show you what he did last month. Need a training partner? Joe Gold would alternate exercises with you every Monday, Wednesday, and Friday at 6:00 P.M. Almost everyone over 30 years of age was a mentor to someone under 20. That's the way it was at Tanny's and that's the way it was on the weekends at Muscle Beach." And that's pretty much the way it was in gyms and training rooms all over the country in the 1950s, 1960s, and 1970s. **Pumping iron the efficient way was a privilege, a privilege that was passed down from older to younger and from advanced to novice.** This privilege involved a long dose of the basics and hard work; plus simplicity, as opposed to complexity; and *confidence* that what you were doing was going to produce results, and it did! Come to think of it, I believe one of the reasons why you guys at T-Nation have been so successful is in one word: **mentoring.**

Your T-Nation team welcomes the beginning trainee or newbie into the fold with all kinds of helpful guidelines. If he has a question or two, he's encouraged to ask it on your forums, where he can expect a prompt answer.

This final statement from T-nation sums it up nicely;

T-Nation: You know, the more I talk with you the more I realize that the historical aspects of weightlifting and bodybuilding run deep and are indeed meaningful.

In yet another T-nation article, The Tanny's gym manager mentioned in the Darden interview was interviewed himself, and had some fascinating insights about denizens of the Dungeon in his time, and the attitudes of the time;'

http://www.t-nation.com/article/bodybuilding/wider_realman_shoulders&cr

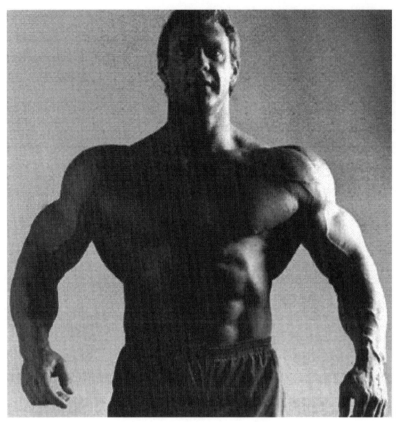 Scott Wilson displays massive width

If you've ever attended a national bodybuilding championships, you know the characters in the audience are often more interesting to watch than the guys on stage. I remember one story in particular about a rather impressive audience member. I first heard about this bizarre incident from several old-time bodybuilders. **Ben Sorenson, a lifter who managed Vic Tanny's famous gym near Muscle Beach,** related the most complete version to me. "It was at the 1948 Mr. USA contest at the Shrine Auditorium in Los Angeles," Sorenson remembered. "Before the start of the show, some of us Tanny's Gym regulars were hanging out in the lobby when a guy walked in with the broadest shoulders I've ever seen. I mean they were freakishly wide — at least 25 inches across. Steve Reeves had some tremendous shoulders on his frame, but they weren't this broad." "What was he wearing?" I asked. "He had on a tan-colored sweater with a two-inch-wide blue stripe that encircled his upper chest and each arm just below his deltoids," Sorenson replied. "Of course, that stripe emphasized the breadth of his shoulders even more. As the guy approached where we were standing, I judged that he was about 20-years old, 6-feet tall, and probably weighed 210 pounds." "Did you get a chance to talk with him?" "No, at the last moment, when he saw us starring in awe," Sorenson said, "he veered to his right and quickly made his way up the stairs. Evidently, he had a seat in the balcony and he didn't want to be confronted. But we watched him go up the stairs and it was obvious to some of us what the kid had done. One of the guys in our group said he got a better look at the guy later in the balcony and he also vouched for what I'm about to explain."

SEVEN SWEATERS

"It seems the bodybuilder went to a shop in Tijuana, Mexico, which specialized in supplying theatrical clothes for Hollywood movies. There he was measured for seven custom-tailored sweaters that he could carefully layer on his upper body to provide the illusion of having extra-wide shoulders. "Visualize this: The first sweater had an extra-large neck hole and a bottom that stopped at mid-torso, and sleeves that ended just past the elbows. Each of the middle five sweaters had a slightly smaller neck hole and a slightly longer bottom and longer sleeves. The seventh sweater had to be very large through the shoulders, chest, and upper arms, but be carefully tailored to fit normally at the neck, waist, and wrist." "I think I understand what you're talking about," I noted, shaking my head in amazement. "It must have been a little like seeing some of those inflatable muscle suits that are used on certain television shows to simulate exaggerated strength?" "You're right," Sorenson said. "At first glance, you're shocked because there's a chance that the size is real. But then you realize that it's a joke, or worse, the guy is actually serious about his desire to project broad shoulders." "Ben, why would a young man want to project extra-wide shoulders?" I wanted to know.

WIDE SHOULDERS MAKE THE MAN

"Because 'shoulders make the man' and 'the wider the better' were common beliefs that were prevalent during and after World War II," Sorenson answered. "Armed forces recruiters frequently made reference to needing *real* men to fight, as opposed to *sissy* men. Boys everywhere wanted to be like the *real-man heroes*, who they saw in both the movies and the newsreels, or heard about on the battlefields." "You mean men like Johnny Weissmuller, Clark Gable, Burt Lancaster, and John Wayne?" I said. "Their broad shoulders always seemed to be emphasized in their movies. Today, you can even see the exaggerated, heroic shoulder width in kids' action toys and cartoons." "Exactly," Sorenson said. "But there's also another angle to this concept . . . because the greatest hero of all — a man among men — at least, for all us guys who fought in the War, was Audie Murphy."

AUDIE MURPHY — A MAN AMONG MEN

"You're so right," I remembered. "I grew up near Houston and Murphy was from north Texas — so he got a lot of publicity around the state. Not only because he was the most decorated US soldier in World War II, but also because of his heroic movie roles. All the kids in my neighborhood admired that serious-styled cowboy he played in his western movies. He was fast on the draw and his Texas twang seemed to speak to our hearts. His movie, *To Hell and Back*, which was also his autobiography, had to have been right up there in popularity with John Wayne's *The Alamo*. "In my neighborhood, most of the kids identified with Murphy because he was short (5 feet, 7 inches), lightly built (145 pounds), and somewhat of an underdog — for approximately half of most of his movies. Then, when he'd had enough, his controlled anger would take over and he'd become what every teenager wished he could become: *A Real Man*, a guy, who when provoked, could become an unbeatable-fighting machine. "It was almost like

Murphy didn't need to lift weights, you know? He was a true 'natural' who had all-around athletic ability. His steely, laid-back, raw ability allowed him to destroy all those Germans in real life and do the same to the bullies or bad men in the movies."

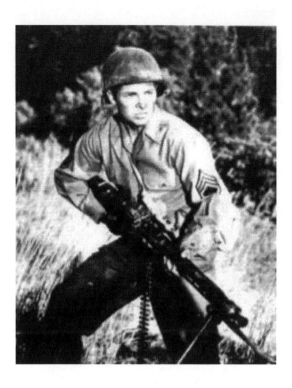

Audie Murphy was a real-life hero to kids growing up in the 1940s and 1950s.

"That does make sense," Sorenson said, "but I'll tell you Ellington, with us mortals, weight lifting was a huge benefit, both during and after the War. There was much truth to *shoulders making the man*. Strong, broad shoulders sure helped me, they helped George Eiferman, they helped Joe Gold, they helped Steve Reeves, they helped all the other soldiers I knew who lifted during and after the War." "Besides Reeves," I asked, "who had the broadest shoulders in Tanny's Gym?"

CHUCK AHRENS AND HIS SHOULDER STRENGTH

"Vic Tanny's younger brother, Armand, was almost Reeves's equal on shoulders," Sorenson answered. "Reeves' shoulders, from deltoid to deltoid, measured with a caliper, were 23-1/2 inches. Tanny's were 23-3/8 inches. And Bill Trumbo was between those two. (1946 Mr California - AAU, Tall, 2nd. But the guy who impressed me the most, was a young **Chuck Ahrens** weighing in at 275 pounds. Six-foot tall Ahrens, actually had shoulders like that guy wearing those seven-tailored sweaters wished he had. "If you've followed the Iron Game for the last 50 years, you'll remember some of the amazing feats of strength that were attributed to Ahrens by the muscle magazines in the late 1950s and 1960s. There was a lot of fiction, no doubt, presented as fact.

But I saw Ahrens, when he was only a teenager, do standing lateral raises with a pair of 90-pound dumbbells in his hands. And he did them in fairly good form. Even then, the boy kept his body covered, and I never heard of anyone ever seeing him without his shirt. But his very broad shoulders and huge arms were undeniable."

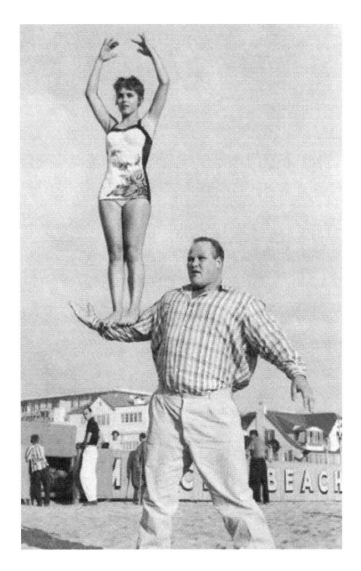

Chuck Ahrens performed this demonstration of shoulder strength in 1957 at Muscle Beach. Ahrens weighed 280 pounds and the girl weighed 75 pounds.

"I remember reading that Ahrens also did seated presses with dumbbells weighing 160 pounds each," I noted. "And I've read several times that his shoulder width, measured accurately with calipers, was 26-5/8 inches. Those are the widest shoulders I've ever heard of. In 1983, I personally measured Scott Wilson's shoulders at 24 inches. His deltoids and overall shoulder width were awesome. I doubt very seriously that Ahrens ever had anything close to the muscularity that Wilson achieved."

"You're right," Sorenson said, "Ahrens was never in hard, ripped condition. And I can't vouch for Ahrens' shoulders ever spanning 26-5/8 inches. My personal opinion would be . . . they were 25-1/2 inches — tops. I've heard from reliable sources, however, that he handled 160-pound, or even heavier, dumbbells on seated presses." "So Ben, dumbbell lateral raises and overhead presses would be a recommended part of your shoulder-development program, right?" "Definitely dumbbell lateral raises, but not dumbbell presses. I always preferred military presses with a barbell to any type of dumbbell press. In my opinion, you can concentrate more with a barbell, than with dumbbells, especially on pressing movements. "At one time, a military press meant that you had to perform the lift using strict military posture: heels together, back straight, chin down, and with only the strength of your shoulders and arms. Within a couple of decades during the middle of the last century, the concept deteriorated into more of a jerk than a press, until the competitive lift was finally discontinued in 1972. It's a shame, you seldom see bodybuilders today doing overhead work. As a result, the shoulder mass of the typical bodybuilder has suffered."

Most gyms in the 1940s and 1950s, according to Sorenson, had an outside caliper handy for this meaningful measurement. Unfortunately, such a tool is seldom seen today. An alternate way of determining shoulder width is as follows:

• Take off your shirt and stand with your back next to a smooth wall.

• Hang your hands in a relaxed manner and touch the sides of your thighs. Do not flare your elbows or widen your lats. (By flaring your elbows you can get another inch or so on the measurement, but you're simply fooling yourself.)

• Have a buddy stand in front, and with a yardstick in his hand, place one end next to your right deltoid and extend it to the front. Have him make a light pencil mark on the wall at the inside edge of the yardstick, which signifies the protrusion of your right shoulder.

• Apply the same procedure, with the yardstick and pencil, on your left deltoid.

• Step away from the wall and measure, with the yardstick or tape measure, the horizontal distance between the two pencil marks.

That horizontal measurement (which includes both deltoids), in inches and fractions of inches, is your shoulder width.

The average man in the United States is 5-foot 10-inches tal, and weighs 172 pounds. His shoulder width is 18-1/4 inches.

Using that as a starting number, if your shoulder width is approximately 18-1/4 inches . . . then, your shoulder width is AVERAGE or NORMAL.

A little bit goes a long way in shoulder width . . . 20-inch-wide shoulders look significantly broader than average shoulders; 21-inch shoulders will get plenty of attention; 22-inch shoulders will draw stares from almost everyone; 23-inch shoulders are super heroic and will get you a ticket on the front row of Mr. Olympia contests; and 24-inch shoulders are as rare as a 500-pound overhead press. The goal of this two-week plan is to add at least 1/2 inch of muscle onto the width of your shoulders.

THE REAL-MAN ROUTINE

Ben Sorenson is correct. Bodybuilders today should definitely NOT ignore overhead pressing. The other key to this routine is the triple pre-exhaustion cycle of dumbbell raises that you do before the overhead press. Also, the overhead press separates into three stages, which adds a different feel to the standard movement. Appreciation goes to Andrew Shortt of Ottawa, Canada, for his assistance in designing and testing this routine.

Here are my deltoid exercises for wider, real-man shoulders:

• Bent-over raise with dumbbells, seated, and immediately followed by:

• Lateral raise with dumbbells, seated, and immediately followed by:

• Front raise with dumbbells, seated, and followed by:

• Overhead press with barbell, standing, performed in thirds . . . middle, top, and bottom.

(During Week 2, add a final set of the regular overhead press.)

Below are the directions for the two workouts that make up Week 1 and the two workouts that compose Week 2.

WEEK 1: WIDER-SHOULDER CYCLE

For the wider-shoulder cycle, you'll need dumbbells, a barbell, and a bench.

Bent-over raise with dumbbells: You won't require much resistance on each dumbbell to get the job done here: 10-20 pounds per dumbbell will work for most trainees on the bent-over raise, and it won't change as you move into the lateral raise and the front raise. The idea is to pre-exhaust the deltoids (posterior, lateral, and anterior) and get a burning shoulder PUMP, before you get into the press. Then, you can use your triceps to force your pre-exhausted deltoids into making a deeper inroad into your starting level of pressing strength. Or, in short, it stimulates your deltoids to grow. Grasp a light set of dumbbells and sit on the front edge of a flat bench. Bend your knees 90 degrees and place your feet together. Lean forward and move your chest near your thighs. Allow the dumbbells to hang near the floor with your arms almost straight. Keep a slight bend in your elbows throughout the movement.

Bring both dumbbells to the sides in an arching motion until the dumbbells are in line with your ears. Pause at the top for 2 seconds and lower smoothly to the starting position. Repeat for maximum repetitions, which should be in the 8 to 12 range. After the final repetition, do not place the dumbbells on the floor. Straighten your torso into a vertical position and go immediately into the lateral raise. Lateral raise with dumbbells: Sit up straight, stabilize your shoulder girdle, and maintain a slight bend in your elbows. Lift the dumbbells laterally until your arms are parallel to the floor. Pause for 2 seconds. Lower slowly while relaxing your neck and face. Repeat for 8 to 12 strict reps. Move immediately into the front raise. Do not place the dumbbells on the floor. Keep holding them. Front raise with dumbbells: Slide forward to the edge of the bench. Bend your knees and place your feet together. Sit upright and maintain a slight bend in your elbows. Raise both dumbbells to the front while keeping your thumbs up. Pause for 2 seconds when your arms are parallel to the floor and lower slowly to the bottom. Repeat for 8 to 12 repetitions. After the final repetition, place the dumbbells on the floor and move immediately to the overhead press with a barbell.

(By now, you should have a burning PUMP throughout your deltoids. Much of the pump is a result of the 2-second pause in the top position of the dumbbell raises. It may be helpful to count to yourself . . . 1-0-0-1, 1-0-0-2 . . . during each rep.)

Overhead press with barbell, standing, performed in stages or thirds . . . middle, top, and bottom: After the triple pre-exhaustion with the dumbbell raises, you won't be able to handle nearly as much as you normally do in the overhead press. I suggest that most trainees try initially from 60 to 80 pounds. Next, visually divide the range of motion of the overhead press into three stages as follows: *bottom,* from upper chest to chin; *middle,* from chin to eyebrows; and *top,* from eyebrows to lockout.

Grasp the barbell with a shoulder-width grip and bring it to the front shoulders. While standing, do 8 reps in the middle third. Then do 8 reps in the top third and a final 8 reps in the bottom third.

Squeeze into each mini-rep and make the movements smooth. Each stage of 8 mini-reps should take approximately 20 seconds. Halfway through, you should feel a deep burn throughout the deltoids. Remain focused and keep pushing. If you don't feel exhausted at the end of the third stage, the barbell is too light and you should increase it for the next session. Finish off the set by performing several full repetitions in the press. Your goal for the fourth session is 12 mini-reps in each stage.

WEEK 2: WIDER-SHOULDER CYCLE

For Week 2, perform the same exercises in the same order, with one exception: On the completion of the overhead press, which is done in stages, take 2 MINUTES REST. Then, perform the overhead press with as much weight as you can, for 8 to 12 repetitions. Keep the form strict, but you can cheat a little on the last several reps.

Review for Week 2, do these five exercises:

• Bent-over raise, immediately followed by:

• Lateral raise, immediately followed by:

• Front raise, immediately followed by:

• Overhead press with barbell, in stages: middle, top, and bottom.

Rest for 2 minutes.

• Overhead press with heavier barbell

The entire shoulder cycle, including the rest period, should take only 7 to 8 minutes. Again, if you do the exercises properly with the correct resistance, you should have a tremendous shoulder pump after 3 minutes . . . and it should become even more pronounced during and after the overhead presses.

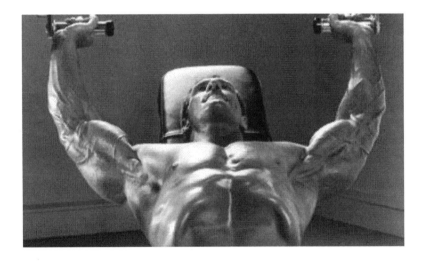

Scott Wilson's 24-inch shoulders do a good job of stabilizing his 18-inch upper arms and 15-inch forearms . . . as he performs an overhead press machine.

Chapter 2   More Culver City secrets

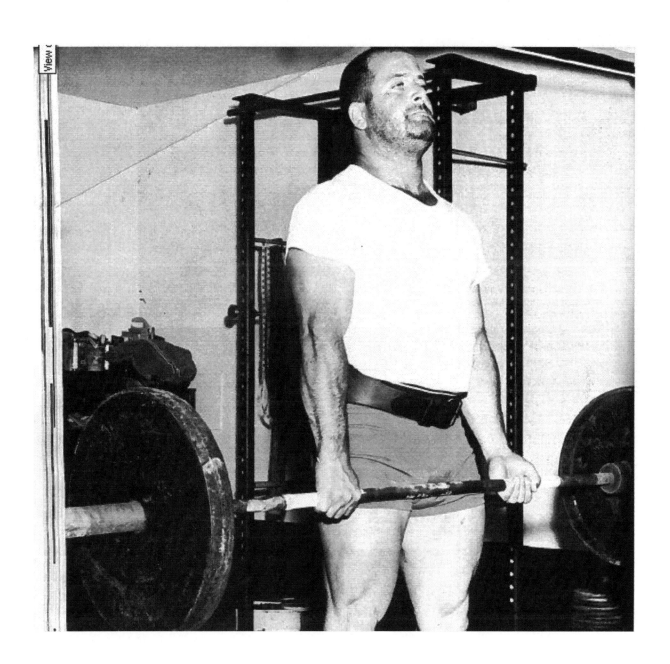

While I covered the original Westside guys pretty well in my "Forgotten Secrets of the Culver City Westside barbell club revealed" book, I have managed to dig up a few more items to create this chapter.

The picture above & the illustrations following are from a Muscle Builder article penned by Charles Smith.

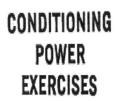
CONDITIONING POWER EXERCISES

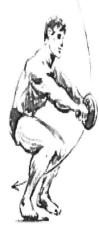
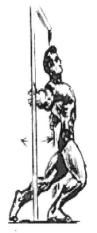
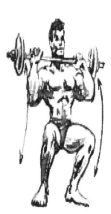
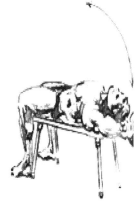

1. Do 10 reps of the Two Hands Swing, to warm up and loosen your muscles for the work to come.

2. DOOR FRAME SWINGS will help your breathing return to normal. Do about 10 or 12 reps.

3. POWER CLEANS can build great endurance; do about 10 complete reps for flexibility and stamina.

4. BREATHING PULLOVERS increase your vital capacity greatly. Do 10 complete reps.

POWER LIFTING

CONDITIONING ROUTINES FOR POWER LIFTERS

BY CHARLES A. SMITH

Member, Weider Research Clinic

★ I remember a statement made several years ago by a well-known Olympic lifter, to the effect that the best way to build up strength in the press was to press. This makes a good deal of sense—as far as it goes. Concentrating on the movement to *improve* the movement is a sound philosophy, but it's far from being the answer to the development and maintenance of great power. So many times we think of a move containing the force of specific muscle groups. We fail to realize that behind every move a whole series of coordinated events had to take place.

Certainly, one of the most important requisites to success in the field of athletics is the proper mental attitude. The nerve force generated by a controlled mental stimulus can exert a power that is almost beyond our imagnation. How many times have you seen a lifter "psyching up" before an attempt. He literally forces strength into his muscles. He consciously controls the nerve forces in his body until all the electricity is turned on "go." Now as he grips the bar the "thing" becomes a contemptible adversary that has challenged his right to lift it. It is like the old saying that "faith could move mountains."

I firmly believe that a man whose mind is disciplined through study, or just plain use, will have a greater opportunity of succeeding in projects where that mind will be needed. Too many people think of lifting as a purely physical endeavor, but I can't swallow that. The strong back and weak mind cliché has more holes in it than a piece of Swiss Cheese.

A good example of what I mean is Terry Todd. Or "Big T" as he's known down Texas way. By any standard he's a giant of a man. Standing next to him is an overpowering experience. This massive man has carved out such lifts as a 500-lb. bench press, 760-lb. deadlift, 715-lb. squat, and a 225-lb. strict curl. He had also done 5 seated behind the neck presses with 300 lbs., cleaned and pressed 400 lbs., power snatched 300 lbs., and power cleaned 400 lbs. It's obvious that Terry Todd is a strong man in many directions.

To the casual observer, Terry Todd is just a big strong man with *(Continued on page 50)*

CONDITIONING ROUTINES

(Continued from page 37)

little else than lifting records to his credit. If that casual observer bothered to do some research he might discover that the muscles of Todd's brain are every bit as strong as the ones you see hanging on his frame. Recently he earned his Ph.D. in physical education. I can safely say that when you see Todd lift, you are seeing the *whole* man in action—and just look at the results.

This doesn't mean that I recommend you earn a doctorate in order to become a successful lifter, but it does mean that I feel that a strong, disciplined mind helps in *any* enterprise and that includes lifting. This, of course, is the emotional side of competition. The physical is something that is a little easier for us to comprehend. As I had stated earlier, very few moves are ever done without the help of several coordinated activities.

Training to reach and then keep in top physical condition is just as important as training for physical power.

but it wasn't too many years ago that the Egyptian lifters were just about the best in the world. Most of the lifters in the club were, or had been, world champions or record holders. Such men as Shams, Hussein, Ibrahim, Nosseir and El Touni would train there for all to see. It was a great thrill for a young strength fan like myself to witness first-hand the training of these amazing athletes.

I had always heard that they trained exclusively on the three Olympic lifts, so you can imagine how surprised I was when I found out differently. A substantial portion of the workouts would consist of free-hand movements such as turning, bending, rotating the trunk and the arms and legs and shoulders. This didn't explain to me how they got the tremen-

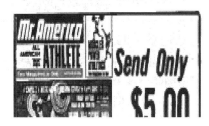

Now it seems almost commonplace to read articles about the Russians and Japanese and so many others doing all types of conditioning training. They have found that by having endurance they can train longer and by having flexibility they can lift better. But, you ask, to what degree does the power lifter need these requisites? Just the same as the Olympic lifter. This is because he handles even heavier poundages, placing a greater strain on the joints and ligaments which, in turn, requires an even greater amount of energy.

Because a power lifter needs far greater staying power than the Olympic man, and because speed is not as important in power lifting as it is in Olympic lifting, the exercises a power lifter must concentrate on must necessarily be different. The power man has to concentrate on those exercises that improve elasticity and flexibility and that build stamina and increase joint and tendon resistance to injury or strain. Here are some examples:

In fact the two are inseparable. One cannot exist in the full without the other. Tip-top condition is the sharp edge to the physical razor. It's the ability to react with maximum efficiency and give your finest possible performance at *any* time; that, to me, constitutes *real* power. I'll bet if someone asked you to define "top physical condition" you'd get about as many answers as there are people. Sure it takes such things as rest and proper nutrition but it also takes joint flexibility, muscle elasticity, a strong heart and lungs and improved respiratory function. While power lifting builds raw power, it doesn't give you the physical conditioning necessary for being the complete strongman. For better conditioning it is necessary to do "assistance exercises."

The first time I came in contact with what are now called "assistance exercises" was during the period from December 1940 to February 1941. I was serving on a cruiser which had been badly damaged at the beginning of the battle for the island of Crete. We had to be towed to the nearest port for repairs. That port happened to be Alexandria, Egypt. While there, I joined the famous Tramway Sports Club on a very "temporary" membership. For the few months I was there I received the reward of seeing one of the finest Olympic lifters in the world. Some of you may not be aware of it,

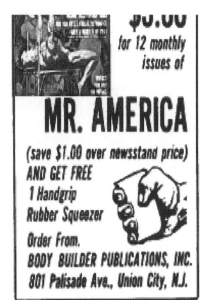

dous endurance they seemed to have. They could go for hours and seem as fresh at the end as they were at the beginning of their training sessions. One day I found out the secret.

I arrived at the gym at a time when all the men were out on a nearby soccer field, so I went over to watch what they were doing. I might say that it was as hot as blazes, which made walking alone a task, much less training. I was shocked by what I saw. One by one the lifters would take a light bar and snatch it, step forward, put it down and snatch it immediately again in a continuous set of reps. He would do this until he had worked himself the full length of the field *and* back.

THE TWO HANDS SWING:

This movement was a great favorite of such strongmen as Herman Goerner, Ron Walker and Charles Rigoulot. Don't worry about style. The important thing in this one is that you breathe deeply and heavily. It is also one of the finest exercises for the lower back and the entire shoulder girdle. First you take a fairly long dumbbell so that the plates won't cut into your wrists. Load it with enough weight to get out ten repetitions. Now place the weight between your legs, which should be about 18" apart. With fingers interlaced around the bar, swing the weight overhead, breathing in at the same time. Without a pause swing the dumbbell back to the starting position as you exhale. After you have completed the ten repetitions, immediately do the following—

DOOR FRAME SWINGS:

Stand about 18" in front of a door frame. Place your hands on the top or sides of the door frame—depending upon your height. With your body rigid and your knees locked, sway forward, inhaling deeply and your head thrust back. Push back to the starting position and do this for 10 repetitions or until the heavy breathing from the swings has returned to normal.

POWER CLEANS:

Most people think of this one strictly as a power builder, not as a great endurance builder. How wrong they are. First choose a weight that will cause you to breathe heavily after ten reps. Dip and clean the weight to the shoulders. Without a pause put the bar back to the starting position and clean it again, using only the lower back and arms and keeping the knees locked. Do ten reps this way then go immediately to the following exercises.

BREATHING PULLOVERS:

Lie on an exercise bench with the head relaxed over one end. Raise the knees—*this is important*—place your feet on the bench flattening your entire trunk. Keep your body glued in this position. Weight is not as important as correct performance and breathing. Grasp a barbell about shoulder width and lower it from an arms-locked-over-the-chest position until it is level with the bench over the head. While moving to that position it is important that you inhale deeply. As you bring the weight back to the starting position, exhale forcefully. Repeat for 10 repetitions.

POWER JERKS:

Take a barbell loaded with your best pressing poundage. Now jerk the weight overhead by just dipping at the knees. You can use the Weider Multi-Power Exerciser on this one for better control. As soon as the weight is overhead drop the weight to the shoulders and repeat until you are breathing heavily. Then do the following—

BENT-ARM BREATHING PULLOVERS:

This is the same as the straight-arm pullovers except that the arms are bent and the weight is passed to the floor. The minute it touches pull it back to the chest, keeping the arms bent. Remember that while you are lowering the weight you must FORCE the air into your lungs; as you bring the weight back, you exhale vigorously.

TRUNK SWAYING:

Use your Weider Multi-Power Exerciser for this one. Trunk swaying is designed to add flexibility to hip the leg joints and elasticity to the hip and lower back muscles. Stand upright between the Multi-Power posts and grasp one in each hand. Sink down into the medium depth split, allowing your hands to stay at shoulder level. Now comes the best part. Sway the body back and forth as far as you can. After a few repetitions change the position of the legs so that the one that was forward is now behind and the one that was behind is now forward. Repeat the swaying moves. Remember that the object of the exercise is to move slowly and without jerking.

FULL BODY CIRCLES WITH A BAR:

Take a 6' empty bar and grasp it as far apart as you can, so that it just clears the top of your head. Standing upright with the bar held out in front, raise it up over and behind your back. Return to the starting position and repeat for 10 to 15 reps. Nothing beats this one for keeping the shoulder muscles supple.

If a layoff from your regular program is indicated by a feeling of staleness, or weariness from your last workout, or if stiffness remains too long in a worked muscle group, use *conditioning exercises* exclusively for a couple weeks. Start off with a single set for each exercise and work up to three. Then take two or three days off and rest before you return to your regular power program.

If you would like to incorporate a few of these exercises into your regular power workouts, then perform them at the end of each workout—start off performing only one set per exercise, and gradually working up to three.

Whether you completely substitute these exercises for your regular workouts, for a short period of time, or perform a few each regular workout, you'll find that your lifts will improve, you'll experience less injury, and you'll be an enduring strongman of supple might and sinew instead of a pile of pain-racked tissue.

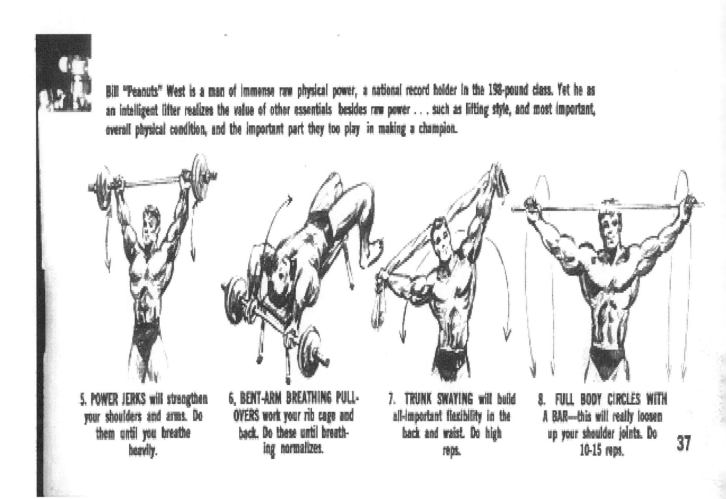

The following page shows another great picture of Bill West clowning around with Arny at Gold's gym, and Dick Tyler and Joe Weider overlooking an up and coming young bodybuilder.

GOSSIP

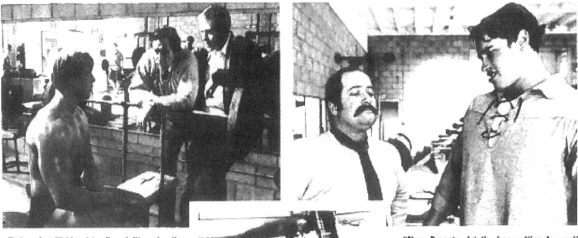

Trainer Joe Weider (standing, left) and writer Dick Tyler frequently make the gym rounds—advising the champs on their training information and gathering new discoveries to report in MUSCLE BUILDER. Here Joe and Dick chat with California sensation Chuck Fautz—a hopeful in the 1969 IFBB MR. AMERICA contest on September 13th. (Zeller)

"Now, Peanuts, dot tie does nutting for you!" says mammoth Arnold Schwarzenegger to his powerlifter counterpart, Bill "Peanuts" West. Arnold's ordinary bodybuilding exercises are practically power records—so he and Peanuts occasionally take a workout together. Big A is all set for the IFBB MR. UNIVERSE and MR. OLYMPIA events on September 13th. (Zeller)

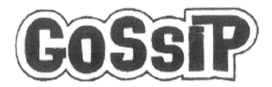

DICK TYLER on the WEST COAST
Gossip from Muscle Beach

ED GIULIANI on the EAST COAST
Muscle Gossip from the East

The text that goes with the picture on the top right follows;

The other day I was waiting in the gym for a man I was to do a story on. That almost seems to be the story of my life. While I was there, in walks this here guy with sideburns and a Charlie Chan-type mustache. Ordinarily it would have been hard to recognize him when he came in but he had the shape of only one man. He looks like four logs stuck in a block of cement and could only be the peanut man himself, Bill West.

"Er . . ." I said with devastating accuracy.

"I know," said Bill. "Why do I look this way. Well, it's because I'm doing a film with Kirk Douglas. It's a Western and I play a convict in prison."

Then I noticed something else. Over his sweat shirt he wore a tie.

"Er . . ." I said again.

"I know," said Bill, "Why am I wearing this tie over my dirty sweatshirt?"

I nodded.

"Well," he continued, "I'm planning to do some great lifting today and I thought I should dress for the occasion."

Maybe that's why he's one of the greatest powerlifters in the world—he's got class.

— — —

Another Gossip column piece covering our boys is this one;

VENICE . . . Pat Casey, 280-pound lifter, did a 785 Squat in training. George Frenn, 242, potentially the greatest hammer thrower in the world, crowded Casey with a 700 Squat. They train together at the West Side Barbell Club in Venice, California. Hal Conelly, top hammer thrower in the world today, does many Stiff Legged Deadlifts to offset the terrific back pull of a rotating hammer.

Here's more from the same column;

GOSSIP FROM DICK TYLER . . . "A few nights ago I dropped by Bill 'Peanuts' West's garage gym. While it isn't large, it's well-equipped. I would say that it has more weight per inch of space than any of your largest muscle palaces in the country. All the equipment is heavy duty and meant to take all the punishment that the men of might who use it can dish out. When I say 'men of might' I should put the 'm-s' in capital letters. Peanuts' gym is undoubtedly the power lifting headquarters of the Muscle Beach fraternity. As an example, when I dropped by this particular evening a giant hulk shaped like a man was sitting on the supine bench. As I got closer I realized it was none other than the strongest supine presser of all-time, Pat Casey. Pat is an unassuming man who hasn't even begun to tap his great power. 'Just take a look at that arm,' said Peanuts about the big things hanging from Casey's shoulders. 'Feel the thing,' he continued. 'Wh-where do I start?' I blurted. This was a problem. I don't think that my two hands even spanned the front surface of the amazing Casey biceps. I was then asked if I would help spot Pat on his supine presses. It took there of us to do the job. Bill West was on one side, Armand Tanny was in the middle and I was on on the other side. All this was needed to get the weight up to the starting position. I have never seen so much weight lifted so easily in my life. These presses were in the best of style. The hand spacing was at the required 32 inches. There was no touch and go, belly tossing or collar-to-collar stuff. All was 'legal' and a beautiful exhibition of real power. So much weight was put on the bar that I thought it would break. Every time I turned around I was asked to put on more plates. Finally 'we' had 560 pounds on the bar. Pat took the weight and pressed it about as easily as you can put a spoonful of food into your mouth, and that's pretty easy. He looked like he could do reps with that heap of iron. Feeling strong, he asked for 585 pounds. That was his personal record, which, of course, is a world record. Just was his personal record, which, of course, think, every time Pat Casey starts to practice his supine presses he lifts more than anyone else in the world. We lifted the 580 pounds up to the big man. Slowly, he lowered the enormous thing to his chest. After a pause, the weight started to rise. His left side (the side I was on) wasn't going up as fast as I thought it should. I thought he was going to lose the lift. So, I touched the bar to help. This, of course, would disqualify any lift. After seeing what he had done earlier — I believed him. I now make a fearless prediction that Pat Casey will do a supine press of 600 pounds, within the year. Nothing like safe predictions, I always say. That's the safest one I've ever made since I bet someone he'd be bored at an AAU contest."

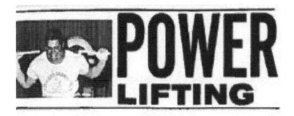

POWER LIFTING

WHAT HAPPENED THIS MONTH, AND WHAT TO EXPECT TO HAPPEN IN THE POWER LIFTING WORLD IN COMING MONTHS. NEWS — LIFTING REPORTS — RECORDS — GOSSIP

Compiled by Power Editor JON TWICHELL,
Member of the Weider Research Clinic

YOU will note accompanying this article are up-to-date listings of both the American Amateur Power Records and the top American power lifters. These continuing charts will be kept each month by Power Editor Jon Twichell, and all officials running power contests are invited to send their results in for publication and entering of records and top totals.

These two charts will be joined next month by a complete listing of IFBB Power Records. At this writing 4 IFBB power contests will be conducted in the next 5 weeks, including IFBB Eastern States Power Championships and IFBB Power Championships in Nashville, Tennessee. With these results in we will set up a preliminary *(Continued on page 65)*

POWER LIFTING PANORA

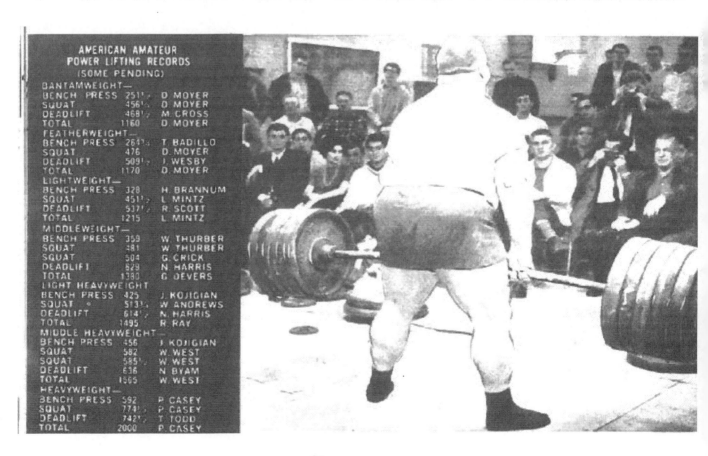

AMERICAN AMATEUR POWER LIFTING RECORDS (SOME PENDING)

BANTAMWEIGHT—
BENCH PRESS 251½ D. MOYER
SQUAT 456½ D. MOYER
DEADLIFT 468½ M. CROSS
TOTAL 1160 D. MOYER

FEATHERWEIGHT—
BENCH PRESS 261½ T. BADILLO
SQUAT 476 D. MOYER
DEADLIFT 509½ J. WESBY
TOTAL 1170 D. MOYER

LIGHTWEIGHT—
BENCH PRESS 328 H. BRANNUM
SQUAT 451½ L. MINTZ
DEADLIFT 537½ R. SCOTT
TOTAL 1215 L. MINTZ

MIDDLEWEIGHT—
BENCH PRESS 359 W. THURBER
SQUAT 481 W. THURBER
SQUAT 504 G. CRICK
DEADLIFT 629 N. HARRIS
TOTAL 1390 G. DEVERS

LIGHT HEAVYWEIGHT
BENCH PRESS 425 J. KOJIGIAN
SQUAT 513½ W. ANDREWS
DEADLIFT 614½ N. HARRIS
TOTAL 1495 R. RAY

MIDDLE HEAVYWEIGHT—
BENCH PRESS 456 J. KOJIGIAN
SQUAT 582 W. WEST
SQUAT 585½ W. WEST
DEADLIFT 636 N. BYAM
TOTAL 1565 W. WEST

HEAVYWEIGHT—
BENCH PRESS 592 P. CASEY
SQUAT 774½ P. CASEY
DEADLIFT 742½ T. TODD
TOTAL 2000 P. CASEY

Again, the Muscle Builder Powerlifting Panorama depicts more accomplishments of the original Westside boys, as shown above & below;

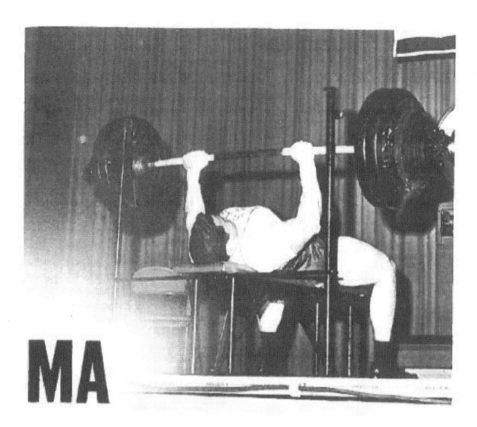

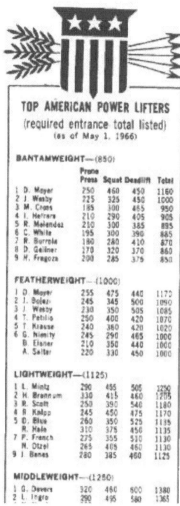

Titans of the power world! LEFT, you see the one and only Paul Anderson Deadlifting over 700 pounds at a recent power show. What sort of a total Paul could have made in his prime is only conjecture. ABOVE, Ronnie Ray of Dallas recently set up a new Mid-Heavy total mark of 1495. BELOW, George Frenn Squatting with 685 in Bill West's garage. Frenn set up a 1700 total, also just broke his leg and now continues power work, cast and all!

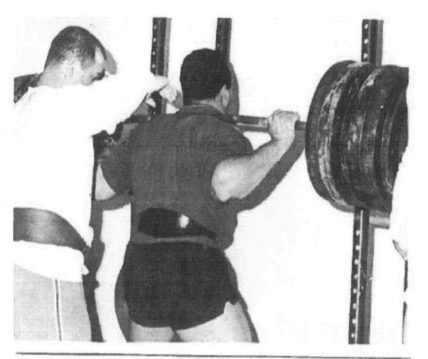

This next picture shows Bill with 3 of the greatest lifters of all time, on Muscle Beach;

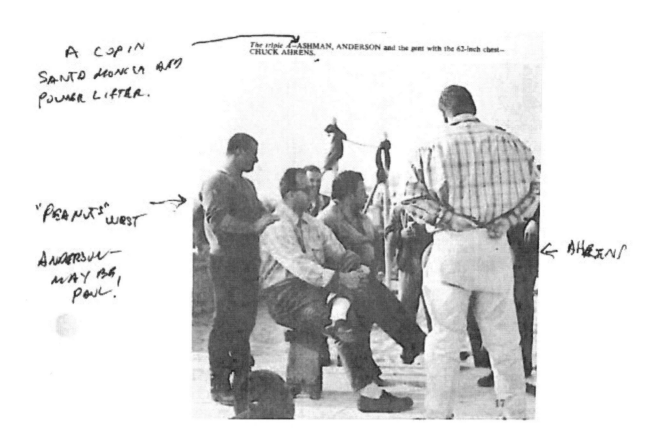

This picture was from Sam Calhoun's collection

The next article is about a guy that had a chapter dedicated to him in my Culver City secrets book, but this article is a new one;

DAVE DAVIS

POWER LIFTING + SHOT PUTTING = SUCCESS

A personal interview with Dave Davis, Power Lifter—Shot Putting champ, and how he uses Power Training to build up his athletic prowess. As Told by Dave Davis to Armand Tanny, MR. USA and Power Editor

★ A few years ago the Muscle Beach Gym in Santa Monica became a showcase for several of the nation's greatest shotputters. Nobody threw any shotputs, but everybody lifted a lot of weights. To the reporters of a big national sports weekly magazine who had come to do a story on the heaving heavies it was perfectly baffling. At that time the word was out that weight training was the sure way of making long throws with the shot, and it surprised observers to see these men spending so much time in the barbell gym. When one reporter asked Dave Davis how often he trained with the weights, Dave replied, "Every day." How often did he throw the shot then? The answer floored the magazine man. "Once a week," said Dave.

At that time the young Dave Davis might have submitted to over-enthusiasm for the weights, and if military service happened to interrupt his swift advance in the shot, he had proved the value of weight training up to that point. Almost overnight he had advanced his throws to nearly 65 feet, a gain of seven or eight feet. That gave him a spot on the 1960 U.S. Olympic team, but a last minute hard luck injury prevented him from going to the games.

"Whenever I have a good year with the weights, I have a good year with the shot," says Dave. He had a particularly good year in 1960 because that was when Dave Sheppard, champion weightlifter, suggested to Davis that he do heavy incline barbell presses because he would build power at the same angle at which he put the shot. It proved to be correct.

The state of mind required for a maximum top performance by an

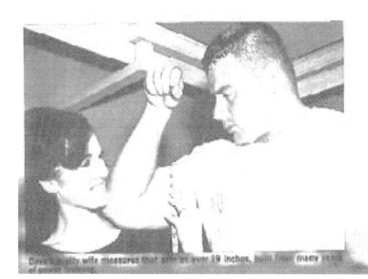

Dave's lovely wife measures that arm at over 19 inches, built from many years of weight training.

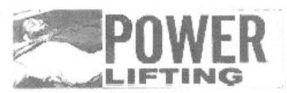

POWER LIFTING

DAVE DAVIS' BIG 3 FOR BUILDING POWER & SIZE

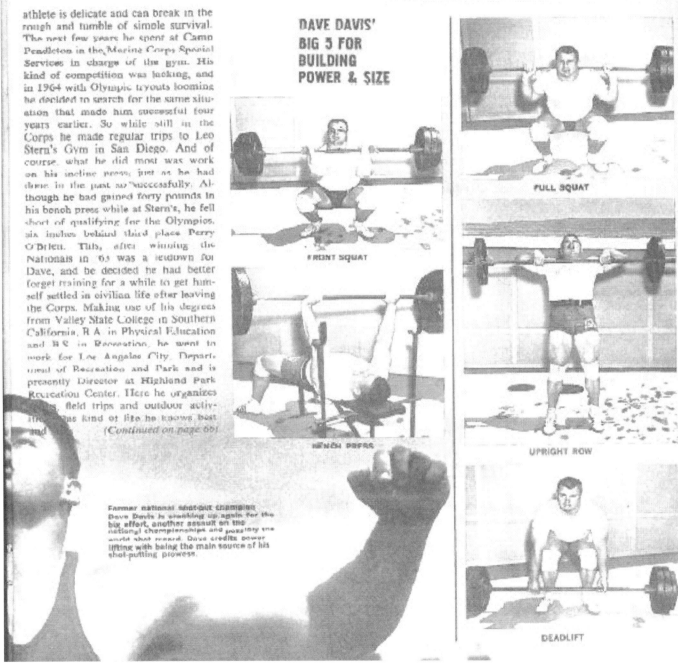

athlete is delicate and can break in the rough and tumble of simple survival. The next few years he spent at Camp Pendleton in the Marine Corps Special Services in charge of the gym. His kind of competition was lacking, and in 1964 with Olympic tryouts looming he decided to search for the same situation that made him successful four years earlier. So while still in the Corps he made regular trips to Leo Stern's Gym in San Diego. And of course, what he did most was work on his incline press, just as he had done in the past so successfully. Although he had gained forty pounds in his bench press while at Stern's, he fell short of qualifying for the Olympics, six inches behind third place Perry O'Brien. This, after winning the Nationals in '63 was a letdown for Dave, and he decided he had better forget training for a while to get himself settled in civilian life after leaving the Corps. Making use of his degrees from Valley State College in Southern California, B.A. in Physical Education and B.S. in Recreation, he went to work for Los Angeles City Department of Recreation and Park and is presently Director at Highland Park Recreation Center. Here he organizes games, field trips and outdoor activities — the kind of life he knows best and *(Continued on page 66)*

Former national shot-put champion Dave Davis is smashing up again for the big effort, another assault on the national championships and possibly the world shot record. Dave credits power lifting with being the main source of his shot-putting prowess.

FRONT SQUAT
BENCH PRESS
FULL SQUAT
UPRIGHT ROW
DEADLIFT

The text section above is not super clear, So I blew it up below;

athlete is delicate and can break in the rough and tumble of simple survival. The next few years he spent at Camp Pendleton in the Marine Corps Special Services in charge of the gym. His kind of competition was lacking, and in 1964 with Olympic tryouts looming he decided to search for the same situation that made him successful four years earlier. So while still in the Corps he made regular trips to Leo Stern's Gym in San Diego. And of course, what he did most was work on his incline press, just as he had done in the past so successfully. Although he had gained forty pounds in his bench press while at Stern's, he fell short of qualifying for the Olympics, six inches behind third place Perry O'Brien. This, after winning the Nationals in '63 was a letdown for Dave, and he decided he had better forget training for a while to get himself settled in civilian life after leaving the Corps. Making use of his degrees from Valley State College in Southern California, B.A. in Physical Education and B.S. in Recreation, he went to work for Los Angeles City, Department of Recreation and Park and is presently Director at Highland Park Recreation Center. Here he organizes field trips and outdoor activities. This kind of life he knows best and *(Continued on page 66)*

DAVE DAVIS

(Continued from page 29)

him fine. The work was ideal for an athlete in training, but for a year Dave's off hours didn't offer him much inspiration.

Then one day out of the West Side Barbell Club at 4227 Neosho in Culver City, California, there came some strange rumblings. A dragon breathing smoke and fire perhaps. Dave went down to investigate. It was none other than an old track acquaintance, hammer thrower George Frenn making with heavy power lifts. Frenn very well knew the value of power lifting in throwing the hammer. Champion Hal Connelly was already feeling the heat of the dragon's breath down his back. Frenn's long hammer throws were closing in fast. Dave Davis plunged into the action. Power lifting! Exactly what he needed, the strong gunpowder to cannon out that sixteen pound grape. Frenn's sudden rise with the hammer reminded Davis of his own great gains five years before when heavy weight training lengthened his own shot throws so suddenly.

Although their field events were their main love, power lifting, subtle mistress, has opted for their affection. Yes, the hammer and the shot continue to go out great distances, but the barbells with which they do the bench press, squat and dead lift continue, undisguised, to grow and throwing. His running workout twice a week goes like this:

Jog—2 laps
4—220 yard sprints, approx. 30 seconds each.
Twice a week: Shot Put
Twice a week: Power Lifting
Tuesday—Bench Press
135 10 reps
225 5
315 3
405 1
425 1
445 3 singles
Squat
135 5
225 5
315 3
405 3
475 1
535 1
500 5
Saturday (Following shot put practice)
Bench Press
135 10
225 5
315 1
405 1
425 1
435 1
445 1
450 1
465 1

plosive manner of his art, a 70 feet throw is a strong possibility before long. A conservative, despite his explosive power, he will pass 65 on admission.

Dave was never small. In high school he weighed 215. In college he was 225. Now at 6'3" he goes 285, much heavier and stronger than when he made nearly 65 feet in 1960. Though considerably shorter than record holder Matson 67¼", and 6'6" McGrath—whose heights are a distinct advantage—he plans on his new strength and weight to overcome their present lead.

He feels that age can never be a barrier. Comparatively young himself at 28 he cites Perry O'Brien who at 35 is throwing better than ever, and recently in practice made 64 feet. Perry has always trained with weights.

That he has a saturated program he proved to himself recently when he tried to include incline presses to his training. The first day he was capable of 380, his all time best, but he was drawing on reserve power which soon ran out because of his explosive squanderings. His incline power dropped with each successive workout, and after a few weeks he simply gave it up and decided to stay with the flat bench. However he returns to the lift a couple of weeks before shot flagrantly heavy. In other words they are all very much in love with power lifting.

Show a man a mountain, he'll try to climb it. Show a man a barbell, he'll try to lift it. Show him the three power lifts, and he's also hooked. Dave directly set up a power lifting program for himself. Twice a week he lifts, twice he runs, and twice he throws the shot. He has made running part of his training on the advice of Hal Connelly who coaches at Santa Monica High School, and he seems to regard it with some excitement, a re-discovery of an ancient effort. Running gives him speed, coordination and condition. It adds spice to the steady diet of lifting

WHAT WILL YOU SEE AT THE 1967 IFBB TEENAGE & SR. MR. EASTERN AMERICA SHOW AT THE BROOKLYN ACADEMY OF MUSIC ON JUNE 3rd ?

FABULOUS CONTESTANTS!

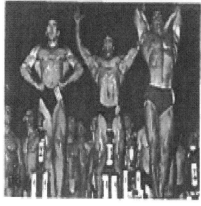

That constitutes his entire power lift program for the week. He must conserve for practice so he does no supplementary exercises. Still his progress is swift and his potential enormous. He has explosive power. He lifts with speed, the same way he throws the shot. Heavy lifts look ridiculously easy. He is a 285-pound mountain of raw material. His strength fluctuates widely because he hasn't had the background of steady power lift training, but time will change that. He has made the following lifts: Bench Press 465; Squat 570; Dead Lift 575. He does not practice the dead lift. Five seventy-five is what he made in the contest. When the current track season is finished he will start dead lift training. Frenn and Connelly, on the other hand, both practice the dead lift for the back power needed to reign up on the whirling hammer with its hundreds of pounds of centrifugal force.

Where he formerly did nothing but incline presses, Dave now does mostly the flat bench presses. A few weeks before a track meet he receives his incline press to strengthen his throwing angle. He keeps at the weights right up to throwing time. He mixes lifting with throwing throughout the track season. When his lifting power is up, his throwing power is the greatest. In fact his first throws for the 1966 season were 62 feet, practice efforts with only weightlifting power behind them. Dave is in the best shape of his life, and knowing the ex- put time.

On occasions he will do front squats and has made 460. The position gives his arms flexibility, just what he needs to hold the shot at the shoulder. Squats give him balance and a feeling of security. For these reasons he continues to weight train during track. Always at the start of each track season his throws are a little stiff, but later on he loosens up. He is careful to fully warm up at all times both in the gym and on the track. In cold weather he is extra cautious. He throws better when it is warm, and claims he does better in meets held during the day rather than at night. Without a doubt, warm southern California is a trackman's paradise.

Dave is big and needs fuel so he stokes about four times a day. He avoids starches and stays with salads and daily portions of meat. He drinks a daily mixture of powdered milk equivalent to five quarts of whole milk.

Measurements:

Neck 19 ½	Thigh 29
Biceps 19	Height 6'3"
Chest 50 normal	Weight 285
Waist 42	

Dave has it in him to be the best shot putter in the world. He could also be one of the greatest power lifters. He is working harder at both now than ever in his life, and like the proverbial Mary's little lamb: Wherever Dave's power lifting goes, his shot put is sure to go also.

PENNSYLVANIA OPEN POWER LIFT MEET-EASTON, PHILLIPSBURG & VICINITY Y.M.C.A., EASTON, PENNSYLVANIA—NOVEMBER 26, 1966

	B.P.	S.	D.L.	TOT
123 lb. class—				
Roman Mielec	230	310	415	955
Ruben Melendez	210	295	385	890
Fred Glass	170	235	430	835
William Stewart	175	220	350	745
Carl Lauer	200	200	340	740
Howard Wasserman	155	235	320	705
132 lb. class—				
John Bojazi	250	355	480	1085
Allen Lord	220	350	500	1070
Jack Kemmerer	220	310	450	980
148 lb. class—				
Frank Bradford	300	400	470	1170
Nick Olzel	270	400	480	1150
Brian Walraley	285	345	475	1105
Stephen Scott	270	360	460	1090
Steven Altamura	225	305	445	975
Lawrence Schlipf	210	300	375	885
165 lb. class—				
William Brokenbaugh	280	395	575	1250
Henry Reed	270	415	520	1205
George Connelly	275	400	500	1185
Eldon Williamson	290	400	460	1150
Lou Kushner	265	640	475	1115
Richard Giandrea	260	360	480	1100
John LeVasseur	210	285	370	865
181 lb. class—				
Felix Gomes	315	485	600	1420
Gene Cameron	280	450	550	1280
David Isaksen	275	415	560	1250
Tony Griger	240	405	520	1165
Sherwood Ellis	280	375	460	1115
Frank Puswald	260	370	450	1080
John O. Fair	250	325	470	1055
198 lb. class—				
William Andrews	410	525	600	1535
Joseph Weinstein	410	500	575	1485
Carlton Smithin	340	490	615	1445
George DeMott	295	460	575	1330
Thomas Laphan	280	400	530	1210
Robert Flyte	260	360	550	1170
William Taylor	270	415	480	1165
James McKenna	330	360	470	1160
Al Tressler	255	370	475	1100
Heavyweight				
Wes Joiner	400	*610	*675	*1685
James Williams	*455	485	635	1575
Hugh Cassidy	435	535	600	1570
Edward Moerlins	350	540	655	1545
Leonard Swarbell	350	480	580	1410
David Tillman	380	460	550	1390
Albert Larson	300	500	525	1325
Jack Groenendael	305	385	500	1190
Simmie Cramer	300	365	450	1115

* Meet Records.

This meet report that shows up in the same magazine that contained the Dave Davis article is of particular interest because it was local to me, and I know Fred Glass personally, who placed 3rd in the 123 class as shown.

Believe it or not, Fred is still actively competing to this very day, and was one of the athletes featured in my just released "Coal, Steel & Iron, Pennsylvania's Golden Triangle of strength"

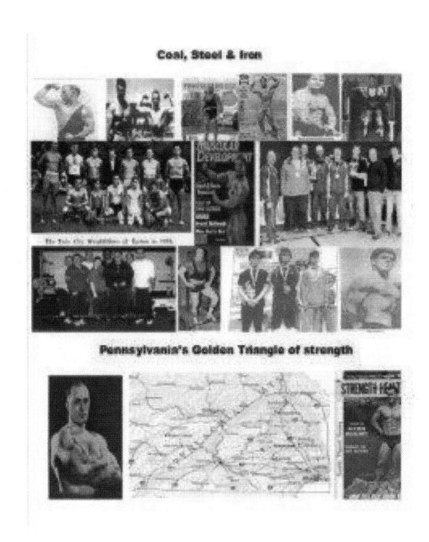

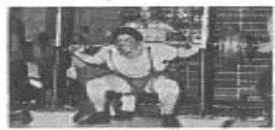

Pat Casey squatting with 800 — for a new American record.

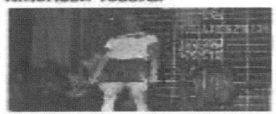

John Kanter performing a dead lift with 610 in the 198-pound class. He won with a total of 1600 for a new American record.

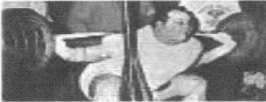

Robert Weaver squatting with 790 at the Sr. National Power Lift Championships in Dallas, Texas.

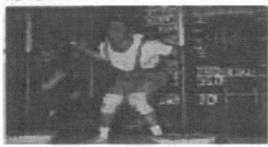

Len Ingro squatting with 503 at 165 pounds —for a new record.

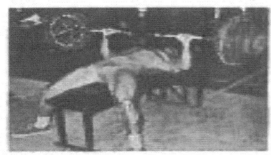

Chuck Coliras attempts a 320 bench press —but failed.

Culver City Westside members Casey, Ingro & Collras featured in the Power Highlights clip above.

Training tip of the month: Many bodybuilders devote a great amount of time to triceps training, but power lifters neglect this valuable adjunct to Bench Pressing. One top lifter who doesn't neglect it is Pat Casey, and we all know how much he can Bench Press! Casey credits his 592-pound Bench Press record to assistance exercises done to strengthen his triceps, and here's his favorite exercise: *Combined Triceps Press and Pullover*. This is done by starting with the weight on the chest, then lowering it into the Pullover position. Bring the bar back up to the face, then Press it to over the chest with the triceps alone. Come back to starting Pullover position, with the weight resting on the chest, and repeat for about 6 reps, 6-8 sets, with maximum wieght.

LATE NEWS HOT OFF THE WIRE ...Bob Weaver now weighing 325, recent training bests are 500-815-715 for a 2030 Total...Bill West out with a shoulder injury, will aim to win back his Total mark from Kantor when he resumes training...When will Pat Casey venture out of his California backyard and enter a contest against top competition?...Light-heavy champ Bill Andrews now lifting a bit as mid-heavy...Russian heavyweight champ Leonid Zhabotinsky was observed barely Bench Pressing 286 for 2 reps, and had to make 2 attempts to get up off the bench!...Paul Anderson still making the rounds, speaking to Christian groups, but his power lifts barely exceed those done by other lifters today...Los Angeles Meet uses 242-pound class for first time.

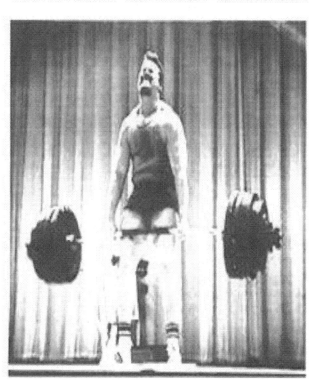

Although Peanuts West bombed out in the bench press his trip to the meet enthusiastically wasn't a total loss. Here, the meet's popular star George Frenn tells the audience how Peanuts' advice and encouragement helped him set three new records.

283-pound Don Cundy almost became first man in history to officially put up 800 deadlift He failed to get shoulders back as shown. Settled for 780 and title.

In my recent book "The Old School Back Training Bible", there was a short chapter dedicated to Don Cundy, who is pictured at right, above. Don was a legendary deadlifter.

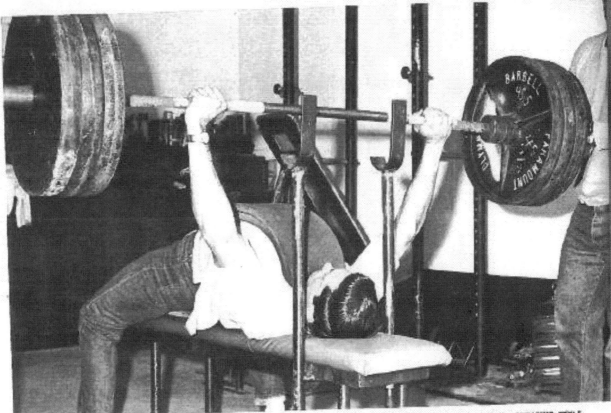

Many new American records... 242-pound class records set up... Anderson on national TV... continued interest in international power contests... 500-pound Deadlift as Bantamweight lost as record, apparently... Novice lifter sets national record!

Lenny Ingro shown doing Belly Toss above

Paul Anderson recently appeared on national TV, in a guest spot on the Johnny Carson show. Unlike many muscle figures on TV, Paul talked very literately, and really impressed Carson with his strength, especially doing 4 reps in the One-Arm Press with a 270 lb. dumbbell. After talking of his Christian work and mentioning his boys' home, Paul finished off with a back lift of 8 members of Carson's orchestra. Anderson also included skipping in his demonstration, and left a better impression than many other muscle figures who get a chance at national publicity.

The 242-pound class saw its first official records set up with results from the recent Surf Breakers meet, but no sooner were they set than broken, first by a Jim Whitt Squat in a Midwest meet, then completely obliterated at the recent California state championships. In addition to this news, it is now reported that Jim Roberson will reduce to the 242-pound limit and now lift in this class. What competition he and George Frenn will make!

Reg Park visited Bill West's muscle factory for a power workout on his recent trip to the West Coast. Also, Park set the record straight on his Squatting ability, saying 605 for two reps was his tops.

RAMA
by JON TWICHELL, Power Editor

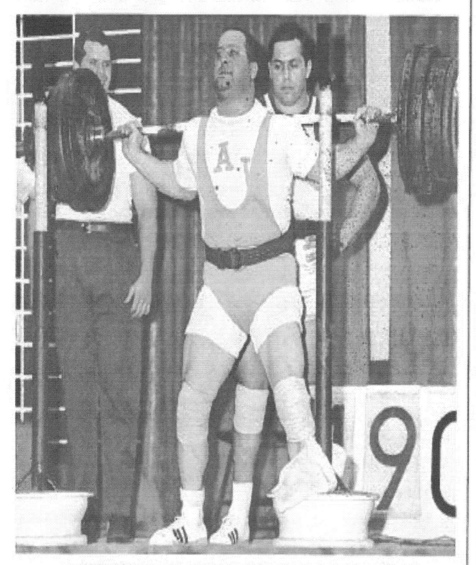

A NEW RECORD! At the recent California Championships, Bill "Peanuts" West Squatted with 603½ lbs. for a new Middle-Heavyweight record. It was 'Sectional Training' as outlined in the special article that appears in this issue that helped Bill build the power to establish this great record. It's the same system that has helped many other power champs break records, too — don't miss it!

I.F.B.B. SPECIAL
JACK DELINGER
(MR. AMERICA/MR. UNIVERSE)

will be a guest poser at the MR. WESTERN AMERICA CONTEST on Aug. 6th (see p. 71 for details). This will be his first posing exhibition in nearly 15 years. He will pose again at the MR. WORLD-MR. AMERICA-MR. OLYMPIA-MISS AMERICANA SHOW on Sept. 23rd (see pg. 55 for details).

&

LARRY SCOTT
(MR. AMERICA/MR. UNIVERSE/TWICE MR. OLYMPIA)

will be a guest poser at the MR. WORLD-MR. AMERICA-MR. OLYMPIA-MISS AMERICANA SHOW on Sept. 23rd, along with Delinger.

At this show you will also see the greatest contest lineup of all-time—including Dave Draper, Sergio Oliva, Frank Zane, Don Howorth, Chuck Sipes, Ricky Wayne, Harold Poole, Glen Kyle, and all the stars you see in this magazine. How can you afford to miss it?

SEE PAGES 55 & 71 FOR DETAILS!

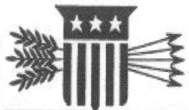

AMERICAN POWER LIFTING RECORDS (some pending)		
BANTAMWEIGHT		
BENCH PRESS	273	E. Hernandez
SQUAT	456½	D. Moyer
DEADLIFT	468½	M. Cross
TOTAL	1160	D. Moyer
FEATHERWEIGHT		
BENCH PRESS	295	E. Hernandez
SQUAT	476	D. Moyer
DEADLIFT	518	J. Bojazi
TOTAL	1170	D. Moyer
LIGHTWEIGHT		
BENCH PRESS	341½	R. Quarty
SQUAT	451¼	L. Mintz
DEADLIFT	556	B. Smith
TOTAL	1255	B. Spangler

The text box is not super legible, so here is the improved version;

A NEW RECORD! At the recent California Championships, Bill "Peanuts" West Squatted with 603½ lbs. for a new Middle-Heavyweight record. It was 'Sectional Training' as outlined in the special article that appears in this issue that helped Bill build the power to establish this great record. It's the same system that has helped many other power champs break records, too — don't miss it!

Partial results from the California power lifting championships show many new American records; Enrique Hernandez Bench Pressed 295 as a Featherweight, Bill West Squatted with 603¼... first past the 600-pound barrier in the 198 class... while Len Ingro just missed a 515 Squat as a Middleweight.

The real news was the 242-pound class for all new American records were set. Paul Yazoline came through with a 448¾ Bench Press and a 1650 Total. George Frenn, fully recovered from his foot injury, established himself as the man to beat in this class, Squatting with 682½, Deadlifting 685, and Totalling 1760! This is almost equal to his best as a heavyweight, so this is his class to have. Full results of this meet will be printed next month.

Only in power lifting! The former record for the Bench Press in this class was 359, held by Bill Thurber. A short while ago Jim Mansfield, a Rocky Mountain area lifter, upped it to 361 (equal to the IFBB record), then Thurber took the record back with a lift of 364½.

However, he's now lost the mark again. To who? Joe Pepi, who Bench Pressed 367½ in a junior power meet! How's that for coming out of the woodwork? Pepi, unfortunately, Squatted with less than he Bench Pressed and also Deadlifted only 10 pounds more than his BP. Back to the gym, Joe. (Continued on page 75)

MIDDLEWEIGHT
BENCH PRESS	367½	J. Pepi
SQUAT	503	L. Ingro
DEADLIFT	630½	N. Harris
TOTAL	1400	L. Ingro

LIGHT HEAVYWEIGHT
BENCH PRESS	446½	R. Ray
SQUAT	517	W. Andrews
DEADLIFT	626	F. Gomes
TOTAL	1530	R. Ray

MIDDLE HEAVYWEIGHT
BENCH PRESS	461¼	W. Sano
SQUAT	603½	W. West
DEADLIFT	659	J. Dzurenko
TOTAL	1600	J. Kantor

HEAVYWEIGHT—242 POUNDS
BENCH PRESS	448¾	P. Yazoline
SQUAT	682½	G. Frenn
DEADLIFT	685	G. Frenn
TOTAL	1760	G. Frenn

HEAVYWEIGHT—UNLIMITED
BENCH PRESS	593	P. Casey
SQUAT	800	P. Casey
DEADLIFT	761	D. Cundy
TOTAL	2035	P. Casey

33

Here are the results of this meet and some more of interest (you will note George Frenn and Len Ingro serving as loaders... how's that for dedication to your sport, and lack of a swelled head?):

LOS ANGELES JUNIOR POWER MEET
Held at Los Angeles YMCA

	Bench press	Squat	Dead-lift	Total
132-lb. class				
Steve Zahn	*230	150	280	695
Robin Hughes	160	185	330	675
132-lb. class				
Wayne Goodman	*210	205	*340	755
148-lb. class				
Rudy Lozano	*285	335	*450	*1070
Bob Plumpton	245	275	415	935
Paul Corley	195	*355	385	935
Frank Patterson	180	245	385	800
165-lb. class				
Willie Kindred	330	*425	*525	*1280
Vito Rotunno	320	350	465	1135
Joe Pepi	**370	345	380	1095
Tom Lincir	265	345	435	1045
Bob McPhetridge	270	330	360	960
Rolf Hunn	220	230	380	830
181-lb. class				
Adam DeLeon	295	*410	*520	1225
Mike Miller	395	390	500	1185
Frank Glover	275	310	415	1000
Robert Hudson	160	235	365	590
Don Walbrecht	250	250	—	500
198-lb. class				
Osmo Kiiha	320	450	500	1270
Ralph Hetzel	350	400	480	1230
James McVay	310	430	470	1200
Jim Waters	310	370	470	1150
Robert Rehmar	240	275	425	940
242-lb. class				
Ernest Ewald	*350	*425	*560	*1335
Jack Hamry	265	400	490	1155
Homer Wilson	235	335	405	975

* Denotes new junior record.
** Denotes new American record, actual weight 367½.

Outstanding lifter of the meet was Willie Kindred of Zuvers Gym.
Judges: John Scott, Ramon Garcia and Ken Yokogawa.
Loaders: George Frenn and Len Ingro.
Announcer: Ken Sommer.
Scorekeeper: Dave Granger.

Here and there: The aforementioned Bill Thurber is reducing to lift as a Lightweight, and has done 340-440-470, Total 1250, weighing 151. This is right about equal to the just-set new Lightweight Total mark.

There are so many changes in the records that rather than mention them all, we suggest you just look over the chart. Take a quick glimpse at the 242-class records, for they will probably change as fast as meets can be held, for a while.

POWERLINES
WEIGHTY HAPPENINGS ON THE WEST COAST

by DICK TYLER
West Coast Editor

• In sports, the most exciting part of any contest is the actual competition—or is it? When you're lucky enough to be backstage during and before the battle, you'll find that some of your greatest memories will be honed from the drama of great athletes preparing for the test. It's actually a study of men under pressure.

• Like drinking, all men react differently. Some are great kidders and release their tensions with laughter while others take their pent-up concerns out on the weights. Some do better in the warmups when nothing is up for grabs than they do when everything counts on the way they lift and how much. Call it jitters or pressure, but the bigger the contest the greater the excitement. Of course, I can just sit back and enjoy it all, 'cause all I gotta do is rest on my gluteus maximus and take in the sights and sounds.

• At the recent California State Powerlift championships things were more exciting than usual. This, in great part, is due to the fact that power lifting is still fairly new as an organized sport and records are continually being created. I now make the lofty prediction that the records of today, as great as they may be *now*, will be small compared to what they will be a few years from now. While feeling so wise, I think I'll go out on a limb and make a 5-year forecast. So get the clippers and cut me out. I mean cut out the *predictions*, save, and then see how close I'll be— *(Continued on page 54)*

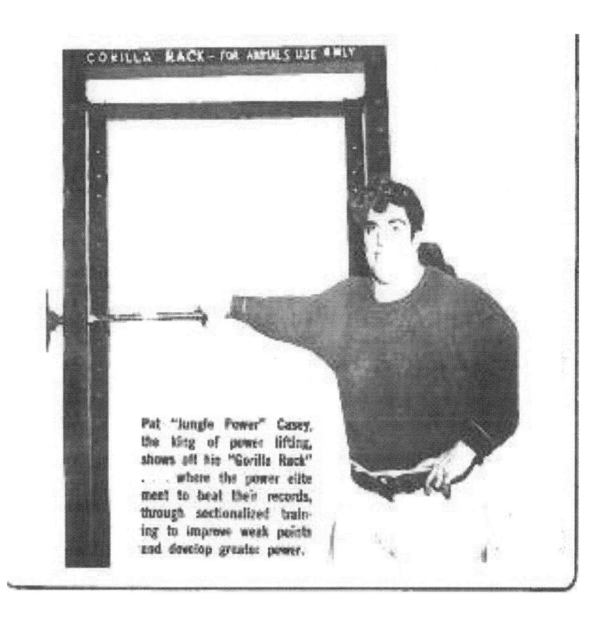

POWER LINES
(Continued from page 81)

Bantamweight Class
Bench Press	375 lbs.
Squat	580 lbs.
Deadlift	590 lbs.
Total	1,325 lbs.

Featherweight Class
Bench Press	400 lbs.
Squat	605 lbs.
Deadlift	620 lbs.
Total	1,425 lbs.

Lightweight Class
Bench Press	435 lbs.
Squat	625 lbs.
Deadlift	650 lbs.
Total	1,600 lbs.

Middleweight Class
Bench Press	460 lbs.
Squat	650 lbs.
Deadlift	715 lbs.
Total	1,725 lbs.

Lightheavyweight Class
Bench Press	550 lbs.
Squat	715 lbs.
Deadlift	725 lbs.
Total	1,875 lbs.

Middleheavyweight Class
Bench Press	610 lbs.
Squat	850 lbs.
Deadlift	870 lbs.
Total	2,125 lbs.

Heavyweight Class
Bench Press	725 lbs.
Squat	990 lbs.
Deadlift	1,000 lbs.
Total	2,500 lbs.

That's what I call nerve or is it just plain stupidity? But gimme a break, if I get 20 lbs. either way I'm doing great. Ooops. The crystal ball just rolled off the table and I won't be able to predict again until I'm drunk —on Super Pro 101. Hic!

Back to the California championships—first I must say that it was one of the best organized and run contests ever presented. This was so mainly through the efforts of Ramon Garcia. He's been a power booster for years. He also happens to be one of those who exercises the "get things done" muscles as well as his mouth. As a result, things do get done better than ever. You couldn't have asked for more equipment or better facilities. And chalk? Why the powder was flying so much that I thought I was in a snow storm in a soft-drink commercial. But the final touch, the crowning glory, was the messenger service. That's right. People were there to aid the lifters by going out for food or making phone calls. I couldn't believe it. I didn't want to leave but I had to face reality and now I'm back to making my own phone calls and walking through the yellow pages with my fingers.

I've found that too many people think of the power lifts as just a demonstration of crude power. This is opposed to the sophistication of the Olympic lifts. The theory is that timing and coordination play such an important part in the Olympic lifts that the slow, deliberate power moves are merely demonstrations of sheer force. I'll buy that. Who wouldn't, and be proud of the purchase! I do think, however, that the power boys are being sold a little short. Sure it takes strength but it also takes great style and control. All moves must be done in the correct form and the lifts, being as slow as they are, are carefully observed and judged.

Believe me, waiting for the clap from the referee when several hundred pounds are helping to engrave a steel bar into your chest can seem like waiting for the wife to get off the phone. Lately, I've seen more and more style appear at the meets. Maybe I'm prejudiced, but I feel that a great deal of this concentration has been due to the efforts of "Peanuts" West. He's everywhere during a meet. Hardly a lift is made without the careful once-over by West. He makes "Evil Eye" Fleegle look like a piker. Here is the consummate athlete and trainer. A man completely absorbed in the struggle of man and weight. Two excellent examples of style are two of the lighter stalwarts, Eric Biswell in the 123-lb. class and Enrique Hernandez in the 132-lb. class. All the moves are slow and deliberate. In fact, I watched them so intently that I was almost hypnotized by them. I think Biswell could have an excellent chance of copping the Junior National title. He's good in all the lifts. Right now he can do a 355-lb. deadlift but "Peanuts" feels he's got an easy 410 in him. The only 410 I might have in me is pennies. As a 132-pounder Hernandez warmed up for the meet with 205 lbs. in the bench press for 10 reps. He also squatted with 255 lbs. for 10 reps and deadlifted 310 lbs. for 5. To think that these men are so light, almost makes you want to die-t.

Years ago I used to go down to Muscle Beach and train. From almost the earliest days, I can remember seeing the exceptional Chuck Collras physique pushing the weights around. In fact, Bill West credits a great deal of his original drive in training to the efforts of Collras. The friendly rivalry has continued through the years until now "Peanuts" is a national power lift champ and record holder. What about Collras? Well, for a while I heard nothing about him and figured he had been lost in the California smog. That isn't too hard to do. This seems to happen to a lot of bodybuilders for some reason. I suspect that it's because the pressures of business and family life consume too much time for the proper amount of training. Whatever the reason—too many promising champions seem to vanish. So here we have Collras, a man in his mid-30's with business and family responsibilities, now making a "comeback." The amazing thing about all this is that he isn't satisfied with just one aspect of weight training. Chuck is competing in both power lifting and physique, in an attempt to prove that a man needn't have to look like an elephant to be as strong as one. Right now he's able to do the same lifts he did ten years ago but then he weighed 165 lbs. while now he competes in the 148-lb. class. He plans on winning a major physique title and power title on the same night. That would be a first and quite possibly a last. I know a lot of guys who can't decide whether they want to enter physique or power competition—so they end up doing nothing.

The amazing Pat Casey did it again. That's right—he made me make a fool of myself. I get this call from "Peanuts." "Dick," he says, "Casey is now incline pressing 250-lb. dumbbells." I yawned. "I can do that," I said. There was a silence from the other end. "What was that?" said West at long last. "I can press two 50-lb. dumbbells while standing," I replied confidently. "Peanuts" broke into laughter. "Lissen, I said Casey could incline a pair of 250-lb. dumbbells." I thought for a second. "No, I can't do that." "I can't either," said Peanuts. "Come to the gym this Saturday and watch him incline 500 lbs." To make a long story short, Pat pushed up a perfect 505-lb. incline press. I leave you with a word of advice. When you hear of something that Casey can do, don't say you can do it too, unless you want to claim yourself as stronger than my arm pits after a workout.

The following article is about another man that trained with the Culver City boys, who was discussed at length and had his own chapter in the book dedicated to the crew;

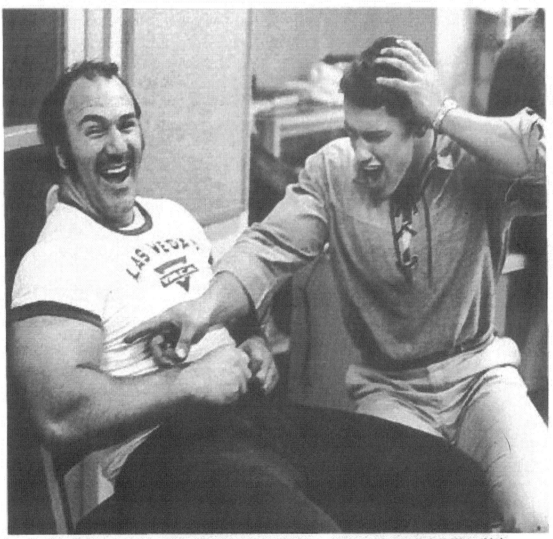

OF ALL THE INFAMOUS WALLS IN THE WORLD, WHETHER IT BE IN BERLIN OR CHINA NEITHER IS STRONGER THAN THE ONE CARVED IN HUMAN FLESH AND CALLED WAYNE COLEMAN.

"Mein Gott!" cries Arnold, "...22"—and he sits while I train!" Not exactly... Wayne Coleman trains his 6' 4" 300-pound body hard—and these arms are capable of putting the shot at 58' 4"!

THE WALL

by Dick Tyler

(Photos by Zeller)

YOU may not believe this but I'm always looking for interesting people. I believe that your eyes should have better exercise than just looking at a bunch of meaningless words. The urbane wit of Santa Monica and camera craftsman Art Zeller knows this and as a result I get many leads from him. A few days ago I got a phone call.

"Dick," asked Art, "how would you like to interview a wall?"

I got the feeling he was trying to tell me something.

"Okay," I said, playing along with a gag.

"Good. Meet me at Gold's Gym at 1:30 on Saturday."

He hung up. He did that on purpose. For at least an hour I tried to control myself. I wasn't going to give him the satisfaction of my calling back to find out what he meant. I couldn't stand it any longer.

"Hi, Dick!" said Art as he picked up the phone. "The 'wall' is what I call anyone who weighs 300 lbs. and stands 6' 4"."

He hung up. I called back again.

35

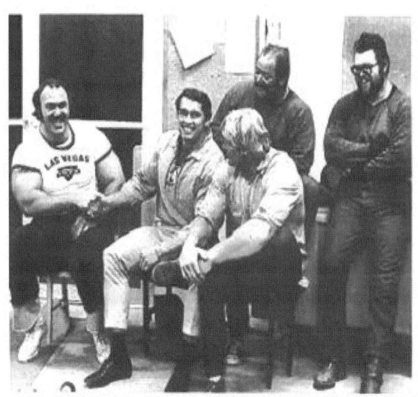

Good-natured Coleman is everyone's pal, and since he has the build of a bodybuilder and the strength of a powerlifter... the guys at Gold's Gym really dig his company. He's seen here with Arnold Schwarzenegger (shaking hands), and—left to right—Dave Draper (sitting), Bill "Peanuts" West, and Jim Hamilton.

"And he has 22" arms," began Art.

"And his name is Wayne Coleman," I continued.

"How did you know?" asked Art.

I told him I had already heard about him from Peanuts West and that I had already planned on doing a story on the guy. With that I hung up.

On Saturday I went to Gold's Gym. For a change I was early. Within a few minutes Peanuts came in. He had grown a mustache and sideburns for a Western film he was going to do.

"What happened to your eyebrows," I asked.

"Huh?"

"They slipped down to your lip?" I laughed.

I was the only one who did.

"Wayne should be here any minute. Wait'll you see him."

Almost as if on cue, in lumbered the "wall" himself. I didn't have to be told who he was. My mouth must have hit the floor.

"This is..." started Peanuts.

"Yeah," said Peanuts, "he doesn't need a sign to tell anyone."

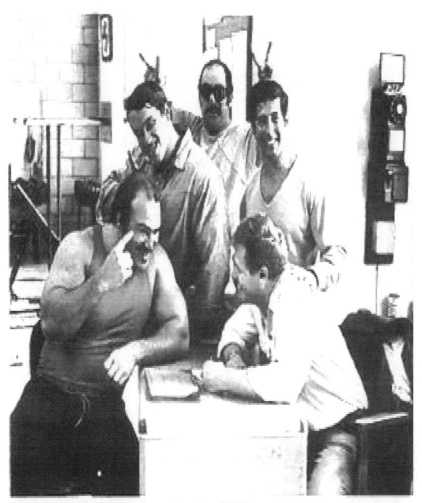

"It's mind over matter," says Coleman to interviewer Dick Tyler. Maybe it is—but it takes more than brain power to Squat with 650, Deadlift 675, and Cheat Curl 350, just a few of his accomplishments. The guys clown it up for cameraman Art Zeller—left to right ... Arnold Schwarzenegger, Bill West, and Chuck Collras.

need a sign to tell anyone.

In talking to Wayne I found out that he wasn't always this big.

"People seem to think you have to be born this way," he said. "The truth of the matter is that I was really a skinny kid who got pushed around just like the ads say."

By the time he was in the 8th grade Wayne was already 6' 1" tall. Unfortunately, that height carried only 135 lbs. on it. He was a beanpole. He'd look at himself in the mirror in disgust. For a while it seemed that he was destined to remain this way. A collection of bones with no one to give him any advice on remedying the situation. As he got closer to high school and the sporting program it contained he got more discouraged with the prospects of his athletic career. One day he picked up a copy of MUSCLE BUILDER he saw on the stands. This sounds like an old story, but there's no other way to tell it. MUSCLE BUILDER has probably inspired more bodybuilders and *(Continued on page 81)*

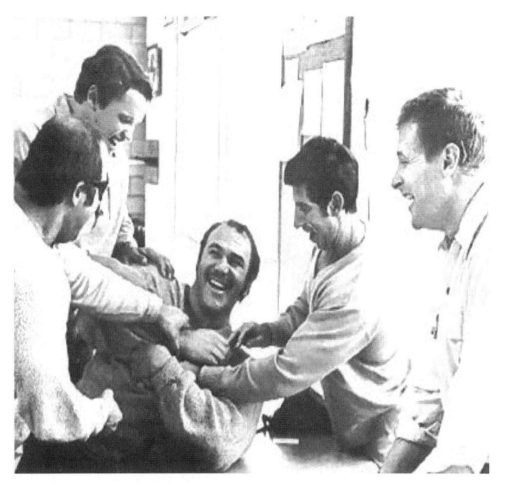

LEFT: It was Bill West (left foreground) who convinced Coleman that power lifts would aid his football career—and now that they have Coleman wouldn't trade the weights for all the pigskin in China. Arnold and Chuck are trying to get a look at that massive 55" chest—while Dick Tyler shares in the laughs.

BELOW: Coleman's favorite lift is the Bench Press and has done 550 with a triceps grip. His goal is 600—before the football season begins. Chuck Sipes by the way has the same ambition... wouldn't it be great to see a power contest between these giants?

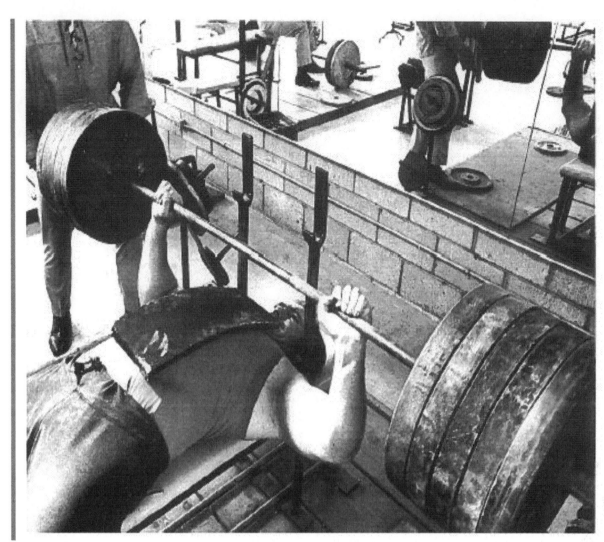

THE WALL

(Continued from page 36)

athletes than any other publication. Wayne was determined to get muscles like those he saw in the publication. The magic word seemed to be *weights*. He located a gym in downtown Phoenix, Arizona. Since he lived a few miles outside of the city and had no car, Wayne would hitch-hike into town three times a week to take his workouts. His dedication began to pay off as he began to grow *out* as well as up.

By the time he reached high school he had the makings of a bull. By his sophomore year he had broken the national sophomore record in the shot and the discus with tosses of 58' 4" and 174' 8" respectively and came within a few points of taking the national decathlon. He looked like one of the country's best prospects for the Olympics. Wayne, however, had other ideas. He was more interested in physique competition. In 1959 he entered and won the Mr. Phoenix contest. In 1960 he won the title Mr. Arizona and in 1961 he won the Jr. Mr. America title. He had a royal road before him. The potential to become a great bodybuilding champion. Then, for little reason, he lost interest. This wasn't really what he wanted after all. He was "cursed" with too much potential. Potential in every direction. He loved competition. If he had his way he'd compete in everything, but he was only one man and there were so many sports.

Wanting to get a good taste of contact sports he began to practice boxing. It wasn't long before his natural athletic prowess began to stamp him as a promising fighter. After a short period of training he entered the Arizona State Golden Gloves. Guess what? That's right, he became the state heavyweight champion. So impressive was his power that he attracted the attention of the manager of the champion fighter Emile Griffith. His first professional bout was part of a supporting card of a championship fight program in Madison Square Garden. What a beginning! Did he win? He literally battered his opponent into submission. Did he continue? Of course not. The training regimen needed to maintain the best fighting bodyweight was too vigorous. He didn't care enough for the sport.

Still a young man and growing more powerful by the day, he decided to try his hand at football. It was the same success story all over again only this time the ending promises to be different. He likes football so much that he wants to make it a career. He was signed by the Oakland Raiders as a defensive end but due to an injury he had to sit out the season. This year he'll be playing for the Montreal Alouettes in Canada. After that it's Oakland again and what promises to be a career of great importance in professional football.

It was only recently that Wayne was introduced to serious power lifting. He was on a visit to the Southern California area when he met Peanuts West. Peanuts happens to be not only a great lifter but one of the greatest trainers and technicians in the game. It wasn't difficult for him to see the potential in this massive strongman. West convinced Coleman that his football career would be aided by concentrating on power moves. He had no idea, however, just how strong Coleman was. In just a few months the gains made were unbelievable. At the present time Wayne stands 6' 4" tall and weighs 300 lbs. His chest measures 55", neck 20", arms 22", thighs 30" and calves 19½". His lifts are almost as astounding. He Squats with 650 lbs., Deadlifts 675 lbs. and cheat Curls a 350-lb. barbell. His favorite lift is the Bench Press and has Pressed with a triceps grip—550 lbs. He hopes to Bench Press 600 lbs. before the football season begins.

Wayne's program has been carefully worked out and controlled by West to take advantage of his limited time, enormous potential and his football needs.

THE WAYNE COLEMAN POWER PUSH

As with most power programs the emphasis is not on endurance but on strength. While lifting the concentration is intense but the periods between the lifts can be protracted. Coleman trains three times a week on the following program:

1. *Bench Press*—Wayne doesn't like to leave best things to the last. He starts with his favorite lift. He uses a standard 32" grip and sometimes narrower. Starting with 225 lbs., he does 6 reps, then he jumps to 315 lbs., then 405 lbs. and knocks out single reps with 500 lbs. If he's feeling particularly strong he'll go for limit poundages. Thirteen sets with varied reps are done.

2. *Seated Lat Pulls*—to balance the pushing power generated by the Bench Presses, Wayne does 10 sets of 5 reps with 300 lbs. in the seated lat pulls.

3. *Alternate Standing Dumbbell Presses*—with a 130 lb. dumbbell in each hand, Wayne does alternate Presses for 5 sets of 5 reps.

4. *Preacher Bench Curls*—this is one of the best ways to build 22" arms. Wayne does it by doing 10 sets of 8 reps with a 150-lb. barbell.

5. *Pushdowns*—with a close grip on the lat bar and his elbows held close to his sides, Wayne pressed downward until his arms are locked. He does this for 10 sets of 8 reps with 170 lbs. If his arm ever goes to 23" this exercise will be the boot it needs.

6. *Squats*—Wayne finishes off his program with this exercise by performing 10 sets. He starts off with 225 lbs. for 5 reps and works up to singles with 605 lbs.

Wayne tries to get a full share of his eight hours of sack time. He eats three meals a day and tries to eat steak for every one of those days. He supplements his meals with heavy dosages of protein and with Vitamin E, which he feels is an important endurance factor for his football career. Unfortunately, Wayne has time to train for only five months out of every year. In that time, however, he packs in a year's worth of experience. Wayne is a very likable guy who doesn't seem to know himself just what he's capable of. Bill West knows. If you don't want to see a grown man cry just don't ask West what would happen if Wayne were able to train for a full year.

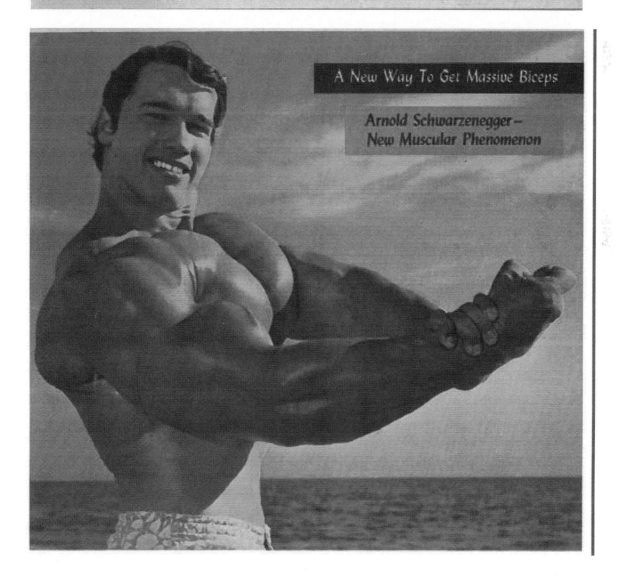

In the late '60s, Arny burst onto the scene and the men of the original Westside crew were the kings of the new powerlifting game

Powerlifting Clinic with Frenn, Casey;

This is the 3rd in our monthly series of questions and answers designed to dispense information to powerlifters on training problems. Because the sport is only a few years old, information on all phases of powerlifting is thin-and not many of our readers and lifters are thoroughly familiar with all the techniques and how to get the most out of their workouts, or how top train properly to smash records. I will tackle some questions myself, and will call on top powerlifters to answer some, because I believe that only powerlifters thoroughly experienced in the sport can truly provide positive answers on training. The answers you will get through this clinic will not be the arm-chair variety provided by phony authorities, but knowledge of the champs themselves. Send me your questions, and I will get one of the top champs to answer them, the one I feel best qualified in the particular area. All your questions will be answered, to help you reach the top rung in power. The address is; Powerlifter's Clinic, C.O. Weider Barbell l Co., 801 Palisade ave, Union City NJ, 07087.

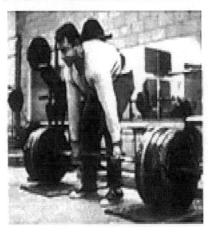

Newcomer Bob Reamer "psyching up" for a 525-pound Deadlift. This advanced form of preparation—pouring all your thoughts into the lift about to be made and visualizing the successful execution of that lift—can often spell actual success. Top athletes in every field are realizing the power of positive thinking. (Zeller)

PSYCHING UP FOR RECORDS

Dear Joe:

I am anxious to know how champion powerlifters psyche up for a competition. I have heard that George Frenn does some pretty strange things to get himself ready for a meet. I remember seeing him at the York Nationals in 1967, and he was a real show. Does Frenn plan to compete anymore?

Thank you.

Doug Hennington,
Harrisburg, Pa.

Dear Doug:

You're right; Frenn has done some pretty strange things to get himself psyched up for a contest. He figures if any particular "thing" will help you lift more, use it. What does it matter how silly it may seem if it works! While he was powerlifting as a 242-pounder he remained undefeated for three years. Frenn has used music and created impossible mental challenges to encourage himself before a meet. But a big bet really stimulates him to fight. Then his blood boils and he really pushes. Bill West, Harold Connolly, and Pat Casey have always inspired Frenn greatly—because they all represent a real challenge. He expects to compete in a few power meets this year, but will concentrate on the hammer for the most part.

Best of luck,
Joe Weider

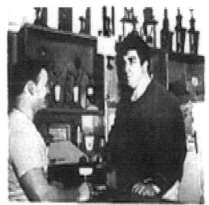

Powerhouse Pat Casey has "momentarily dropped out of the power scene" to concentrate on his duties as a policeman for the Seal Beach City Police Department. Imagine being whacked by a night stick in Pat's fist!

FULL SQUAT TECHNIQUE

Dear Joe:

Would you please outline a good Full Squat routine? I have read conflicting reports of good techniques, George Frenn's included. I have seen his technical analysis published, and I want to know what is best in order to improve myself.

Thanks for your help.

Homer Jones,
St. Louis, Mo.

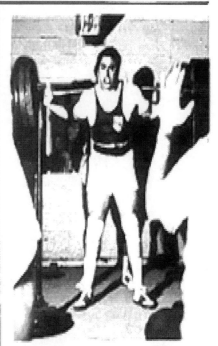

Every top powerlifter has his own unique method for increasing lifts—and George Frenn's for Full Squats is detailed in this month's "Clinic." Here you see Jon Cole about to Squat with 750.

Dear Homer:

George Frenn's Full Squat technique is a good example for you to follow. It has been published several times, but here it is—outlined for you.

Frenn lifts on Tuesdays and Saturdays. On Tuesdays he does heavy Bench Squats and low Box Squats. The Bench Squats are as follows: 255 x 5; 345 x 3; 425 x 3; 525 x 2; 615 x 2 to 5; 705 x 1 to 5; 775 x 2 or 3; 850 x 1; 910 x maybe.

The low box routine is similar; he does the following: 345 x 2; 435 x 2; 525 x 1 for 2 to 3 singles; 615 x 1; 665 to 690 x maybe.

The bench is 18 inches high up the floor, while the low box is 14 inches high. On Saturdays he uses the (Continued on page 70)

POWERLIFTERS CLINIC

(Continued from page 41)

same Bench Squat progression except that he stops at 705 pounds and does singles with a possible attempt with 740 to 750 pounds, depending on whether he feels good. His best training Squat is 800 pounds below parallel at a bodyweight of 236 pounds.

Best of luck,
Joe Weider

IT'S LIKE SWIMMING... YOU NEVER FORGET

Dear George Frenn:

I have been powerlifting for several years now and I have discovered that my strength does fluctuate if I do not train, but, depending upon the food I eat and the amount of sleep I get, my strength does not drop more than 10 percent even if I do no lifting for long periods of time. However, I must do running and stretching of the muscles. I was wondering if you have had any experience in this area, or is it just my imagination? I would appreciate hearing your ideas on the subject.

Thank you,
Pat O'Callahan
Bellflower, Calif.

end of 1967 I have noticed that you and other champs have been competing less and less. Is the Club still active and will you compete again?

Thank you,
Al Burger
Edmonton, Alberta, Canada

Dear Al:

Due to a back injury followed by another and another, I have been forced to take a layoff of sorts—but I'm almost ready to get started again. Frenn has been active in the hammer throw, and, as a consequence, has spent less time powerlifting. Bill Thurber had to stop lifting because of family obligations.

This year Frenn will compete in the Los Angeles City Meet, but that will be it—as he plans to go to Europe with the U.S. Track and Field team. I do believe the Club will regenerate itself and work up a strong team late next year; Frenn promises to return then, and so do I.

Best of luck,
Bill West

WHERE HAVE THEY GONE?

Dear Joe:

Dear Pat:

First, I would like to say that you have the same name of a famous athlete who was active back in the 30's. He was Pat O'Callahan, the Olympic Champion Hammer Thrower from Ireland.

About your question, I must say that I have had similar experiences. I have laid off the Bench Press for as long as a year and a half and have been able to make 90 to 92 percent of my best lift in the first workout. The only explanation I can offer is one of learning. Apparently, you have learned the technique so well and you are so confident that you can perform the feat. Many times one actually learns more about certain techniques if he quits practice for a time. I hope this answers your question.

Best of luck,
George Frenn

THE CLUB'S JUST "RESTING"

Dear Bill West:

I have followed the exploits of the Westside Barbell Club since 1965 when it first came into contention. Since the

Several years ago the weightlifting news was filled with headlines about such notables as Terry Todd, Gene Roberson, Pat Casey, and Paul Yazalino—to name a few. Have you any idea what these giants are doing now?

Thank you,
Jerry Skolsky
Pittsburgh, Pa.

Dear Jerry:

Terry Todd, as far as I know, is still coaching at the University of Texas, in Austin. As you might know, he completed his doctorate. I do not have any information concerning Gene Roberson. I would appreciate learning his whereabouts—and ask readers to send information. Pat Casey is now a policeman for the Seal Beach City Police Department. As for Paul Yazalino, he has retired and gone into business with his father up in Northern California. Paul eventually made a 500-pound Bench Press. Again, if readers have any information on these and other greats of former years—we'd appreciate hearing from them so that we may spread the word.

Best wishes,
Joe Weider

George Frenn, key member of the Culver City club, ended up having a regular powerlifting column in Muscle Builder for a while;

AMERICAN POWER SCENE

By GEORGE FRENN

IN Phoenix, Arizona the bottom fell out of the record book for the 198- and 242-pound classes—as John Kantar and Jack Barnes stole the spotlight from yours truly in what proved to be a highly successful powerlifting competition—the Phoenix Open Power Meet.

At first it didn't seem as if the meet would come off, what with Ronnie Ray and Jon Cole declining, but thanks to John Kantar, Jack Barnes, and the fact that I *gave in* at the last minute—the lift took on meaning. Ronnie had to forego the competition due to financial problems; Jon had to be at the Orange County Track and Field Invitational to throw the discus; and I was set to throw the hammer the next day, in Hayward, Calif., and didn't care to exert myself.

I weighed in at 244½ pounds so I lifted in the heavyweight division. Jack went into the 198-pound class, and John, the 242½-pound division. It went something like this:

The light classes did their lifting in the morning. Greg Stewart, a 132-pounder, set a state Squat record of 305, another with *(Continued on page 57)*

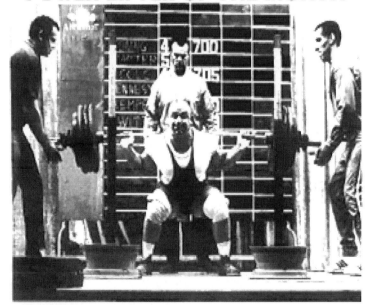

POWER LIFTER OF THE MONTH

JOHN KANTAR. Congratulations to John Kantar on his Squat of 764½ pounds—a lift which definitely ranks him among our "Powerlifters of the Month." As most of our readers know, John has been lifting for many years on the national level, and has won the 198-pound crown, a silver medal in the 198-pound class, and last year placed second to Jon Cole in the 242-pound class. This year John should win the 242-pound class, for it was Jon Cole's record he broke. When breaking the National Squat Record, John also established a 2,000-pound Total in the 242-pound class. Keep up the great lifting, John Kantar!

NEW AMERICAN POWERLIFTING RECORDS
(some pending)

123-LB. CLASS
- Bench Press ... 272 ... E. Hernandez
- Squat ... 456½ ... D. Meyer
- Deadlift ... 440 ... M. Cross
- Total ... 1160 ... D. Meyer

132-LB. CLASS
- Bench Press ... 319½ ... E. Hernandez
- Squat ... 476 ... D. Meyer
- Deadlift ... 543 ... A. Lord
- Total ... 1175 ... A. Lord

148-LB. CLASS
- Bench Press ... 355½ ... B. Thurber
- Squat ... 525 ... D. Blue
- Deadlift ... 580 ... D. Blue
- Total ... 1525 ... D. Blue

165-LB. CLASS
- Bench Press ... 378 ... R. Burnett
- Squat ... 516½ ... L. Ingra
- Deadlift ... 668 ... R. Burnett
- Total ... 1550 ... R. Burnett

181-LB. CLASS
- Bench Press ... 450½ ... R. Ray
- Squat ... 676½ ... J. Barnes
- Deadlift ... 650½ ... P. O'Brien
- Total ... 1595 ... J. Barnes

198-LB. CLASS
- Bench Press ... 486½ ... R. Ray
- Squat ... 674 ... T. Overholtzer
- Deadlift ... 688½ ... J. Ostrosko
- Total ... 1675 ... T. Overholtzer

242-LB. CLASS
- Bench Press ... 542½ ... M. Hennessy
- Squat ... 764½ ... J. Kantar
- Deadlift ... 770½ ... J. Young
- Total ... 2000 ... J. Kantar

HEAVYWEIGHT CLASS
- Bench Press ... 617½ ... P. Casey
- Squat ... 800 ... P. Casey
- Deadlift ... 784 ... D. Cundy
- Total ... 2040 ... R. Meyer

Text box clarified: Congratulations to James Kantar on his squat of 764 ½ pounds- a lift which definitely ranks him among our "powerlifters of the Month" As most of our readers know, John has been lifting for many years on the national level, and has won the 198 crown, a silver medal in the 198 class, and last year placed second to Jon Cole in the 242 class. This year John should win the 242 class, for it was Jon Cole's record he broke. When breaking the National Squat Record, John also established a 2,000 lb. total in the 242 class. Keep up the great lifting, John!

INTERNATIONAL POWER SCENE

by Oscar State, Secretary International Weightlifting Federation

WORLD RECORDS I regret to report that once again the bureau of the International Weightlifting Federation has postponed their official recognition of the definitions of the Strength Lifts and the adoption of a list of world records. They have supported the decision of their Technical Committee to refer the subject to the FHI Medical Committee. They will await the opinion of the doctors who will meet to discuss these lifts and the proposed definitions in September during the world championships in Warsaw.

However, in order to satisfy the numerous lifters and officials who write to me with claims or queries about records on these lifts, I think it only fair to them to publish the lists that I had drawn up for submission to the FHI bureau. At least these lists should help to prevent any false claims. I hope that these lists will also serve as incentives for those lifters who have ambitions for trying to set up world records. Knowing what they must beat might just provide the extra encouragement needed in some hesitant cases. I must emphasize that until the FHI bureau officially accepts these lists, they must remain unofficial.

I am quite sure that you will have immediately observed that all but four of these records belong to the U.S.A. Some cynics have *(Continued on page 56)*

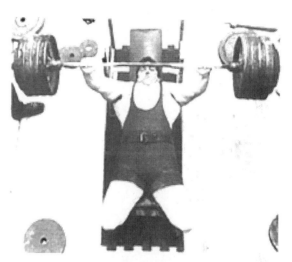

In spite of his retirement, Pat Casey still remains a threat to would-be Bench Press record setters in the super heavyweight division. His 616 still ranks as one of the greatest power lifts in the world.

BANTAMWEIGHT		
Squat	D. Moyer, USA	455
Bench Press	P. McKenzie, Great Britain	279 ¼
Deadlift	M. Cross, USA	497 ½
Total	D. Moyer, USA	1160
FEATHERWEIGHT		
Squat	D. Moyer, USA	475
Bench Press	E. Hernandez, USA	319 ½
Deadlift	A. Lord, USA	542
Total	A. Lord, USA	1215
LIGHTWEIGHT		
Squat	V. Acari, Great Britain	487
Bench Press	W. Thurber, USA	345 ¼
Deadlift	B. White, Australia	610 ½
Total	D. Blue, USA	1325
MIDDLEWEIGHT		
Squat	R. Judge, Great Britain	541
Bench Press	R. Burnett, USA	375 ¼
Deadlift	R. Burnett, USA	667 ¼
Total	R. Burnett, USA	1560
LIGHT-HEAVYWEIGHT		
Squat	T. Overholtzer, USA	665 ¼
Bench Press	R. Ray, USA	449 ½
Deadlift	R. Jackson, USA	672
Total	J. Barnes, USA	1595
MIDDLE-HEAVYWEIGHT		
Squat	T. Overholtzer, USA	673 ½
Bench Press	R. Ray, USA	485
Deadlift	J. Dzurenko, USA	688 ½
Total	T. Overholtzer, USA	1675
HEAVYWEIGHT		
Squat	G. Frenn, USA	731 ¼
Bench Press	M. Hennessey, USA	535 ½
Deadlift	G. Young, USA	769 ¼
Total	G. Frenn, USA	1900
SUPER HEAVYWEIGHT		
Squat	P. Casey, USA	799
Bench Press	P. Casey, USA	616
Deadlift	D. Cundy, USA	783 ½
Total	R. Weaver, USA	2040

Chapter 3   the Dungeon

Before we go in -depth about the dungeon, let's take a look at this nice little piece about Tanny;

http://www.iron-age-classic-bodybuilding.com/vic_tanny.html

Vic Tanny

"From Immigrant to King of an Empire".

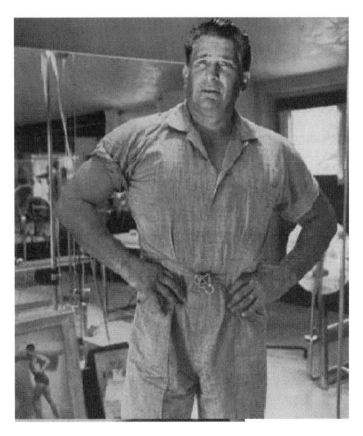

Vic Tanny was born Victor Tannidinardo in Rochester, New York on February 18, 1912. He would become a pivotal figure in the history of bodybuilding. Vic's father, a tailor, and the rest of the family, changed their last name to Tanny sometime in the late thirties or early forties due to anti-Italian sentiment at that time.

Go West Young Man!

Vic Tanny, who had always been interested in physical strength and conditioning, opened his first gym in his parents' garage in 1935. Eventually, he would move to a larger building in Rochester but was disappointed with his volume of members.

Vic had always admired the early American pioneers and their struggle to move west so, in 1940 with $700 in savings, he moved to Santa Monica, California.

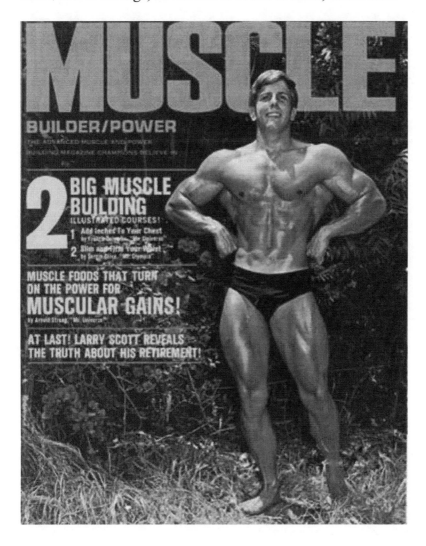

A young Vic Tanny Junior, son of Vic, nephew of Armand and nephew of Bert Goodrich

Struggle and Success...

Tanny's first attempts at operating a gym were a struggle, especially during the war years. Many of his potential customers joined or were drafted to defend the nation.

The prosperity that followed the end of the war saw Vic's gyms skyrocket in popularity. With chrome plated weights, his brightly lighted, colorfully painted establishments welcomed women and men to an almost country club atmosphere. Tanny's gyms were clean and bright as opposed to the dimly lit, smoky and dirty boxing gyms he had visited as a youth. Between 1950 and 1959 Tanny went from one gym to over 60 nationwide with 650 employees and hundreds of thousands of members.

Below Vic surveys one of his gym locations as a member works out

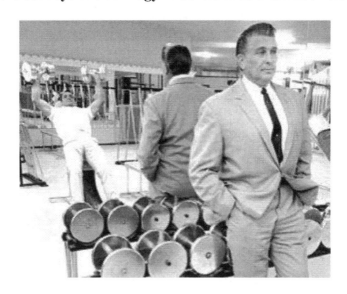

"Take It Off. Build It Up. Make It Firm."

Vic Tanny's gym motto was "Take it off, build it up and make it firm". This was accomplished by lifting weights but every member was cautioned against overstraining and grunting and groaning. Members were put on an initial 3 day a week program of 30 minute duration which included 24 Tanny approved exercises. Memberships were $60 per year on the west coast and $125 per year in New York due to higher costs there. A lifetime membership could be purchased for $339.

"Reducing Salon....Increasing Wealth"!

Vic Tanny was not the creator of the popularity of exercising at that time. There were over 750 "reducing" salons nationwide in 1958 with such names as "Silhouette" and "Slenderella", but he was one of the leaders of the movement. Vic accumulated quite a fortune from his gyms. In 1958 he and his family lived in a $220,000 mansion with 12 phones! Vic Tanny's name became synonymous with gyms, muscle building and fitness. A parody of his gym is seen in the 1963 movie "The Nutty Professor" with Jerry Lewis. Don Rickles plays a trainer of bodybuilders, "Jack Fanny", in the movie "Muscle Beach Party" and "Mad" magazine has even parodied Vic in their "Vic Tinny" issue.

The dream and the fall...

Vic Tanny dreamed big and achieved even bigger! His dream was to spread his gyms all over the world. Tanny may have dreamed a bit too big. Eventually, Tanny's business fell into bankruptcy due to "over-expansion, poor management and lack of capital" according to those in the know. Vic retired to Florida and many of his gyms became part of the Bally gym chain.

All in the Family...

Many of Vic's family were also interested in the health and fitness industry. Vic's mother, **Angela Tanny**, was a lifelong health advocate. She followed her son to California and worked out regularly at his Santa Monica club. It worked well for her. She lived to be 94 years old, passing in January of 1986. **Armand Tanny** was Vic's younger brother. Armand competed in weightlifting early in his career but later turned to bodybuilding and wrestling. He had a career of writing for the Weider publications. Armand appeared in 2 films in 1944,"Lady in the Dark" with Ginger Rogers and "Frenchman's Creek" with Basil Rathbone. Armand died on April 4, 2009. He was 90 years of age. **Vic Tanny Jr.** was a successful Iron Age bodybuilder in the seventies. **Mandy Tanny**, Vic's niece, wrote for Joe Weider's "Muscle and Fitness" magazine for 10 years and penned 2 health food cookbooks. She and her husband developed a chain of gyms between 1990 and 2003. Sadly, Mandy passed away from breast cancer in April of 2010. She was 60 years old.

Vic Tanny, the young immigrant boy who grew a bodybuilding empire, died of heart failure on June 11, 1985. In spite of how his empire may have ended, he will always be remembered for his contribution to the health and fitness industry and the Iron Age era of bodybuilding.

Rest in peace , Vic Tanney.

This next brief excerpt is from an older (1961) time magazine ad on Vic & his gyms: The biggest chain of sweatshops in the U.S. is owned lock, stock and bar bell by wedge-shaped Californian Vic Tanny, 48, an ex-weight lifter whose sell is every bit as hard as his muscles.

Capitalizing on the fetish of physical fitness, Tanny has lured more than a million Americans into some 80 chrome-and-red-carpet Vic Tanny gyms scattered across the U.S., signed them up to membership contracts of six months (typical East Coast price: $185) to "permanent" (seven years: $360) on the pay-as-you-perspire plan.

The forward to the Joe DiMarco chapter in my Culver City book provided a brief description of the Dungeon;

Joe met Bill West at the famous Vic Tanny's gym, A.K.A "The Dungeon"

Here is a brief excerpt from the Oldtimestrongman website about the gym;

Just a stone's throw from the original Muscle Beach in Santa Monica, California, was Vic Tanny's Gym. Shortly after World War II, Tanny converted a 7,000-square-foot USO center, which was located in a basement on 4th Street, into the best-equipped gym in the United States. It was huge, with 15 foot ceilings and all kinds of training equipment.

Vic Tanny's was affectionately known as "The Dungeon" and was *the* place to train during the 1940's and 1950's -- regular members included Steve Reeves, George Eiferman, Joe Gold (of Gold's Gym fame) and Arthur Jones, Bill McArdle (movie actor and bodybuilder), Irvin "Zabo" Kozewski, Spellman, Olympic greats Tommy Kono and Dave Sheppard, one of the movie actors from Wagon Train (James Arness?), along with a whole host of others. It was where Bob Hoffman and the York gang trained on West Coast trips.

This website had a nice little story on Tanny's;

http://www.musclesofiron.com/774/most-impressive-at-vic-tannys-gym/

Most Impressive at Vic Tanny's Gym

July 11, 2011

Several months ago I came across a terrific book titled, *The New Bodybuilding for Old-School Results*. It was written by renowned author Ellington Darden, a protégé of Arthur Jones and advocate of High-Intensity Training (HIT).

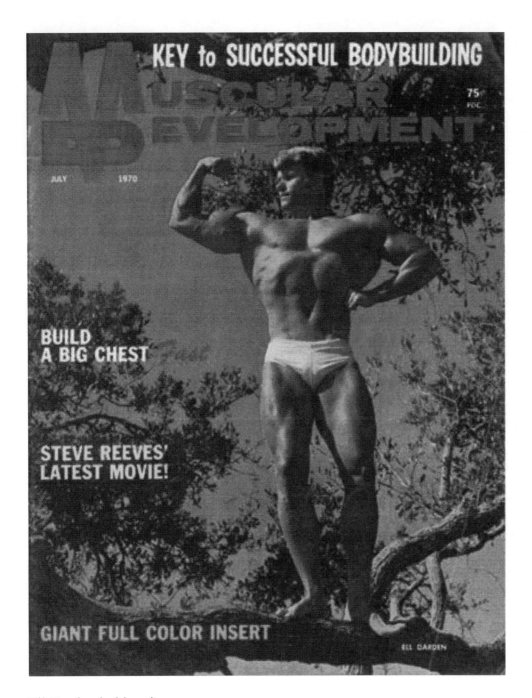

Ell Darden in his prime

In Chapter 1 of Ellington's book, the author presents a "chat" he had with Ben Sorenson. **Sorenson was once the manager of Vic Tanny's Gym, a 7,000 square foot exercise and barbell facility the bodybuilder opened shortly after World War II. This gym, which became known as the "Dungeon", was located in the basement of a building at 4th and Broadway in Santa Monica.** For many years, many of the world's best physique stars and weightlifters trained at or visited Tanny's Gym, including **Steve Reeves, George Eiferman, John Farbotnik, Armand Tanny (Vic's Brother), Malcolm Brenner, and Eric Pedersen.**

In his interview with Sorenson, Darden asked the former manager who, among the many greats he saw at Tanny's Gym, impressed him most. Here was his answer: But you know who impressed me most? It was **Marvin Eder**. He visited for a couple of weeks the last summer I was there. At the Muscle Beach training area, Eiferman and I handed him a barbell loaded to 440 pounds and he bench pressed it for several reps, easily. Then, he did a behind-the-neck press, seated with a 330-pound barbell – and dips with 250 pounds hanging from his waist. His arms also measured a solid 18-1/2 inches.

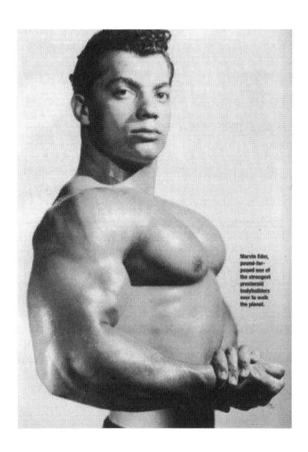

Marvin Eder, pound-for-pound one of the strongest greatest bodybuilders ever to walk the planet.

John Davis, Olympic weightlifting champion in 1948 and 1952, impressed me as well. I saw him unofficially clean-and-jerk 400 pounds, when the world record was only 375 pounds. His physique was right up there with any Mr. America of that era. Eder and Davis, each weighing about 195 pounds, both did several one-armed chin-ups with either arm. That was something to see. What amazing power both Marvin Eder and John Davis possessed! Furthermore, both of these lifters built their extraordinary strength with nothing more than hard training, perseverance, and a fighting spirit. If you have these three things at the forefront of your muscle-building program, you too can become mighty and powerful.

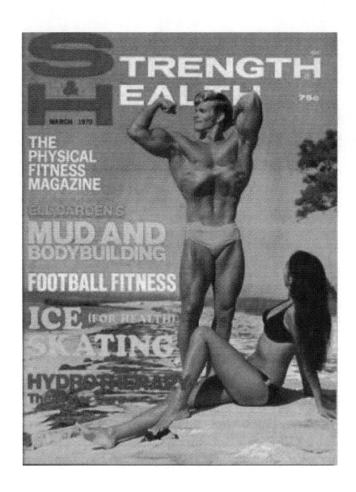

Darden with a pretty young lady on the beach

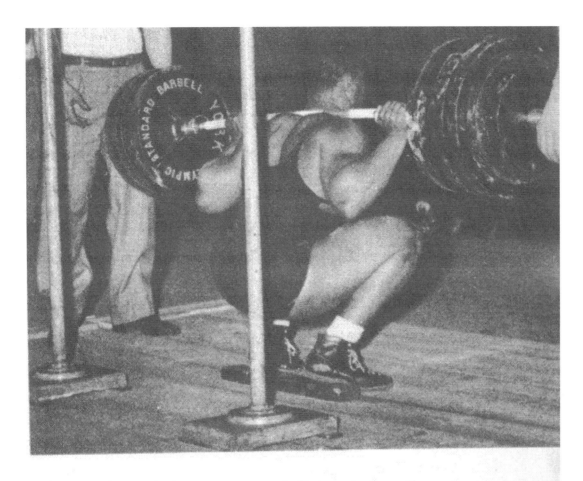

Squatting with heavy weights, five sets of five reps with 450, is an important part of John Davis' training for power. Here he shows his style with 500 pounds at an exhibition staged by John Terlazzo in New York. (Ralph Mazzaro photo)

Tanny's gym was the butt of jokes back in those days, and even a song;

[SICK MANNY'S GYM{1}] Written by: Al Kooper Performed by: Leo DeLyon & the Musclemen First released: Single: 1960.

Appears on:

Singles: Leo De Lyon & the Musclemen A-side: "Sick Manny's Gym" B-side: "Plunkin'" (Musicor, 45rpm, #1001)-1960;

Albums: Rare Novelty, Vol. 1 [Various Artists] (CD, #NO-1955)-2008{2};

{1}The title, "Sick Manny's Gym," is a play on words for Vic Tanny's Gym. Victor "Vic" Tanny (c 1912-June 11, 1985) was a pioneer in the creation of the modern health club. Tanny's gyms played a part in the evolution of the all-male gym to the modern fitness club of today.{2}Transcribed from the track on this album.→ Sick Manny's Gym Lyrics by Leo DeLyon & the Musclemen → All Leo DeLyon & the Musclemen Lyrics / Discography

One of the promising young guys you might have run into in the early days of the Dungeon was this guy;

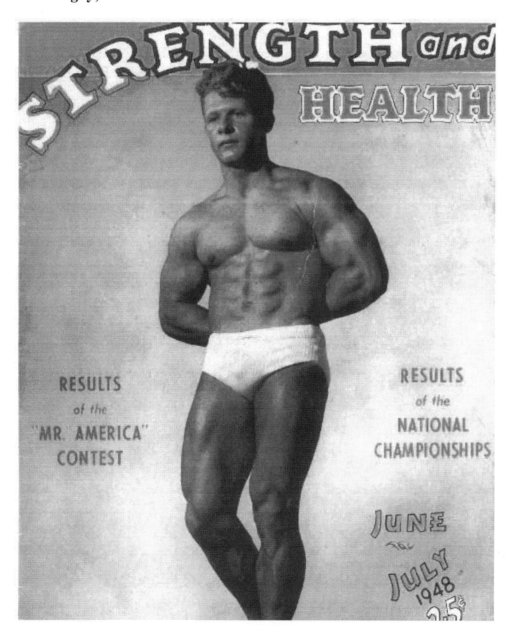

THE MAN ON THE COVER

By George Eiferman, "1948 Mr. America"

GENE MYERS is one of the youngest fellows ever to gain nationwide recognition for his muscular development. At the very tender age of 14, Strength & Health carried a picture of this youthful hercules showing immense physical possibilities and phenomenal development, taken less than a year after starting weight training.

His improvement was always steady and nothing short of amazing. His arms formerly were referred to as "banana arms," but now they are thicker, rounder and more muscular. His scrawny, bony back suddenly seemed to sprout wings, while his shoulders got bigger and broader with each training day, often mistaken for "barn doors!" In spite of his youthful appearance Gene has often been mistaken for some All-American football player, usually by people who are not familiar with the results possible through barbell training.

Several months ago I left York to go to the west coast and, like most of the York champions, I trained at Vic Tanny's gym which I felt would afford me the best possible training surroundings. It was while training in this spacious gym I became acquainted with Gene Myers. I was immediately impressed by Gene's shapely physique. His arms, chest, back and legs were wonderfully developed and the more I studied his proportions the more I realized this boy really has "plenty on the ball."

It didn't take us long to become acquainted for Gene is a sort of easy going fellow and easy to get along with. His constant friend and training companion, whose development is truly amazing, is none other than Pepper Gomez who placed second in the Mr. Los Angeles contest. They train sincerely and have but one purpose in mind: to develop their bodies to the highest degree possible. No personal rivalry exists between them. Each attempts to help the other in every way possible. Rarely do they miss a workout. They train four to five times a week—every week.

We made up a threesome while I was there and went through quite a grind several times. Although I've worked out with many barbell men in my life, I don't think anyone can be more enthusiastic than these two fellows. They train diligently and in earnest. When one scrutinizes their developments, they can realize they have rightfully earned what they have. It's really a pleasure to workout with someone like Gene and Pepper for they serve to inspire everyone who watches them.

Gene's efforts have been recently rewarded when he entered and won the Mr. Los Angeles contest several months ago, while his good friend Pepper Gomez came in second. Now they have another goal in mind: to see who will win the Mr. America contest first. Each felt they were not fully prepared to enter
(Continued on Page 86)

One of the finest physiques in the nation, GENE MYERS of Los Angeles, our coverman. The above photo shows Gene at the age of 18 while the smaller one at the right shows the phenomenal build he attained while only 14 years old. Here is convincing proof for you young chaps—it is never too early to start body building. (Photos by Athletic Model Guild of Los Angeles, Cal.)

By George Eiferman, "1948 Mr. America"

GENE MYERS is one of the youngest fellows ever to gain nationwide recognition for his muscular development. At the very tender age of 14, Strength & Health carried a picture of this youthful hercules showing immense physical possibilities and phenomenal development, taken less than a year after starting weight training.

His improvement was always steady and nothing short of amazing. His arms formerly were referred to as "banana arms," but now they are thicker, rounder and more muscular. His scrawny, bony back suddenly seemed to sprout wings, while his shoulders got bigger and broader with each training day, often mistaken for "barn doors!" In spite of his youthful appearance Gene has often been mistaken for some All-American football player, usually by people who are not familiar with the results possible through barbell training.

Several months ago I left York to go to the west coast and, like most of the York champions, I trained at Vic Tanny's gym which I felt would afford me the best possible training surroundings. It was while training in this spacious gym I became acquainted with Gene Myers. I was immediately impressed by Gene's shapely physique. His arms, chest, back and legs were wonderfully developed and the more I studied his proportions the more I realized this boy really has "plenty on the ball."

It didn't take us long to become acquainted for Gene is a sort of easy going fellow and easy to get along with. His constant friend and training companion, whose development is truly amazing, is none other than Pepper Gomez who placed second in the Mr. Los Angeles contest. They train sincerely and have but one purpose in mind; to develop their bodies to the highest degree possible. No personal rivalry exists between them. Each attempts to help the other in every way possible. Rarely do they miss a workout. They train four to five times a week—every week.

We made up a threesome while I was there and went through quite a grind several times. Although I've worked out with many barbell men in my life, I don't think anyone can be more enthusiastic than these two fellows. They train diligently and in earnest. When one scrutinizes their developments, they soon realize they have rightfully earned what they have. It's really a pleasure to workout with someone like Gene and Pepper for they serve to inspire everyone who watches them.

Gene's efforts have been recently rewarded when he entered and won the Mr. Los Angeles contest several months ago, while his good friend Pepper Gomez came in second. Now they have another goal in mind; to see who will win the Mr. America contest first. Each felt they were not fully prepared to enter *(Continued on Page 86)*

The Man on the Cover

(Continued from Page 8)

this year's Mr. America contest which I was fortunate in winning, but I can't help but believe that Gene will be a hard man to beat in any best built man contest in the future.

Gene has shape, strength, bulk and plenty of muscle. His fine development appears fully matured although his extremely youthful facial appearance belies his age. He will be 19 years old this August and at the rate this boy is improving, it's hard to conceive the terrific development he will possess in another year or two.

Normally people do not credit a barbell man for his efficiency and feel most of them cannot do anything else but lift weights. Gene, however, is an exception as many other barbell men are. He has placed second in an A. A. U. Flying Ring Championship and is rated as a top man in this field. When one sees Gene execute some of the difficult flying ring routines one is amazed at his timing, ability and skill.

Gene and his buddy Pepper have another secret ambition . . . they want to own and operate a large and fully weight equipped gym somewhere in California so they can help others to improve their health, strength and body development. Yes, it's hard to beat such enthusiasm and I feel certain they will reach this goal as well. If they do succeed in opening a gym they are bound to be a great success in this field too.

Some of their favorite exercises are curls, chins, dips, and presses, but a large variety of exercises are included in their training schedule such as the pullovers, squats (note Gene's exceptional legs), rowing movements, etc. Some of Gene's amazing strength feats are doing a curl one hand with an 80 pound dumbell. He has also performed an incline bench press with 105 pound dumbells in each hand, repeating each ten repetitions.

His ideal is and has always been John Grimek. A number of people believe he looks like Grimek in body proportions. There is no doubt as he gets more matured he will develop even shapelier and huskier proportions than he has at present and should go down in the best built man

Armand Tanny was mentioned in that last section. Here is a great little interview with him in his advanced age; Iron Game History Volume 6 Number 4

Armand Tanny remembers Steve Reeves

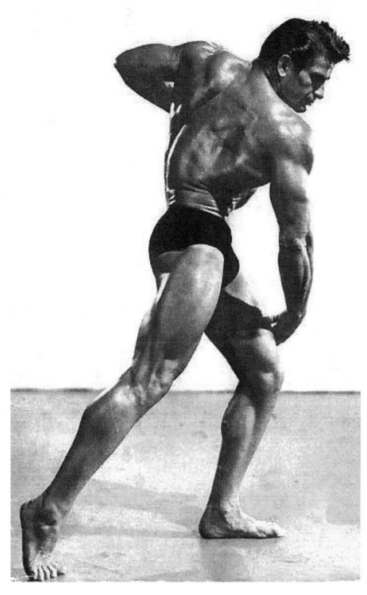

Armand in his prime

Terry Todd conducted this interview in June of 1999, near Armand Tanny's home in Woodland Hills, California. Tanny has lived in southern California for over 60 years and has made significant contributions to the iron game as a competitive weightlifter, a bodybuilder, and a prolific writer for many physical culture magazines, including *Muscle & Fitness.*

TT: Am I wrong? It seems like I remember somewhere that there was a time when you and George Eiferman and Steve Reeves were all living pretty close to one another near Muscle Beach.

AT: Oh yeah, that's right.

TT: That was kind of amazing that three guys who'd have such big reputations would be so close. I'd guess those were kind of your salad days.
AT: Really. We all lived there at the same place for awhile. We paid a total of $60 a month or something like that, you know? We were right on the water. I could jump off the balcony onto the sand of Muscle Beach. It was the life. I got there in '39 and was in the Beach area down to 1958, so it was about 20 years that I was there most of the time when I wasn't rambling around.
TT: When were you and Reeves and Eiferman all there together at the same time?

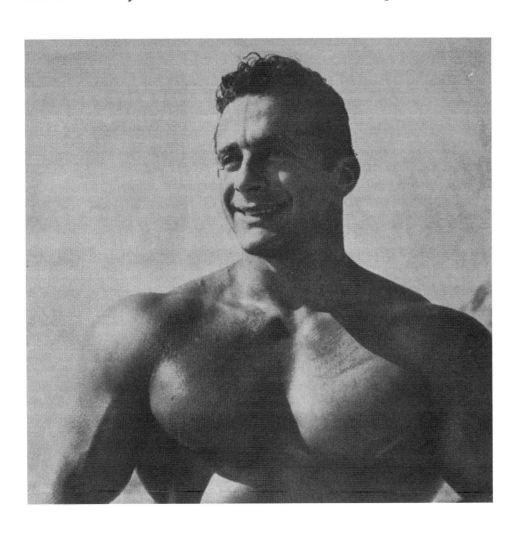

George Eiferman

AT: It was in the late 40s because we were all competing, you know, and all three of us competed in the 1949 Mr. USA show. That one show had Grimek, Clancy Ross, Reeves, Eiferman, me, and others, too. So those of us who lived out here had a lot of opportunity to watch one another and train together.
TT: Where did you do most of your training, on the beach or in the gym?
AT: In the gym. The Tanny Gym. Fourth and Broadway. (AKA the Dungeon)

TT: So if you'd do something at the beach with the weights it would be just light stuff, or maybe a little arm work?

AT: Yeah, right. But I might do some odd lifts, too. I used to have a little trick I'd do. I'd pull maybe 300 pounds or so to my shoulders in a power clean and jerk it overhead and then walk down through the sand holding it over my head.

TT: I don't imagine you had too many people trying to match that.

AT: No.

TT: Old George was a great presser, though, wasn't he?

AT: He had tremendous pressing power. He wasn't a talented weightlifter, but he was really strong, particularly in the pressing movements.

TT: I know he's told me he wasn't very good in cleaning or things like that.

AT: No, he didn't have that speed, you know, that quickness that a top lifter needs.

TT: I remember seeing photographs of him playing a trumpet and at the same time pressing a person or a 145 pound barbell over his head with one hand.

AT: Yeah, that was one of his stage tricks. After he was out here in the late 40s there was a time when he travelled around the country speaking to school systems, you know. He gave lectures and told jokes and did strength stunts. He'd always take one of the students and press him or her over his head while he was blowing on his trumpet.

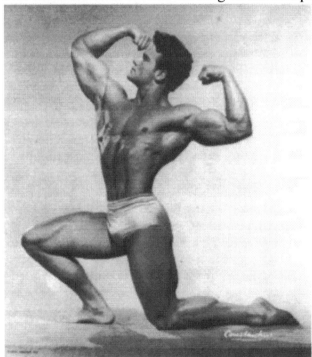

Steve Reeves more or less as he looked the first time he came to Muscle Beach and was seen by Armand Tanny.

TT: I guess Reeves must've been amazing, too, in his own way. He always looked to me like what an artist might have created if someone told the artist, "Okay, let's see you make a physically perfect man." I've always thought that most artists with imagination and real skill would have come up with something a lot like Steve.

AT: Oh, he was so pretty.

TT: [Laughing.] Yeah, that's right. He had real beauty. In all seriousness "beauty" may be the best word for someone made like he was. Everything about him seemed to fit the other parts, with perhaps the most defining parts being his face and those big calves.

AT: Yeah, everything was to perfection. It was just amazing. Yeah, Steve. He used to poke a little fun at himself, you know. He loved to joke. He'd hold out his foot and he'd say, "Isn't that foot perfect?" And it was perfect. Or he'd open his mouth and say, "Not a cavity." And it was true, there wasn't a cavity in his mouth and all we could say was, "Reeves, you dirty dog." You know? But he knew he was special and he was easy with it. He always seemed to be in good spirits and had a lot of fun. He really enjoyed being around everybody at the Beach, you know?

TT: He and his lady friend Deborah came out and visited us at the library a few years ago. He wanted to look at our collection of books and magazines and photos and things. But he had another reason, too, which is that he was thinking about getting a ranch out in central Texas where we live. He said he was serious about moving because everything was getting too crowded where he was.

AT: I could believe that.

TT: And so they came out and stayed a few days with us. That was the first time I'd been around him for any length of time and I found him to have a truly pleasant nature. In a way, he seemed almost shy at first, or at least reserved.

AT: He was a bit shy. But he had a good sense of humor. Loved jokes and fun, you know? A pleasant kid.

TT: But did he have an impact on the beach with the general public?

AT: Oh, man, let me tell you. I think it was about 1945 when I first learned about him. The war was still on and I went up to San Francisco to see Jack LaLanne's gym there, you know, and he said, "Armand, look at this picture." So here was this kid, you know, and he's only about 16 years old in the shot. Here's this 16 year-old kid with this perfect structure. So, Jack says, "Anyway, he's down in the Philippines in the service but he'll be back soon." I thought. Jesus, man. Wow. Great body and he already looked like a man. Anyway, about two or three years later, you know, I'm sitting there at Muscle Beach one day and this fellow comes walking down the beach. He's got a tailored shirt, and when he gets on the sand and starts to strip down, you know, and he's standing out there and we're all watching him I say, "Holy #@#$t! Look at that body. That's Steve Reeves."

TT: I guess when the big crowds were there, he must have had a big impact. I mean, people must have. . .

AT: They followed him around like dogs. Like, for instance, groups of women, middle-aged or older women, would walk by him. He'd be walking down the boardwalk in his trunks and they'd see him coming and then they'd make a U-turn and just follow him. He had a lot of fun with that body, but he never took himself too seriously. He was a hell of a guy.

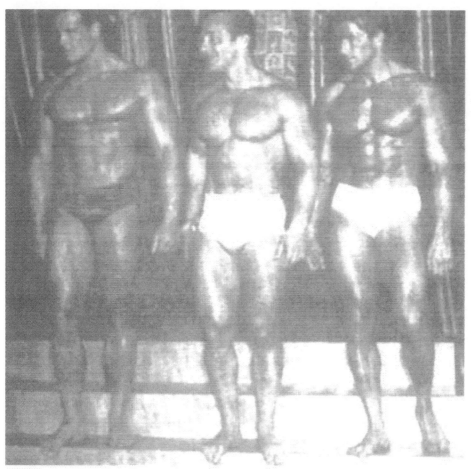

Muscle Beach buddies—Steve Reeves, George Eiferman, and Armand Tanny on stage in the 1949 Mr. USA, which was won by John Grimek.

The following is a nice article written shortly after the unfortunate demise of Armand, and while it may reiterate some information that has already come up, I thought it would make a nice addition here;

Bodybuilding legend Armand Tanny dies at age 90...

Bodybuilding legend **Armand Tanny** died on Saturday April 4, 2009 at an assisted living facility in California at the age of 90.

"Armand began his 70-year physical-culture odyssey at the age of 12, when his **big brother Vic gave him a set of barbells for his birthday**. Unable to control his enthusiasm, he exercised all day long-which caused him to spend the next week in bed recuperating from the resulting soreness. From that point on he trained under Vic's guidance and made excellent progress. Armand excelled at high school sports, but weightlifting captivated him. As a teenager he clean-and-jerked 300 pounds. In 1938 he became the first man in the state of New York to officially perform a 300-pound clean and jerk. He was awarded a trophy for this feat by Arthur Gay, a prominent weight-training authority and gym owner. After a year of premed studies at the University of Rochester in New York, he moved to the West Coast and completed his premed work at the University of California at Los Angeles. He later studied at the Children's Hospital School of Physical Therapy. **The first time Armand appeared at Santa Monica's Muscle Beach, everyone was amazed at the poundage he could lift.** Soon thereafter he won the Pacific Coast Light Heavyweight weightlifting title, and he took the Heavyweight title the following year. He was training hard for the 1940 Olympic Games when they were canceled due to the war. While competing in a college wrestling match, Armand suffered a severe knee injury that eventually caused him to quit weightlifting. He switched to bodybuilding with spectacular success. **His training buddies Pepper Gomez, Joe Gold, Gene Meyers and Malcolm Brenner** urged him to compete, but it wasn't until 1949 that he entered his first contest. Because he had wrestled professionally to pay his college tuition, he wasn't eligible for amateur events. He entered **Bert Goodrich's Professional Mr. USA contest** and finished fifth-behind **John Grimek, Clancy Ross, Steve Reeves and George Eiferman**. Joe Weider was quick to recognize Armand as a future star and invited him to guest pose at a physique show in New York. Weider asked Armand to write some articles for his magazines. Given his premed and physical therapy education and his iron game experience, Armand brought unique qualifications to the field. In 1949 Armand won an unusual open contest, the Mr. 1949, in Los Angeles. The winner was determined by an applause meter mounted in an eight-foot-high receiver. Soon afterward, he was interviewed by movie producers who were searching for a new Tarzan to replace Johnny Weissmuller. Edgar Rice Burroughs Jr.-whose father created Tarzan-was impressed with Armand's rugged good looks, tremendous physique and athletic grace and wanted him for the role. He was overruled by MGM's execs, who selected Lex Barker. Armand did, however, work in a few movies as an extra or bit player. **He and Vince Gironda worked together for several months on the classic "Frenchman's Creek."** His bodybuilding career reached its zenith in 1950, when he won both the Professional Mr. America and the Professional Mr. USA titles. The Mr. USA was the highest title in the world in those days, the equivalent of today's Mr. Olympia.

In the early '50s Vic Tanny opened a chain of gyms featuring state-of-the-art equipment that revolutionized the gym business. Armand helped develop most of the advanced equipment and modern training systems used in all 84 of those gyms. He also devised weight-training courses for the combat crews of the Strategic Air Command. **In 1954 he became a member of Mae West's cabaret show, along with Eiferman, Zabo Koszewski, Joe Gold, Chuck Krauser, Richard Dubois, Dominick Juliano, Les Shaffer and Harry Schwartz.** The nightclub act set attendance records all over the country, topping even Frank Sinatra's. During his 50-year tenure as a feature writer for Weider publications Armand has helped develop dozens of training and nutrition concepts.

He is presently a senior writer for Muscle & Fitness and a member of the Weider Research Group. His daughter Mandy described him as a "true Renaissance man-with a bit of caveman thrown in." He was certainly a living legend."

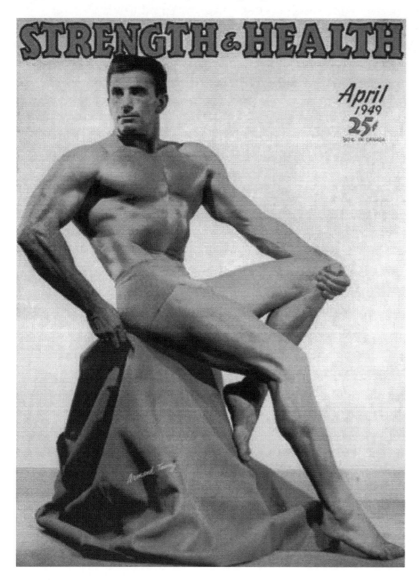

Armand in April of 1949.

LA TIMES ARTICLE:

"Armand Tanny, a pioneering figure in bodybuilding who won national titles in 1949 and 1950 and was a popular figure on Muscle Beach in Santa Monica during its heyday in the 1940s, has died. He was 90. Tanny, the younger brother of gym pioneer Vic Tanny, died of natural causes Saturday at a nursing facility in Westlake Village, according to his daughter, Mandy Tanny. He had been fairly active until last year and was still driving last summer. Originally a weightlifter,

Tanny won the Mr. 1949 title, the 1949 Pro Mr. America title and the 1950 Pro Mr. USA titles in bodybuilding. **In the days before steroids, he credited his wins to diet and hard work.** He was a firm believer in the benefits of raw foods, including tuna, beef, liver and lobster as well as nuts, seeds, fruits and vegetables. **During the 1950s, he was one of the original nine bodybuilders from Muscle Beach who were part of Mae West's traveling nightclub act. According to the book "Remembering Muscle Beach" by Harold Zinkin with Bonnie Hearn-Hill (Angel City Press, 1999), the nine were known as Mae's Muscle Beach Men. They included such prominent bodybuilders as Joe Gold, George Eiferman, and Richard DuBois, whom Zinkin and Hearn-Hill called "the star" of the group, Harry Schwartz, Dom Juliano, Lester "Shifty" Schaefer, Irvin "Zabo" Koszewski, Chuck Krauser and Tanny.** According to Hearn-Hill, Tanny organized a strike with Gold when West cut their $250-a-week salaries in half to boost the take at a New York club. "Armand and Joe were ready to board the plane," Hearn-Hill told The Times on Wednesday. "Mae quickly caved in and they got their full salaries." Tanny also turned to professional wrestling in the 1950s. But for much of his life, the quiet and studious Tanny made his living writing about physical fitness and bodybuilding for his friend Joe Weider's publications, including Muscle Power magazine. Tanny was born March 5, 1919, in Rochester, N.Y. In his early teens, he was competing in weightlifting competitions. In 1941, he placed second in the heavyweight class in the Junior Nationals competition in Akron, Ohio. In that competition, he managed 230, 250 and 330 pounds in the three Olympic lifts (press, snatch, and clean and jerk). He was able to clean a 300-pound barbell one-handed. He attended the University of Rochester before moving to Los Angeles in the late 1930s, where he enrolled at UCLA. But World War II intervened, and Tanny joined the Coast Guard and served until he suffered a knee injury. He left the service and went back to school in Westwood, earning a degree in physical therapy. He also had unaccredited parts in some Hollywood films, including "Lady in the Dark" (1944) and "Frenchman's Creek" (1944). Meanwhile, he kept perfecting his body for the emerging sport of bodybuilding. **When he wasn't at the beach with early bodybuilding pals, including Steve Reeves, Tanny was at the gym in Santa Monica started by his brother, Vic, who years later pioneered the creation of modern health clubs, which were a big part of the Southern California fitness scene in the late 1940s and early 1950s. Vic Tanny's fitness empire eventually included gyms across the country.** In 1949, Armand Tanny married Shirley Luvin, whom he had met at Muscle Beach. His daughter was born in 1950. Tanny left Santa Monica and Muscle Beach in the late 1950s and lived in Hawaii for a decade before moving to the San Fernando Valley and going to work for Weider. In addition to his daughter, Mandy, who is also a bodybuilder and writer, Tanny is survived by his grandson, Mario, a bodybuilder."

The following Muscle Builder article from Mr. Draper mentions the dungeon & I thought it would make a nice addition here;

Muscle champ Dave Draper teams up with wrestling champ Chuck Fish for a shoulder routine guaranteed to build size and classic shape.

FIVE-STEP SCHEME OF TRAINING FOR COMPLETE SHOULDER DEVELOPMENT

BY DAVE DRAPER
Mr. America/Mr. Universe

★ It was early morning and the famous California sun was beginning to light the sprawling metropolis of Los Angeles. The sky was blue, the air clean, and it promised to be another one of those spectacular days in the "Land of Sunshine."

As I made my way to the Muscle Beach Weightlifting Club, I drove slowly through the deserted streets of Santa Monica, enjoying the stillness. I reached the gym and unlocked the door just as the chimes on the corner Salvation Army building sounded, indicating it was 6 A.M. I enjoy training in the early morning, and have for 4 years. I find it a relaxing time of day, which is conducive to productive training; the gym is relatively empty, making the facilities instantly available.

I put on the lights, set the clock and tuned in some soft background music on the radio. The Muscle Beach Weightlifting Club isn't much to look at; it didn't get its nickname, "The Dungeon," for nothing. The ceiling leaks, the floor is cracked, and the whole place leaves much to be desired.

It wasn't many years ago, 7 or 8 maybe, that the gym with its homemade equipment was located on the glorious beach of Santa Monica, some 5 blocks away from its present location. Since then the town's do-gooders, somewhat archaic to say the least, have terminated what they believed to be a circus-like atmosphere at Muscle Beach, gym included, causing the Club to move to its present underground location.

But I love it. The area is enormous. The rugged equipment is not homemade, but tailored for its members' special needs, and there are plenty of weights. Practically speaking, there are better gyms in the area —but to me "The Dungeon" is like an old shoe; it fits comfortably.

I began the tedious but necessary task of training the midsection. Because I regard abdominal work as unpleasant, I prefer getting it over with; plus, I find it limbers and warms the body, still a bit stiff from a long night's sleep. I hadn't begun to sweat when the thunder of heavy hoofs echoed through the empty gym. Chuck Fish, alias "The Mighty Atlas," of pro-wrestling fame, like myself, enjoys the freedom of early-bird training.

He's a giant of a man and looks almost terrifying with his shaved head, beard and handle-bar mustache. But a more gentle and gracious bear you could not meet. It was Monday and the two of us   *more* ▶

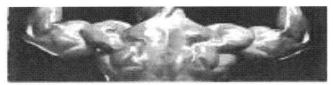

continued

FIVE-STEP SCHEME FOR SHOULDER DEVELOPMENT

planned to combine our training efforts in hopes of making revolutionary progress. In Chuck I saw the size I wanted, and in me he saw the shape and muscularity he wanted. Our mutual knowledge and training instincts, we concluded, would complement each other and the results could well be inspiring.

We soon discovered, as we began working-out and sharing views on weight training, that we both had a particular passion for deltoid development. It is this muscle group, we agreed, that bears the accent of body power and body grace. Make the deltoids and arms your strong points and you'll go a far way in exhibiting a championship physique.

As you can guess, with this enthusiastic frame of mind, we paid special attention to the shoulder area; Chuck, expounding the ways to build size and strength, and me bringing up the rear by assuring fine muscle shape and hardness. And that is what this article is all about—developing shoulder width and thickness with simultaneous attention to shape and muscularity . . . a 5-step scheme of training for complete shoulder development. *(Continued on page 56)*

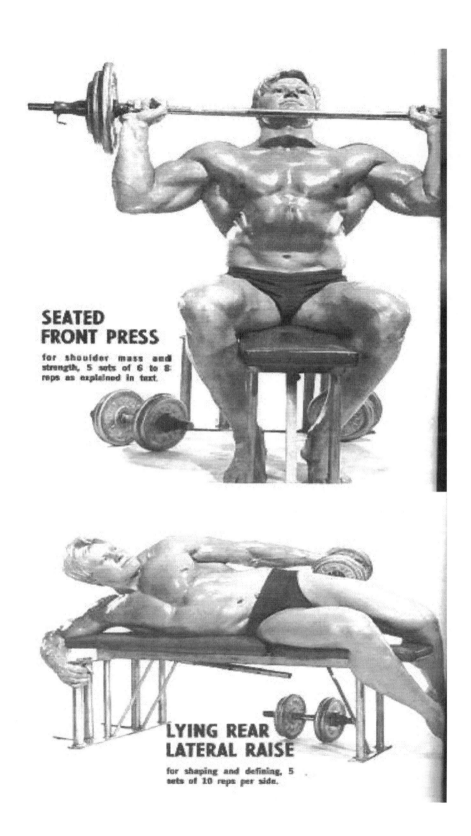

SEATED FRONT PRESS
for shoulder mass and strength, 5 sets of 6 to 8 reps as explained in text.

LYING REAR LATERAL RAISE
for shaping and defining, 5 sets of 10 reps per side.

FIVE-STEP SCHEME OF TRAINING FOR COMPLETE SHOULDER DEVELOPMENT

(Continued from page 10)

EXERCISES

1. Seated Front Press
2. Steep Incline Dumbbell Press
3. Dumbbell Clean and Press
4. Lying Deltoid Raise—Front
5. Lying Deltoid Raise—Rear

1. Seated Front Press. This exercise is performed seated, preferably with the back supported so as to prevent any cheating or unnecessary body movement. And, too, in the seated position the lower back (which is so prone to injury) is less likely to suffer damage.

This powerful movement is responsible for developing shoulder mass and strength. It attacks the frontal deltoid area primarily, in which one's pressing power lies. Thus, in performing the exercise, the accent should be placed on power. The barbell is pressed slowly from the chest-shoulder region to an overhead lock-out position for 5 sets of 6 to 8 reps. In an effort to increase your strength slowly and steadily, add one repetition with each workout until 5 sets of 8 reps are completed. At that point increase the poundage proportionately and go back to doing 6 reps. As your power increases, so will your size.

clean the weight to the deltoids, and without hesitation press to an overhead position. For maximum pump and burn be sure not to lock-out the elbows, but maintain resistance continuously. Return the heavy poundage slowly with concentrated effort, and repeat for 5 sets of 6 grueling but gratifying reps.

Though this is a basic power and bulk movement, it will do much to shape and striate the delts as well. This is the original "cannonball maker."

4. Lying Front Lateral Raise. Now—to etch some deep cuts and protruding striations in those thick and powerful globes of steel. Lying on your right side, grasp a relatively light dumbbell in your left hand. With your legs and free right hand arranged in such a position as to stabilize the body, raise the dumbbell slowly and deliberately from your side—and return to starting position. Five sets of 10 reps per side will crown the delts with inspiring definition.

Again, to assure complete muscle development and add variety to the movement, try raising the dumbbell from various positions; for example, in front of the body or in front of the

2. Steep Incline Dumbbell Press. Another exercise with the emphasis on power, the Seated Incline Dumbbell Press works both the front and side deltoids. Here again, the simple system of increased reps, as applied to the barbell press, should be practiced—that is, 5 sets of 6 reps to start, until 8 reps are reached . . . then add weight and go back to 6 reps. This exercise is responsible for rounding out the deltoids, giving them the famous "cannonball" appearance.

For variation, alter the pressing grip with each set; that is, press one set with the palms forward to affect the frontal deltoids, and follow it with the palms facing each other to affect the side deltoids, or "caps." This change of grip not only assures complete shoulder development, but adds interest to the routine as well.

3. Dumbbell Clean and Press. This rugged movement will add new thickness to the entire shoulder area, including the very impressive upper trapezius muscle. Assume a crouched position with the dumbbells resting on the mid-thighs. With each repetition head. I guarantee encouraging results.

The Front Lateral Raise attacks the front and side shoulder muscles, making them stand out like watermelons in a strawberry patch.

5. Lying Rear Lateral Raise. Another exercise for shaping and defining the deltoids—this one is executed in much the same fashion as the Front Lateral Raise. The only exception is that the dumbbell is brought up from a behind-the-torso position. This movement affects the rear deltoids, primarily, giving them that inspiring (and "patriotic") star-like appearance.

Five sets of 10 slow reps per side will complete your search for ultimate shoulder development.

This routine is great—and results are guaranteed—if you have the determination to tackle it. Don't let discouragement become your training partner. This is the bodybuilder's plague, his worst enemy, a sure sign of defeat. Keep up your spirit to succeed—and you will . . . with my 5-step scheme of training for bombing and building the 3 heads of your delts!

Author's note

It is always an author's dream to get firsthand accounts from real, live witnesses of past events, along with personal anecdotes and stories that you just can't find anywhere else. Such was the case when my friend Jeff Aquirre introduced me via email to Joe DiMarco, one of the core guys from the original Westside barbell club of Culver City. Well, Jeff emailed me recently about the following gentleman, who actually was a manager of Tanny's gym(s) for many years. He was a cover man in August,'59 on Muscle Builder magazine which you will see a page or 2 forward of here, and placed 3rd in the IFBB Mr. America contest of that year. While I decide to put Sam's stuff here in the chapter about the "dungeon", it would be fairly equally at home in the Muscle Beach section, as Sam was active, like many in his day, at both of these venues.

Sam Calhoun

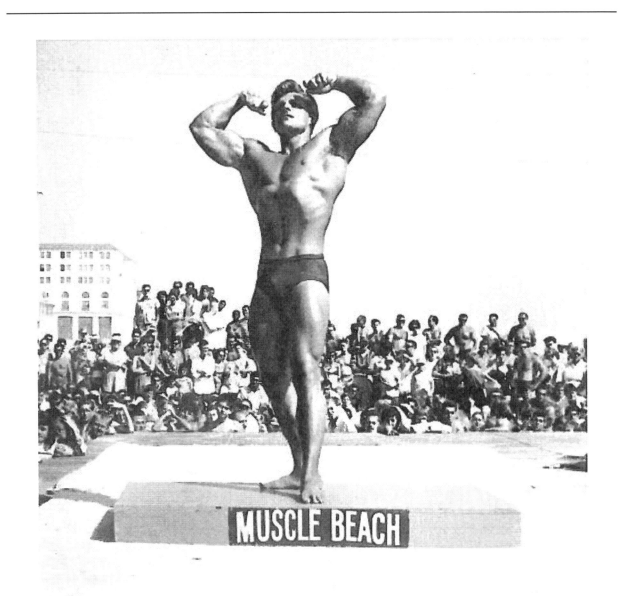

Summer of 1959

Bio

Sam has over 35 years of experience in the fitness industry, starting his career as one of the now famous "**Muscle Beach**" originals; he became "**America's Most Muscular Man", 1959.** He turned his love for fitness into the business of health club ownership for over twenty years. Sam sat on the original "PT Exam Item Writing Committee" for ACE. The consummate personal trainer, he is currently Director of Results Fitness Systems, training for personal trainers and a partner in Progressive Fitness. Sam has been an inspiration to his students because of his dynamic presentation skills, academic depth, his history in club ownership, and his Bodybuilding titles. In 1980 Sam labeled his health clubs "custom-houses" offering "closed-end-training". Sam is the research and development director for Progressive Fitness and a key member of the PF faculty.

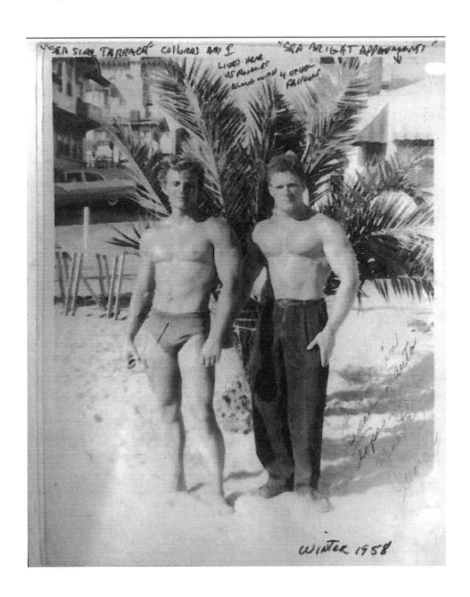

The autograph says; "Success in repairing auto tops, Your Pal, George" (Sheffield) and the hand written notes on the top point out the apartment where Sam & Chuck Collras lived together for a time, as well as the "Seabright" Apartment building nearby.

His industry certifications include: American College of Sports Medicine (ACSM) Exercise Specialist, Personal Trainer, Advanced level, Graded Exercise Test Technologist, and Health and Fitness Instructor, American Council on Exercise (ACE) triple "Gold", Group Fitness Instructor, Personal Trainer, and Weight Management and Lifestyle Consultant, National Strength and Conditioning Association (NSCA) Personal Trainer, National Academy of Sports Medicine (NASM), Personal Trainer, Advanced Level.

Career

- **Ata Fitness**

    Director of Results Fitness SystemsApr-2012

- **Ata Fitness**

    DirectorApr-2012 to Apr-2012

- **Ata Fitness**

    PartnerApr-2012 to Apr-2012

- **Ata Fitness**

    Group Fitness Instructor

- **Ace**

    Fitness Instructor

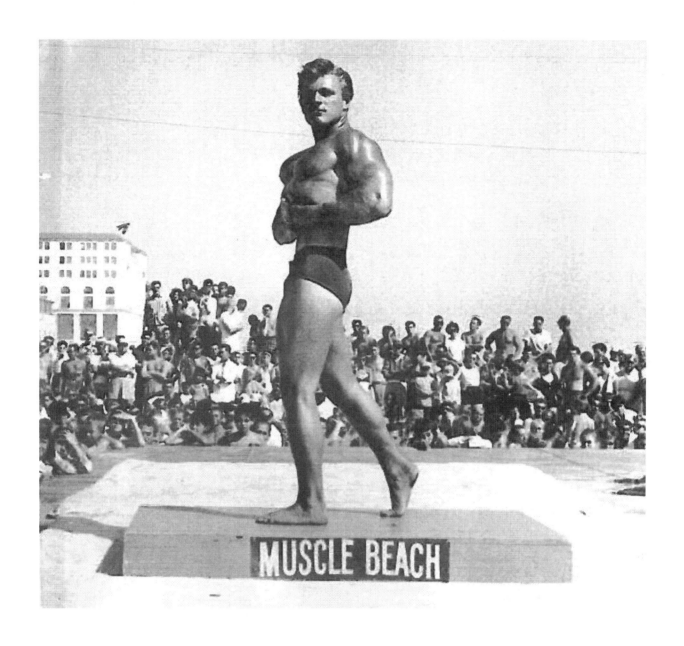

Achievements and Recognition

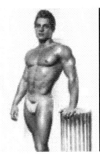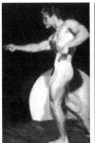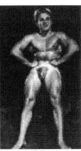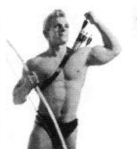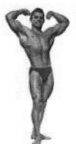

1959 Mr America - IFBB

1 Chuck Sipes
? Luke Adam
? Sam Calhoun
? Torre Larson
? Joseph Simon

1959 August   Vol 9, Num 11   Muscle Builder

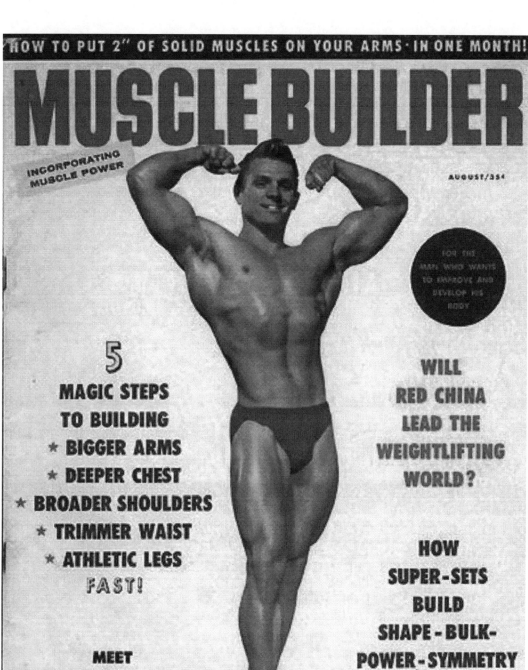

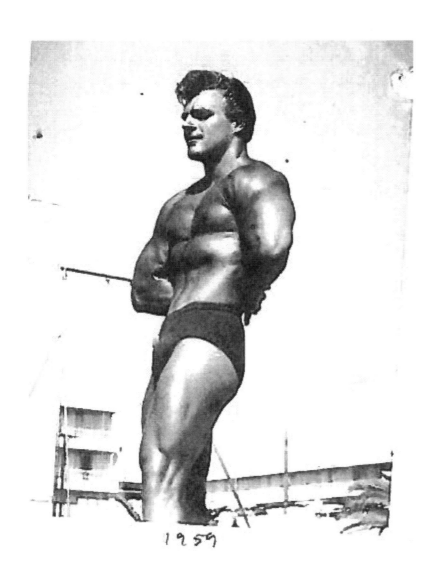

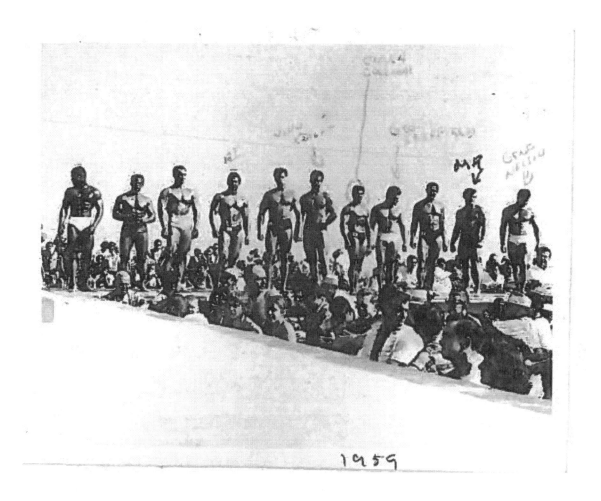

Here is a shot of the rest of the contestants at this 59 contest; Sam has written in a few names of other well known guys from the era including Geoff Nelson, George Sheffield, Chuck Collras, and John Knight.

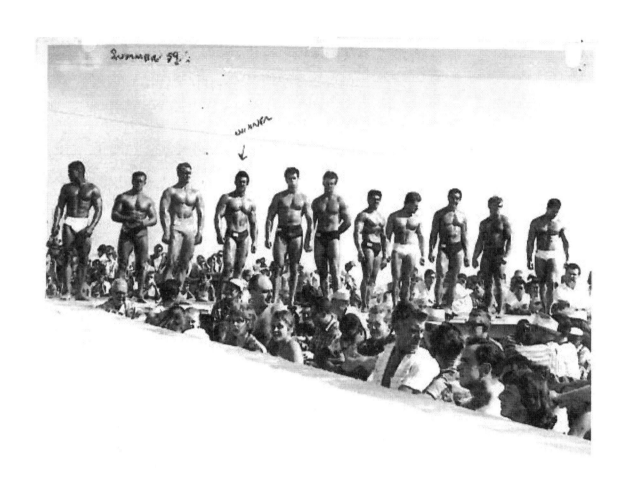

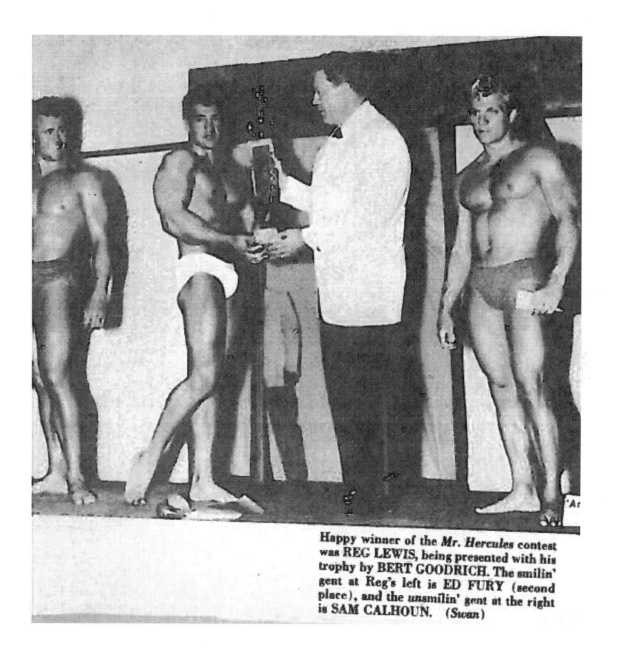

Happy winner of the *Mr. Hercules* contest was REG LEWIS, being presented with his trophy by BERT GOODRICH. The smilin' gent at Reg's left is ED FURY (second place), and the *unsmilin'* gent at the right is SAM CALHOUN. (Swan)

The following Muscle Builder article penned by Sam was focused on his then roommate Chuck Collras, who happens to also have later become a key member of the Culver City Westside barbell club.

"TAKE AN UPPER BODY WORKOUT WITH

Says SAM CALHOUN

The best thing that ever happened for the bodybuilder with limited time to train are the Weider Super-Set and Muscle Priority techniques used according to the Weider Split-Routine method. Here's how a famous bodybuilder keeps his magnificent physique in peak condition the year round, with just 'week-end' workouts at Muscle Beach!

★ "Take it from me, Sam . . . the Weider *Split-Routine* method has not only *built* some of the world's finest physiques . . . it's also *saved* quite a few good ones from 'going to pot' . . . don't you agree?"

DELTOIDS—Super-Set 1   DEI

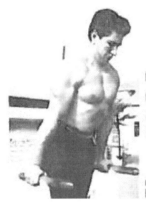 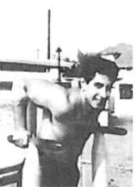 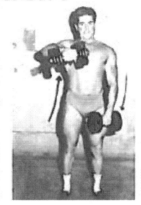 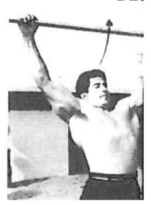

DIPS (beginning and midway point)   CHEATING FORWARD RAISE   CHIN BEHIND NEC

BACK-CHEST Super-Set 3   BAC

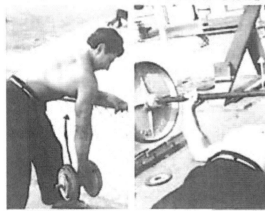 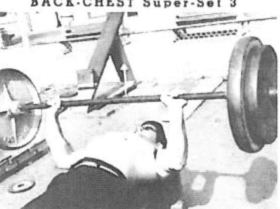 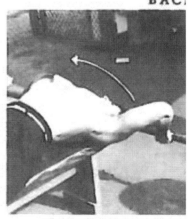

ONE DUMBBELL ROWING MOVEMENT   MEDIUM GRIP BENCH PRESS   HEAVY BENT-ARM PULLOVER

CHUCK COLLRAS"

America's Most Muscular Man

"How do you mean, Chuck?"
"Oh, you know how it is, Sam. A young fellow who's single either going to school or working an eight-hour job—has unlimited time to train. If he's smart, he'll spend two (Continued on page 55)

TOIDS—Super-Set 2

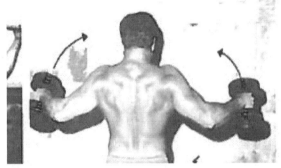

CHEATING LATERAL RAISE

CHEST Super-Set 4

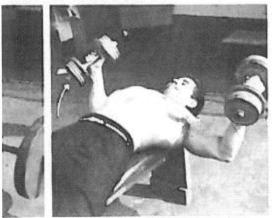

HEAVY BENT-ARM LATERAL RAISE

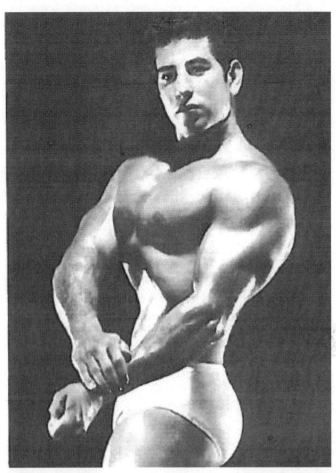

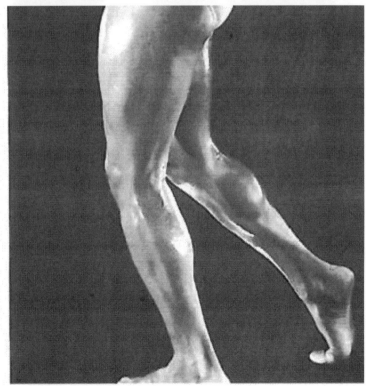

or three hours each day using a Weider **Spilt-Routine** . . . working **upper** body **one** day, then **lower** body the **next**—until he's racked up a total of **three complete workouts** for the **entire** body each week. Training with this effective Weider technique will assure any bodybuilder of a first-class physique in a very short time. He just can't fail!

"I think I'm beginning to get what you mean, Chuck."

"Yes . . . so the fellow builds a good physique, then he falls in love. And you know how easy it is for a barbell man to attract beautiful girls, Sam! I know . . . believe me, for one of the prettiest of them married me! Well . . . once married, a fellow has a lot more than weights to think about. You've gotta make an extra buck or two to take care of extra household expenses, and that takes time.

"Then you have all sorts of extra duties that must be done, and that takes **more** time. Finally when you have a pretty little daughter to come along like mine—well, you've got your hands full, I can tell you!

"Doesn't leave much time to train any more, does it, Chuck?"

"No, it sure doesn't, Sam. But when a fellow has worked hard to build a muscular body and doesn't want to see all his work go for nothing, he can still use the Weider **Split-Routine** method to not only **maintain** his physique at peak condition, but to actually build **greater muscular size, shape and definition.**

"How's that, Chuck?"

"Well . . . take my case, for instance. With my job and all my other duties taking up most of my week-day hours, I save Saturday and Sunday for my very own and apply the **Split-Routine** technique by taking a terrific **upper**-body workout on Saturday, and a really knocked out **leg** routine on Sunday. And believe me, I give each workout everything I've got!"

Chuck really **does** give his workouts every ounce of power, energy and concentration he has. With just two such workouts per week his physique is simply amazing. You'll find him every Saturday and Sunday on Muscle Beach, and you can bet that his charming wife and young daughter won't be far away . . . probably sunbathing on the nearby sands. And he certainly knows how to "budget" his time. In between sets when he's breathing hard, Chuck keeps on the move by walking over to his young family— to play with them . . . kid with them . . . laugh with them—then he's back to the equipment for another set. And he keeps going like this for most of the day!

When you see Chuck Collras walking along at a distance, he looks like a young giant! Yet he's really just a little guy, standing about 5' 4", but appears to be much bigger merely because his weight-trained body has been developed to such fantastic proportions.

At a maximum bodyweight of just under 160 pounds, Chuck can make a Bench Press of 325 pounds! When he Chins, he performs seemingly endless sets of reps, then makes "singles" with a dumbbell weighing almost as much as he does—tied to his waist.

Chuck also does Parallel Bar Dips with a 100-pound dumbbell suspended from his waist. In fact, he is marvelously powerful in all heavy weight-training exercises. But as you watch him working out, you are fascinated with how he ties-in the different exercises for his upper body. **First,** he works his **deltoids.**

"Why do you put delt work at the beginning of your program, Chuck?"

"Because when I exercise other body parts with the various lying Presses, Laterals, Chins and so on, I give the delts a lot of **work** but **not** a lot of **direct exercise.**

"Working out as hard as I do, if I scheduled my deltoid work later in my program I would not be able to handle the heavy weights such exercises require. So by putting it first, it not only pumps my delts terrifically, but makes all my other upper-body work seem to go much more **easily.**

"Then there is a double benefit from placing deltoid work first. Once you've pumped the delts up to melon-size, you can keep them that way throughout the rest of your workout by the continuous exertion given **other** exercises of which some effect is felt in the shoulders. Naturally, this is putting the Weider **Muscle Priority Plan** into action by working the stubbornest muscles first in each workout. Then, with the extra stimulation of the delts through exercises for other body parts, they stay pumped up for an **entire week!**"

"I note that you do a lot of compound exercises, Chuck. Do you generally follow this practice?"

"Indeed I do, Sam. In every workout —whether it's leg day or torso day—I make the workout 100% more effective by using Weider **Super-Sets** for the **most** in muscle flushing. Here's how a typical upper-body workout goes for me, Sam:

DELTOIDS (Super-Set 1)

Exercise 1. Parallel Bar Dips.

Exercise 2. Cheating Forward Raise.

"That's my first deltoid **Super-Set.** I do a set of the Dips with a weight suspended from my waist . . . just heavy enough to permit 10 reps. After the Dips, I grab my dumbbells and dive right into my Forward Raises. Here the weights that one set.

"Then—with just time enough to grab my dumbbells—I go into a set of 8 reps with the Side Lateral Raise, using just enough cheat to get the dumbbells started. That completes one **Super-Set**, and I walk over and play with my daughter for a minute or so until I've caught my breath. Then it's back to the second **Super-Set**, and so on, until I've done five complete sets of **each exercise** alternately—or five complete **Super-Sets**. Needless to say, my deltoids feel like coconuts, my biceps seem as big as volleyballs, and my lats feel as wide as a barn door! That's what **Super-Set** flushing technique will do for you!

"Next, I begin to tie-in back and chest work, just as I tied-in work for deltoids, arms and back. Here again I Super-Set my exercises, as follows:

BACK—CHEST (Super-Set 3)

"I think that working opposing muscle groups is the fastest way to building a superior physique. There's no time lost, and when you do a set of reps for your **back**, then work the opposing **chest** muscles for an equal number of reps, you do not make a terrific drain on your energy since **one** muscle group **rests** while the other **works**.

"Nevertheless, the entire back-chest area keeps terrifically pumped up, with a resultant growth to each. My tie-in of back-chest exercises begins with Super Set 3 . . .

BACK-CHEST (Super-Set 4)

Exercise 1. Bent-Arm Pullovers.

Exercise 2. Bent-Arm Lateral Raises.

"There is nothing like a heavy set of Bent-Arm Pullovers to lengthen the rib cage . . . build wide, flaring pecs . . . and at the same time give the lats and entire back a terrific workout. I use all the weight I can handle in the Bent-Arm Pullover, and with a slightly wider than shoulder width hand spacing, I pull the bar **up** and over to the chest, just barely grazing the nose in doing so . . . using **pectoral power only**. Then, as I lower the weight to starting position, I do so with **back and lat power only**.

"I just **think** the tension into the pectorals as I pull the weight up . . . and I **release** the tension from the pectorals and **think** it into the back as I lower the barbell. In this way, both muscular areas are strongly worked for the 10 reps-per-set of this fine exercise. It requires a heavy weight to really stimulate these two hugest-of-all muscle areas of the body, and I give the exercise everything in mental and muscular power I have to offer.

"Then, without pause, I grab my dumbbells and do 8 reps in the Bent-Arm Lateral Raise. This carves the entire side outline of the pectorals into championship shape and makes it stand out as though carved from rock! After a short breather I go on with the second, third, fourth and a final fifth **Super-Set** of these fine

over the world will soon be hard at work on it . . . that I **guarantee** you!"

—MB

MORE
FORMULA FACTS!

(Continued from Page 23)

the lift. But if he weighed-in at the **absolute limit** of 181¾ pounds, his performance represents a new bodyweight-efficiency performance never equalled in any other class-weight division until now!

Paterni's Formula rating for his Press was 211.816 points . . . that of Zhetetsky equals 212.454 points. And if Zhetetsky's bodyweight were less than the limit, his performance merits an even higher rating.

The interesting fact about Formula lifting performances shows that the **heavier** bodyweight classes are improving at the expense of the **lighter**. Years ago it was assumed that these lighter classes would lift more **proportionately** than their heavier lifting brothers. We here at Weider take great joy in this fact, since years ago we predicted the very things that are occurring with such regularity now!

—MB

Sam sent some pictures with hand written notes, such as this one, which shows just how close he & Chuck were;

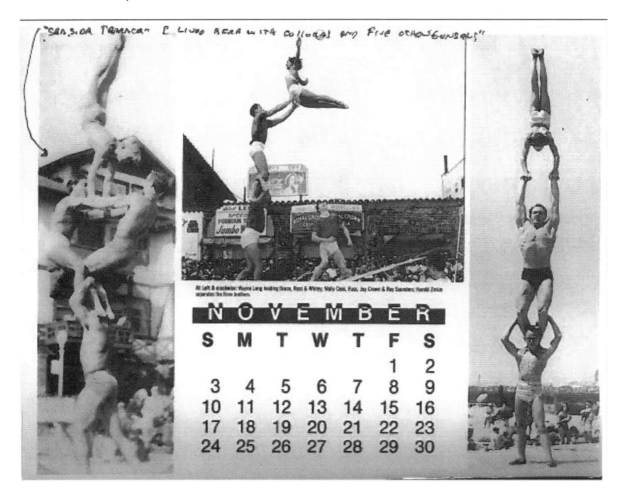

Sam's note is not very legible, but he is pointing out the apartment building where he & Chuck roomed together.

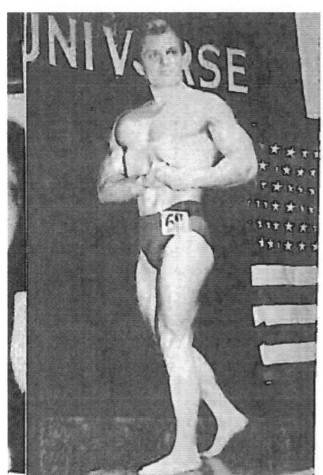
"America's Most Muscular Man" title was taken by SAM CALHOUN.

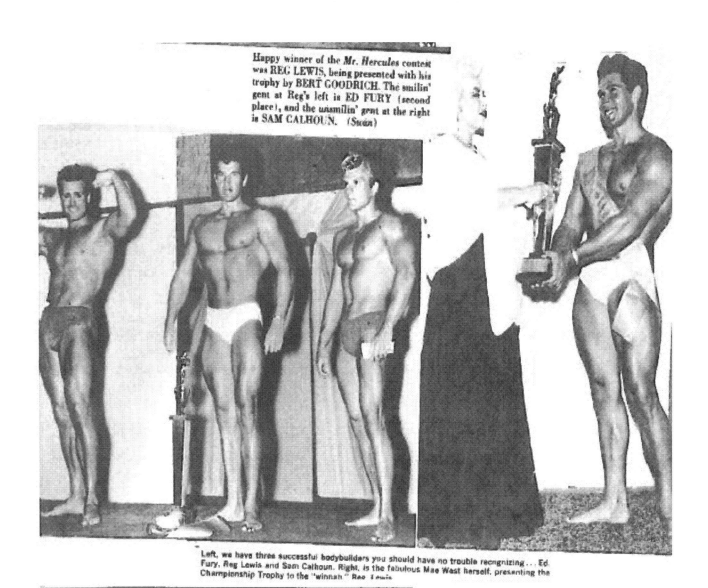

Happy winner of the *Mr. Hercules* contest was REG LEWIS, being presented with his trophy by BERT GOODRICH. The smilin' gent at Reg's left is ED FURY (second place), and the unsmilin' gent at the right is SAM CALHOUN. (Swan)

Left, we have three successful bodybuilders you should have no trouble recognizing... Ed Fury, Reg Lewis and Sam Calhoun. Right, is the fabulous Mae West herself, presenting the Championship Trophy to the "winnah" Reg Lewis.

You see Reg Lewis sharing the stage with Sam in the pictures above; the two were good friends, says Sam.

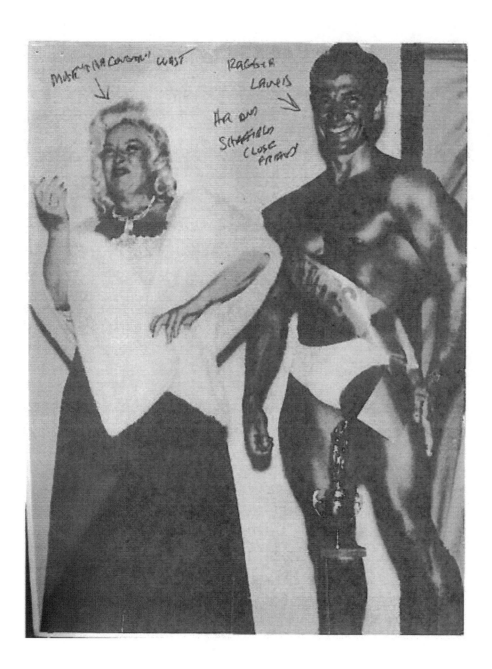

The following pictures are of more of Sam's friends from Tanny's and/or Muscle Beach;

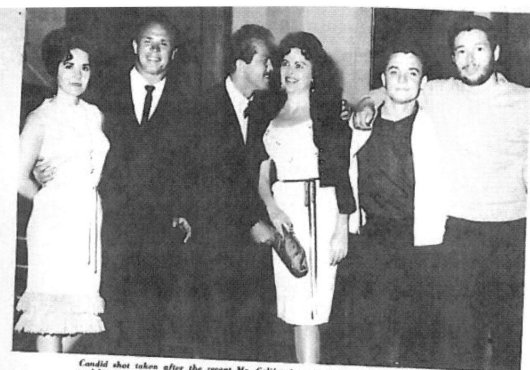

Candid shot taken after the recent Mr. California contest shows ZABO KOSZEWSKI and his girl friend... WES JOHNSON (President of the Muscle Beach Club) and his one-and-only... and two members of the club. (Below) Some of the members of the club on a Sunday afternoon at Muscle Beach... you'll recognize Mr. Abdominals — ZABO KOSZEWSKI — TERRY TRAMMEL — CHUCK MAHONEY — WES JOHNSON (with banana) — and Mr. California — GEORGE SHEFFIELD. (Wolf Schramm)

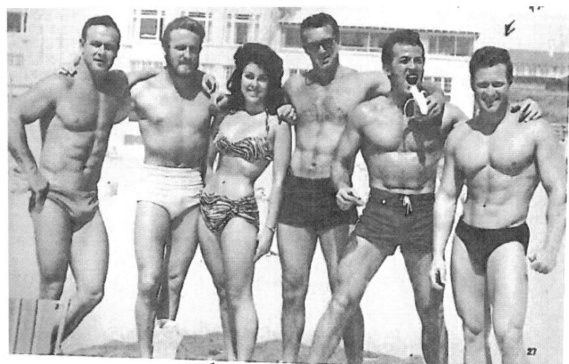

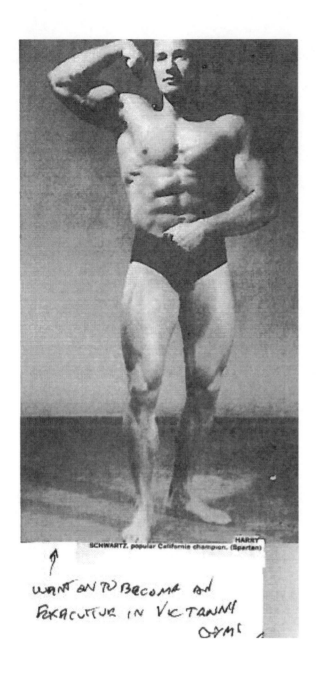

Yet another of Sam's friends.... One of Mae West's 7 Adonises at one time. Harry Schwartz

Doug Strohl was another bodybuilding friend & contemporary of Sam's;

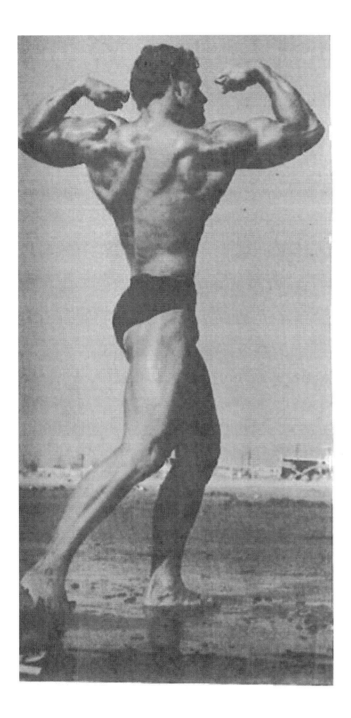

Doug Strohl

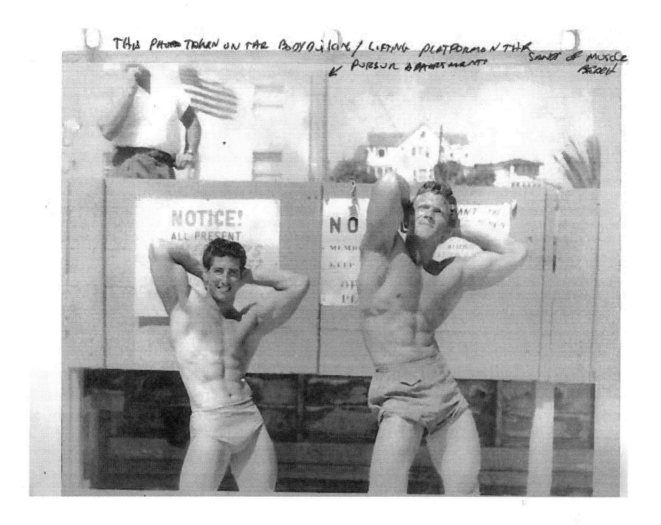

Sam's old roommate Chuck Collras and Doug Strohl on the beach

One more of Doug, on the beach lifting platform;

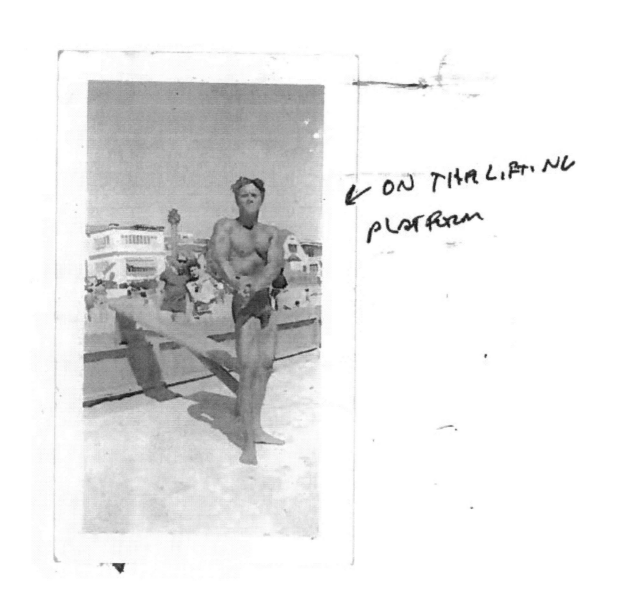

← ON THE LIFTING PLATFORM

Doug Strohl

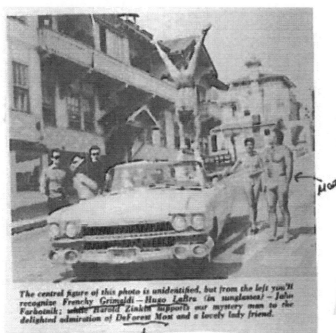 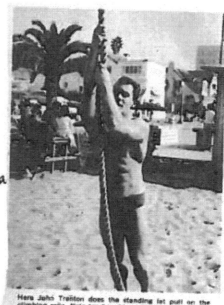

The central figure of this photo is unidentified, but from the left you'll recognise Frenchy Grimaldi – Hugo LaBro (in sunglasses) – John Farbotnik; while Harold Zinkin supports our mystery man to the delighted admiration of DeForest Most and a lovely lady friend.

Here John Trenton does the standing lat pull on the climbing rope. Note too how his abdominals stand out.

Some of Sam's personal notes... poor Sam's hand writing is as bad as mine!

Sam's note clarified; the "Beach Manager of the weight stakes while the club occupied the beach; some 30 ft. or so off the asphalt "boardwalk". Underlined names were beach regulars. Zinkin left the beach taking Bruce Conner's wife with him some years prior to my arrival. Bruce Conner had a club/gym on little Santa Monica blvd in West L.A., a block or two off Westwood blvd.

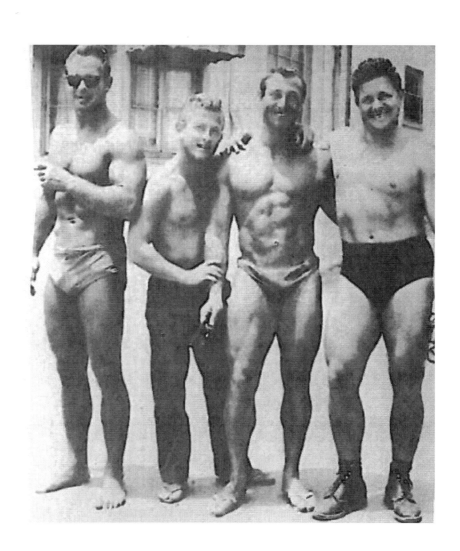

KNEW THREE OF THESE GUYS WELL JOHN ISAACS WAS A RECENT ARRIVAL TO THE AREA

Here is a great contrast shot of 2 great lifters vs. 2 great bodybuilders of the time.

I have had some conversations with Sam Calhoun, and it was great to get some firsthand perspective on Tanny's Dungeon & Muscle Beach that came "straight from the horse's mouth" (no offense, Sam,) Sam was not working for Tanny at the time, but he trained at the dungeon in the early to mid '50s and had some interesting things to relate about his experiences there. He said there were several different "cliques" that trained there in those days. One group was the "old-timers", meaning anyone over 30 and from the "Old School; bodybuilding/lifting days, like Armand Tanny and his cronies. (Sam was a teenager when he started training there) Another group was the wrestlers, many of whom were known as the "villains" of the ring in those days. One name that rung a big bell was "**Gorgeous George**".

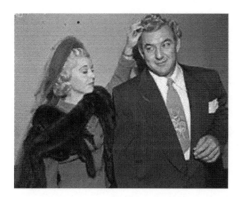

George in 1950, with wife Betty

Having heard the name, but not being too familiar with the specifics on George, I looked him up on Wikipedia, which had some interesting factoids about him;

George Raymond Wagner was born March 24, 1915 in Butte, Nebraska

At 5'9" and 215 pounds, Wagner was not particularly physically imposing by professional wrestling standards, nor was he an exceptionally gifted athlete. Nevertheless, he soon developed a reputation as a solid in-ring worker. In the late 1930s, he met Elizabeth "Betty" Hanson, whom he would eventually marry in an in-ring ceremony. When the wedding proved a good drawing card, the couple re-enacted it in arenas across the country (which thus enlightened Wagner to the potential entertainment value that was left untapped within the industry). Around this same time, Vanity Magazine published a feature article about a pro wrestler named Lord Patrick Lansdowne, who entered the ring accompanied by two valets while wearing a velvet robe and doublet. Wagner was impressed with the bravado of such a character, but he believed that he could take it to a much greater extreme. What he needed was a new professional persona. Later, In Portland, Oregon, Betty (George's wife) told Dean Higinbotham, the nephew of Betty's sister, Evangeline "Eva," how George got the name Gorgeous George. In the early 1940s George had a wrestling match at the Portland Oregon Armory. As he walked down the aisle to the ring, there were two mature women on his right, two rows back from the ring. One of the women loudly exclaimed: "Oh, isn't he gorgeous." That word "gorgeous" struck George and he immediately felt he had found his new professional persona. He would be "**Gorgeous George**." As Elsie Hanson, Betty's mother, was a skilled seamstress, George asked her to make him some resplendent capes that would accentuate his new persona. George wore those capes in all his future matches. Subsequently George debuted his new "glamour boy" image on a 1941 card in Eugene, Oregon; and he quickly antagonized the fans with his exaggerated effeminate behavior when the ring announcer introduced him as "Gorgeous George." Such showmanship was unheard of for the time; and consequently, arena crowds grew in size as fans turned out to ridicule George (who relished the sudden attention).

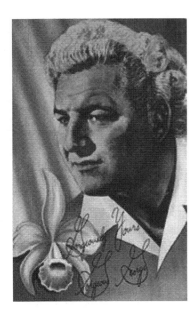

Photo postcard of Gorgeous George, "the Human Orchid" and the "Toast of the Coast", circa 1940s.

Gorgeous George was soon recruited to Los Angeles by promoter Johnny Doyle. Known as the "Human Orchid," his persona was created in part by growing his hair long, dyeing it platinum blonde, and putting gold-plated bobby pins in it (which he deemed "Georgie Pins" while distributing them to the audience). Furthermore, he transformed his ring entrance into a bona-fide spectacle that would often take up more time than his actual matches. He was the first wrestler to really use entrance music, as he strolled nobly to the ring to the sounds of "Pomp and Circumstance," followed by his valet and a purple spotlight. Wearing an elegant robe sporting an array of sequins, Gorgeous George was always escorted down a personal red carpet by his ring valet "Jeffries," who would carry a silver mirror while spreading rose petals at his feet. While George removed his robe, Jeffries would spray the ring with disinfectant (which reportedly consisted of Chanel No. 5 perfume), which George referred to as "Chanel #10" ("Why be half-safe?" he was famous for saying) before he would start wrestling. Moreover, George required that his valets spray the referee's hands before the official was allowed to check him for any illegal objects, which thus prompted his now-famous outcry "Get your filthy hands off me!" Once the match finally began, he would cheat in every way he could. Gorgeous George was the industry's first true cowardly villain, and he would cheat at every opportunity, which infuriated the crowd. His credo was "Win if you can, lose if you must, but always cheat!"

This flamboyant image and his showman's ability to work a crowd were so successful in the early days of television that he became the most famous wrestler of his time, drawing furious heel heat wherever he appeared. It was with the advent of television, however, that George's character exploded into the biggest drawing card the industry had ever known. With the networks looking for cheap but effective programming to fill its time slots, pro wrestling's glorified action became a genuine "hit" with the viewing public, as it was the first program of any kind to draw a real profit. Consequently, it was Gorgeous George who brought the sport into the nation's living rooms, as his histrionics and melodramatic behavior made him a larger-than-life figure in American pop-culture. His first television appearance took place on November 11, 1947 (an event that was recently named among the top 100 televised acts of the 20th century by Entertainment Weekly) and he immediately became a national celebrity at the same level of Lucille Ball and Bob Hope (who personally donated hundreds of chic robes for George's collection) while changing the course of the industry forever. No longer was pro wrestling simply about the in-ring action, but George had created a new sense of theatrics and character performance that had not previously existed. Moreover, in a very real sense, it was Gorgeous George who single-handedly established television as a viable entertainment medium that could potentially reach millions of homes across the country (in fact, it is said that George was probably responsible for selling as many TV sets as Milton Berle). In addition to his grandiose theatrics, Gorgeous George was an accomplished wrestler as well. While many may have considered him a mere gimmick wrestler, he was actually a very competent freestyle wrestler, having started learning the sport in amateur wrestling as a teenager, and he could handle himself quite well if it came to a legitimate contest. The great Lou Thesz, who would take this AWA title away from Wagner, and who was one of the best "legit" wrestlers ever in professional wrestling, displayed some disdain for the gimmick wrestlers. Nevertheless, he admitted that Wagner "could wrestle pretty well," but added that, "he [Wagner] could never draw a fan until he became Gorgeous George." On March 26, 1947, he defeated Enrique Torres to capture the Los Angeles Heavyweight Championship. Then on February 22, 1949, George was booked as the feature attraction at New York's Madison Square Garden in what would be pro wrestling's first return to the building in 12 years. By the 1950s, Gorgeous George's star power was so huge that he was able to command 50% of the gate for his performances, which allowed him to earn over $100,000 a year, thus making him the highest paid athlete in the world. Moreover, on May 26, 1950, Gorgeous George defeated Don Eagle to claim the AWA (Boston) World Heavyweight Championship, which he held for several months. During this reign he was beaten by the National Wrestling Alliance World Champion Lou Thesz in a highly-publicized bout in Chicago. However, perhaps Gorgeous George's most famous match was against his longtime rival Whipper Billy Watson on March 12, 1959, in which a beaten George had his treasured golden locks shaved bald before 20,000 delighted fans at Toronto's Maple Leaf Gardens and millions more on national television. In one of his final matches, Gorgeous George later faced off against (and lost to) an up-and-coming Bruno Sammartino, though he would lose his precious hair again when he was defeated by the Destroyer in a hair vs. mask match at the Olympic Auditorium on November 7, 1962. This would ultimately be his last match, as advanced age and extended alcohol abuse had taken their toll on his body; and his doctors ordered him to quit wrestling. In 2002, he was inducted into the inaugural class of the Pro Wrestling Hall of Fame (PWHF.org) by a committee of his peers. On March 27 he was inducted into the WWE Hall of Fame class of 2010. His 97 year-old former wife, Betty Wagner accepted the honor on his behalf, answering questions and telling the story of how he became Gorgeous George.

Retirement and death

As his wrestling career wound down, Wagner invested $250,000 in a 195-acre (0.79 km^2) turkey ranch built in Beaumont, California, and the wrestler used his showman skills to promote his prized poultry at his wrestling matches and sport shows, popular during his heyday. He raised turkeys and owned a cocktail lounge in Van Nuys, California, which he named "Gorgeous George's Ringside Restaurant".

In 1962, Wagner was diagnosed with a serious liver condition. On advice of his doctors, he retired. This, combined with failed finances (due to bad investments) worsened his health. He suffered a heart attack on December 24, 1963 and died two days later, at age 48.

A plaque at his gravesite reads "Love to our Daddy Gorgeous George".

Legacy

Muhammad Ali and James Brown acknowledged that their own approach to flamboyant self-promotion was influenced by George. A 19-year old Ali met a 46-year old George at a Las Vegas radio station. During George's radio interview, the wrestler's promo caught the attention of the future heavyweight champion. If George lost to Classy Freddie Blassie, George exclaimed, "I'll crawl across the ring and cut my hair off! But that's not gonna happen because I'm the greatest wrestler in the world!" Ali, who later echoed that very promo when taunting opponent Sonny Liston, recalled, "I saw 15,000 people comin' to see this man get beat. And his talking did it. I said, 'This is a gooood idea!'" In the locker room afterward, the seasoned wrestler gave the future legend some invaluable advice: "A lot of people will pay to see someone shut your mouth. So keep on bragging, keep on sassing and always be outrageous."[1] In September 2008, the first full length biography of Gorgeous George was published by Harper Entertainment Press. The title of the 304 page book is *Gorgeous George: The Outrageous Bad Boy Wrestler who Created American Pop Culture* by John Capouya. In the 2005 book, *I Feel Good: A Memoir in a Life of Soul*, James Brown said he used many of Gorgeous George's antics to "create the James Brown you see on stage".[1]

Bob Dylan said meeting George changed his life. In Dylan's book *The Chronicles: Volume One*, Dylan recounts a story of meeting Gorgeous George in person. He wrote, "He winked and seemed to mouth the phrase, `You're making it come alive.' I never forgot it. It was all the recognition and encouragement I would need for years."[1][3]

The 1951 Warner Brothers *Merrie Melodies* cartoon *Bunny Hugged* featured the one-shot character "Ravishing Ronald", modeled after Gorgeous George. The Bowery Boys also lampooned Gorgeous George (with Huntz Hall as a much-heralded wrestler) in the 1952 feature *No Holds Barred*. Musical performers such as Liberace, Little Richard, Elton John and Morris Day show signs of the George meme. Some consider George to have been an early example of camp.[*weasel words*]

The 1978 motion picture *The One and Only* starring Henry Winkler was loosely based on his career.

So George was quite an interesting guy, and it must have been fun to train in the same gym with a guy like that... one of a host of colorful characters that trained at the dungeon. Apparently one section of the dungeon in those days was devoted to the wrestling & boxing genre, with a real official style ring and everything. Yet another group was the Olympic lifters, such as **Ike Berger and Dave Sheppard** of York Barbell, who were "subsidized" by Hoffman so that they could continue to train hard through the winters in the more pleasant climate found in Southern California as opposed to that of York, Pennsylvania. Of course, as members of the AAU, they were not really supposed to be the beneficiaries of such gifts, but as I talked about in my recent book, **"Coal, Steel & Iron, Pennsylvania's Golden Triangle of Strength"**, Hoffman bent the rules in his favor pretty much as it suited him. Representing another group at Tanny's, there were also powerlifters, though powerlifting was not really organized at the time, and then there were the dedicated young bodybuilders such as Sam and his contemporaries (**George Sheffield and Hugo Labra** being a couple notable names), and the homosexual crowd that seemed to gather in places where bodybuilders did. Sam had a funny story about Dave Sheppard; it seems Dave was seeing a very beautiful lady bodybuilder for a while, and had been seen around town with her quite a bit. A popular and charming bodybuilder named Burt started hanging around and eventually stole Dave's girlfriend from him, which as you might guess put him in a poor state of mind for a while. Dave was convinced that Burt's superior physique was what drew the gorgeous gal away from his arms, and thus decided to train more like a bodybuilder and less like an Olympic lifter, despite the fact that the latter was his very bread & butter. Training for hypertrophy by doing high reps, and doing new exercises like the bench press did indeed start to fill out Dave's physique, to the point where he bumped up a weight class in the lifting realm, which had a very negative effect on that side of things, as Dave was not nearly as competitive in the new class. Whether this helped Dave win back the apple of his eye or any other damsel in distress is a question I can't answer at this point. Sam said a lot of the more popular bodybuilders would come around to the dungeon and/or Muscle Beach to take a workout or 2 and hang around, but many were not regulars at the club. Calhoun confirmed the stories told elsewhere about the not-so-prissy conditions in the dungeon, having lots of spots where the tiles had long since been worn away to the underlying concrete, and even the rebar bars that formed the concrete's skeleton were showing in some areas. Cleanliness and hygiene were after thoughts for the most part at the dungeon, with black & green mold growing inches thick in the locker room and bathroom area. Sam said there was a section of the basement where there were some sort of large septic holding tanks of some sort, and every once in a while, there would be back-ups of one or more of these, and there would be puddles of foul water containing who knows what in the lower parts of the gym, but this did not deter the stalwart men who trained there. They were determined to get there workout in regardless of conditions. Equipment was not fancy or sophisticated, but solid and built to take a beating. Lots of free weights abounded, and there were some heavy wooden "a-frame" style benches that served as sort of dual incline benches, as well as heavy planked flat benches, too. While the denizens of the dungeon slaved away under these Spartan conditions, Tanny was trying to lure the more well-healed clientele to his pricier new facility on Wilshire boulevard, which was the type of gym from which many of our more modern "spa-like" facilities arose.

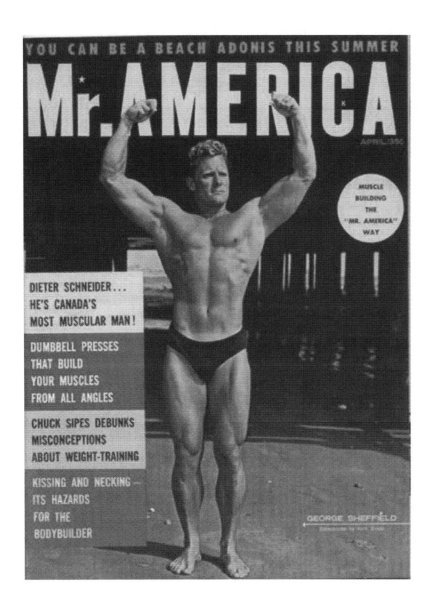

George Sheffield

Here is a shot of George right before winning yet another Venice Beach contest;

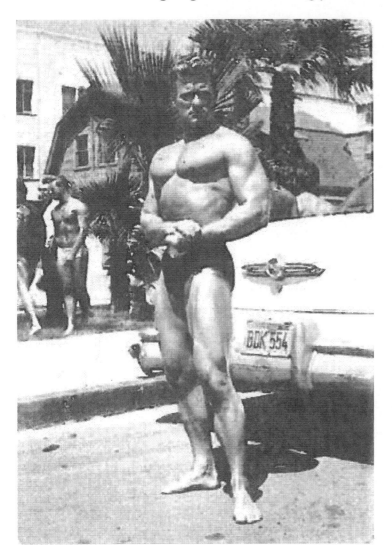

George & Carol;

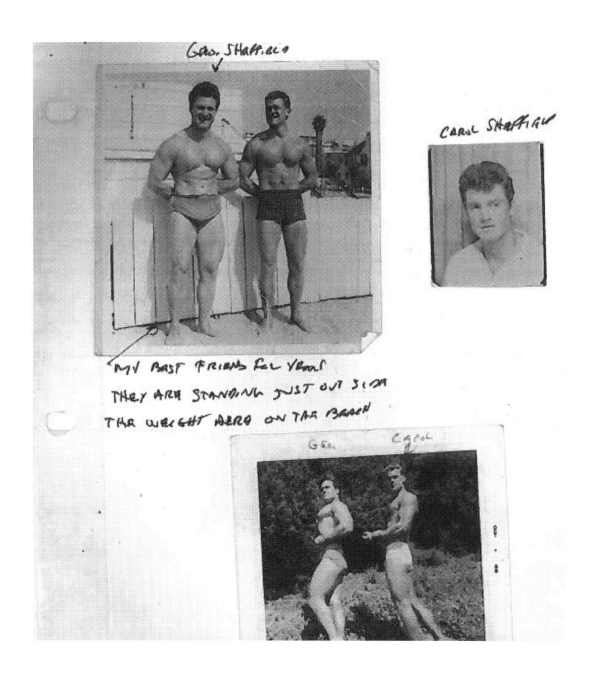

Here is another with George on the beach, in the background is "Silent Len's" grease pit on the left, and the Purser apartment building on the right.

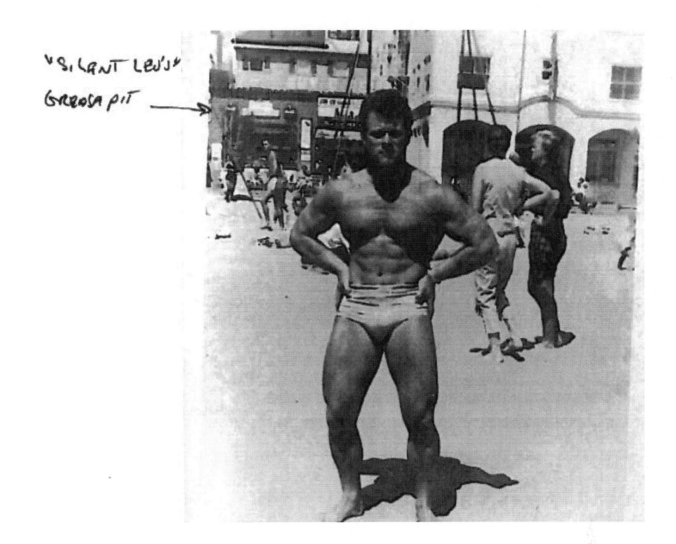
"Silent Lou" Grbosa pit

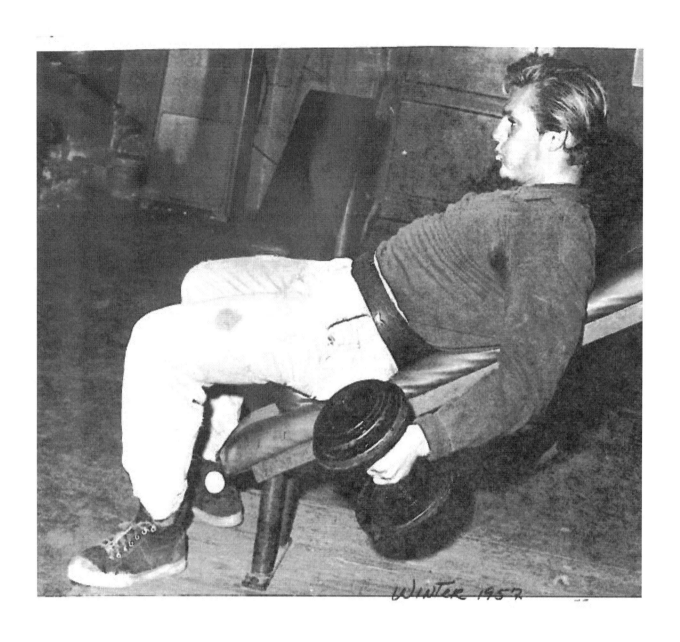

Here's a nice training shot of Sam at the Dungeon

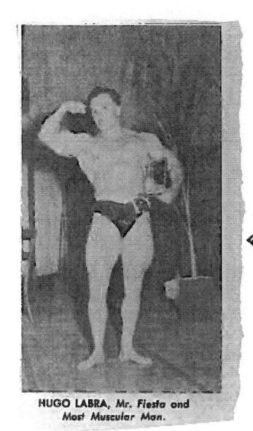

HUGO LABRA, Mr. Fiesta and Most Muscular Man.

Hugo another close friend ←

Hugo was also a friend of Sam's that trained at the Dungeon.

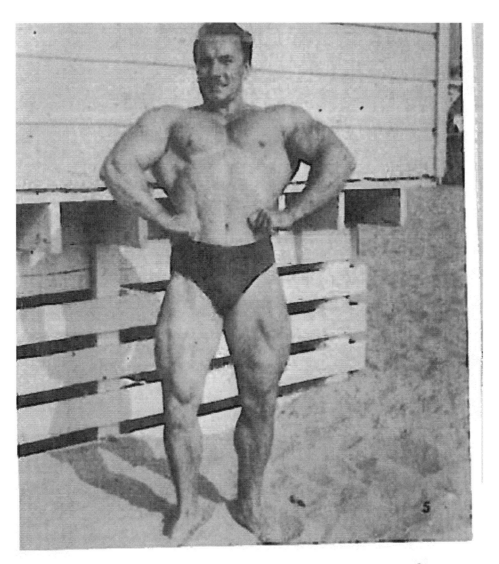

HUGO CABRA - A LIFTER FROM PERU. SUPER SWELL GUY.

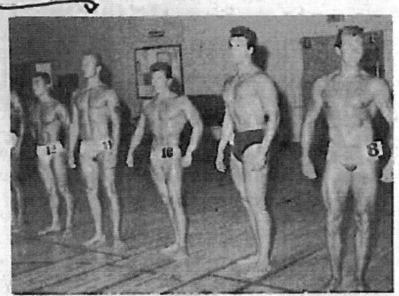

Contestants line up before the judges. The bemused young man on the right is BERNIE ERNST who placed second in the tall men's class.

Here is another great lifter that Sam was friendly with;

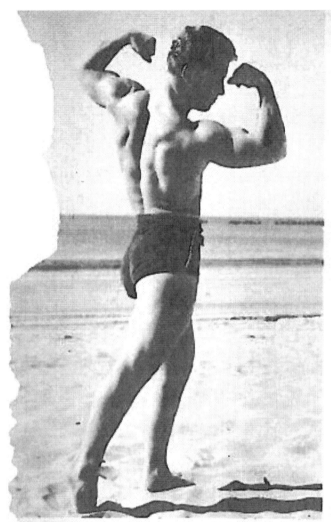
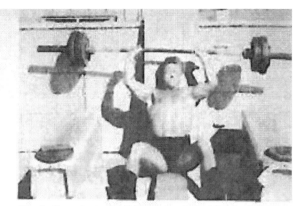

How has Berger developed his amazing Pressing power? Through handbalancing—and Seated Supported Angle Presses.

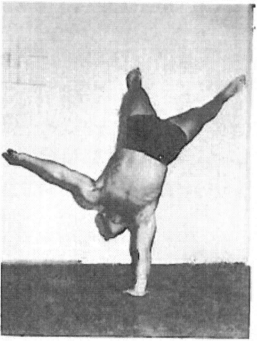

nd champion bodybuilder. Artie Zeller has photographed him dramatically as both.

THE ISAAC BERGER
the lifting world doesn't know

THE ISAAC BERGER
the lifting world doesn't know

by CHARLES COSTER

The story of a great champion doesn't begin with his appearance on the competitive platform. There are special reasons why he has achieved world fame; there have been events leading up to it that have cast their shadows before. In this story we reveal the events in ISAAC BERGER's early life that played such an important part in moulding him into the champion weightlifter he is today!

★ They call him 'Betcha" Berger. He's the guy who'll always take a dare – who'll bet you dollars to doughnuts that "anything you do, I can do better!" He does it too – he's done it since he was eight years old'!

When Ike was just a tadpole-of-a-boy he noticed some other kids in school *(Continued on page 60)*

I knew Isaac + Dave Sheppard well they lived in S.I. and trained in the dungeon and the [?]

My friend Joe DiMarco also has lots of memories about Ike Berger and Dave Sheppard.

This next guy was also a friend of both Sam & Joe;

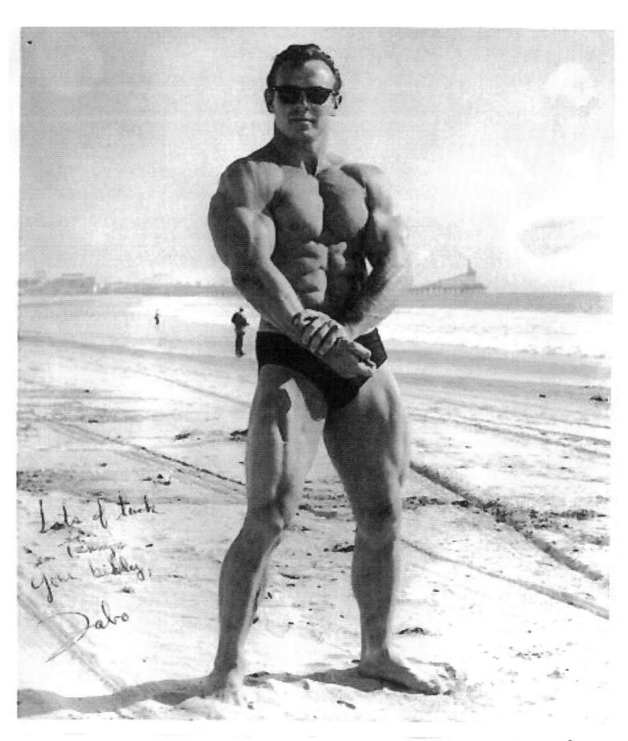

ZABO ANOTHER FRIEND FROM THE BEACH

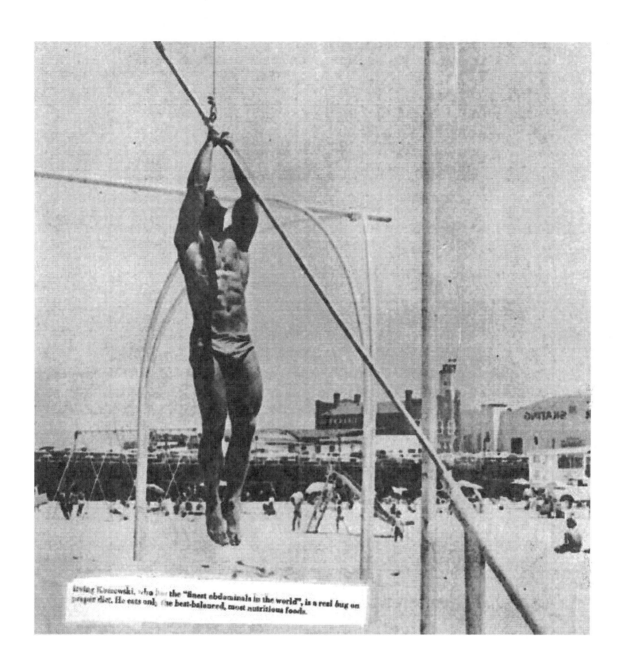

Zabo training those famous abs on the beach.

Here is another Pro Wrestler that trained at Tanny's;

Ray "Thunder" Stern

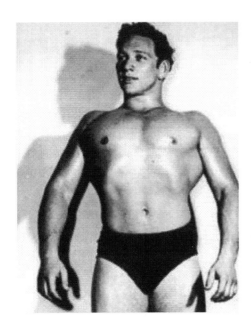

Walter Bookbinder was born in Brooklyn, New York on January 12, 1933. His family circumstances were extremely modest and at the tender age of thirteen, he joined the Merchant Marines using the name Paul Davis. While in this civilian branch of the United States Coast Guard, he began to become very serious about bodybuilding. He even used to carry a PAIR of fifty-pound dumbbells in his duffel bag to be certain he could exercise as desired. In 1949, **Walter went to California's famed Muscle Beach to continue his bodybuilding endeavors**. When his unemployment benefits ended, he planned on leaving the land of perpetual sunshine. **Joe Gold, of Gold's Gym fame, and Armand Tanny, of bodybuilding fame, convinced Walter to stay in California and make a living as a wrestler. Both Gold and Tanny had grappled professionally themselves.** A promoter told Walter that he needed to change his name for commercial reasons. Bookbinder was changed to his mother's maiden name of Stern. The promoter wanted a one-syllable first name so Walter became Ray. The Thunder was added due to the spectacular aerial maneuvers in the ring for which Ray became famous. The Dusek brothers, who were wrestlers-turned-promoters, help to start Ray's New York wrestling career in 1950. Ray wrestled in approximately thirty-six hundred matches over a nearly twenty-year career. He held versions of the World and Tag Team titles. In-ring flying techniques were not the only aerial activities for which Ray became well known. A friend introduced him to flying a plane and Ray went for pilot training and received a pilot's license after only two weeks instruction. Thus began a life-long passion and tremendous financial success for Ray.

He founded Stern Air and his company became recognized as a reliable transport system around the world. Ray also became proficient at acrobatic flying. Stern also became hugely successful in the health club business. He started America's first coed health club and had the first health club with a child's nursery in it to allow the parents to exercise. In 1958-59, a club of his in San Francisco was taking in $100,000.00 PER MONTH! He also had phenomenal success developing real estate and rental properties. We hope that Ray's business ventures will allow him to join us for the 2005 PWHF Induction weekend. If he is able to attend the ceremonies to accept his award in person, please note the quarter-million dollar watch that he wears. A 1994 biography entitled "The Power of Thunder" outlines Stern's principles of business success. We are proud to include Ray Stern as a 2005 PWHF honoree.

The following contains more memories from the great Dave Draper;

Dave Draper remembers the Dungeon

(An excerpt from the awesome Irononline site)

Each of us has a story to tell, whether we're 14 or 40, 18 or 80. Many are complicated but none is simple. Some are packed, not one is empty. Everyone is worth telling but few are heard. Our story is our own. Do you have a favorite tale from your oft-vague life story, one that stirs you and retains its drama and emotion, its colors, scents and sounds? Of course you do, if you think for a second. You're not sure anyone wants to hear it, yet you recall it and relive it from time to time. I, too, have such a favorite recollection from my dizzy life. Ordinary is its most outstanding feature. Life is largely composed of ordinary stories and somebody's got to tell them. If you stood on the corner of 4th and Broadway in Santa Monica, California, 45 years ago and looked north toward Wilshire Boulevard in the early morning and spotted a big young dude with blond hair lumbering in your general direction, chances are it was me. If this guy had east coast stamped on his forehead and carried a motley gym bag and was clueless, you should bet on it.Dum-dee-dum... "Hey mista... ya know weah da dungeon is?" You win... that's me. Who else would be searching for a dark, smelly subterranean dungeon at the crack of dawn within a short walk of the alluring Pacific palisades? Who else sounded like a Jersey hood on the run? It was June of 1963 when I arrived in LAX seeking muscle and might.

George Eifferman, later to become a good friend, picked me up at the budding LA airport, dropped me off at my temporary warehouse digs (couch is in the back... it's getting late... see ya bright and early) and gave me the low-down on the Muscle Beach Gym. He called it the Dungeon, said it was four blocks away and the door was always open. Make yourself at home. Just as he described it, the door was one of a set of two: sky blue, very tall and dragged when you opened it. I was in, and there I stayed until the gym moved in '66. One stepped in, dragged the door shut in chilly weather or at the night's end, and immediately descended 14 broad steps, turned right and descended another 8 in the opposite direction. You've arrived: A basement, no windows, little light, less cheer, tons of weight and gobs of atmosphere. Ready? About-face and walk 10 feet and turn 90 degrees left and walk 15 paces to the locker room, AKA the Trap. Deteriorating 12 by 12 reddish-brown floor tiles shift and scrunch occasionally beneath your feet. It was two weeks before I dared enter that particular dank inner sanctum. It required hardening of the heart, a gathering of courage, much risk and a little madness to step fully into the grimy trap and another week to chance the shower, and this only after observing my new friend, Mike Bondura (ex-Navy), penetrate the murky cubicle morning after morning and emerge alive, well and clean. 40-watt light bulbs have their advantages, failing to cast generous light and reveal the details of one's surroundings. The place was large and a proper choice of locations after the original beach-version of Muscle Beach was required by the city councilmen and women to relocate the broad-shouldered nuisance "somewhere else, not upon our white sands for all to see." It was also dim and grim. White gone gray covered the crumbling plaster walls and half a dozen strategically placed pillars the size of Roman columns held up the place. Other than three or four scattered 60-watt incandescents, the only light that illuminated the Dungeon was a four-by-twenty-foot stretch of block-glass skylight inserted in the Broadway Ave. sidewalk above the far wall. The light was silver-white and harsh and abundant, but only when the California sun was high in the sky. Beneath the skylight were arranged two 12' x 12' lifting platforms, grains of Muscle Beach sand still scrunched between layers of hard rubber mat. Drop a marble and it would roll to their centers, where heavy iron was dumped regularly and mercilessly for decades. The designated lifting areas no longer gathered crowds of admiring onlookers. Rather, you could sit upon a reclaimed section of discarded, over-stuffed movie-theater seats arranged at the now-subterranean platforms' edge and doze off. No one would notice, no one would care. Pausing at the keyboard (computer, not piano) during my recollections, I plotted the length of the Dungeon counting 30 easy paces, or 75 feet, in my mind's eye. Who's gonna argue a foot or two or ten? And the width amounted to 25 paces, or 60 feet. The ample height of 15 feet floor to ceiling forgave the Dungeon its dungeon-ness, accenting the sense of space -- room to reach, to stretch, to expand, to groan and grow. The temperature was always 68 degrees, no matter what time of day or year. And the smell was as consistent: foul with moldy mustiness and the tang of sweat, but well mixed with oxygen and clean ocean air. Sensory adjustments were painless and quick; you could see, breathe and feel, and in silence most anytime. Joy is found in strange places. Opposite the front door and clinging to the wall at a 45-degree angle was a second staircase that opened to the rear parking lot. A narrow, thin-stepped contraption, it sagged in the middle and threatened to collapse should it be disturbed. Those who chose the dilapidated structure to enter or escape used it only once, knowing they had pushed their luck. Beneath the ill-stacked stairway was the small mystery room behind a crooked, time-stained yellow door. Alone one morning, which was often the case, I managed to stir up some endorphins with a volley of PBNs supersetted with side-arm laterals.

I dragged a slug of water from the corroded water fountain eight feet from the entry to the ominous mystery room. Feeling pumped and dangerous, I yanked the door open to expose broken wood furnishing, cracked ceramic toilet fixtures, lightless lampshades and framed pictures of someone's long-silent family -- all covered in deathlike dust, damp, moldy and thick as cotton. Spiders and rats (and spirits) retreated in startled wisps. Imprisoned for decades the dust and stink and blackness fought to escape its confines. I shut the door with lightening swiftness, not my place to release voiceless, yet hysterical captives from the past. Most of the gym's equipment was handmade and clustered in one particular quarter of the cavernous basement. Overhead stood five stories of old hotel and rented rooms and aging occupants in total ignorance of the activities below. We could lift and win and lose and die and no one would care, especially those tipping shots of cheap booze in the saloon above the squat rack. Diluted whiskey and warm beer dripped from soggy plaster overhead to form a puddle beneath the nasty, oversized rack. One slip too many and you're an alcoholic. I loved the dumbbells (10s to 150s) that sat on splintery 2 x 10s supported by milk crates -- when milk crates were milk crates. They were comprised of plates of every manufacturer collected by every musclehead in Southern California over 25 years, and they were welded together in handy heaps resembling... well... dumbbells. They rattled and pinched and made a monkey of ya one day and a strongman in time, if you persisted. The benches were bulky and perilous and less attractive and were pieced together by the same guys who welded the dumbbells... and repaired the leaky pipes, hung the front door and decorated the mystery room. There must have been a sale on sky-blue paint at the local hardware. The only color in the gym was the blue of the benches and the red splotch of their oilcloth coverings. Two movable flat benches, two bench presses, one incline bench, one steep-incline bench, one preacher curl and one beer-soaked squat rack -- what more could an authentic musclehead ask for, besides a pump and burn and a weekly unemployment check? Other bare necessities included a chinning bar and a set of dipping bars made of galvanized pipe and covered with layers of chalk; an overhead pulley setup for free-swinging plate-loaded cable pull-downs and a long cable and pulley for seated lat rows -- these, the most primitive and effective back-builders in the world. Oh, yes, and one mobile hunk of mirror broken from a larger hunk served anyone who needed to see himself. There was the homey touch, a couch in a serene area where no equipment but a crudely crafted Roman chair and a scored tumbling mat bursting at the seams were tastefully arranged. Ambiance and modern art. The couch was of the stained and contagious variety you'd hastily circumvent in any frightening alley. At the inside edge of the left front leg my training partner and I hid our chalk. Only we knew it was there. That's about it. The rest of the place was strewn with Olympic bars of varying degrees of curvature and malfunction and plates that never bent or broke. Impression, imperfection and improvising were the Dungeon's foremost muscle building features. Not to mention Zabo, Dick Dubois, Armand Tanny, Gene Shuey, Sam Martin, Peanuts West, Hugo Labra, Joe Gold, Artie Zeller, Chuck Collras, Chet Yorton, George Eifferman, Reg Lewis, Dick Sweet, Zeus and Thor...

Time to head for the Weight Room to inflate and ignite, pump and burn, soar and fly...

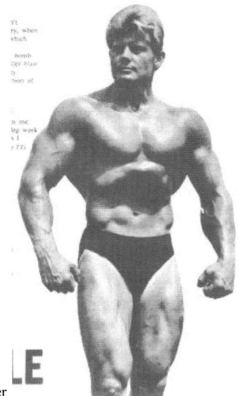

Go... Godspeed... Draper

Here is another Muscle Builder excerpt featuring the memoirs of another guy that worked for Tanny and was mentioned in the Draper piece above;

MUSCLE MEMORABILIA

By GEORGE EIFERMAN — Mr. Universe

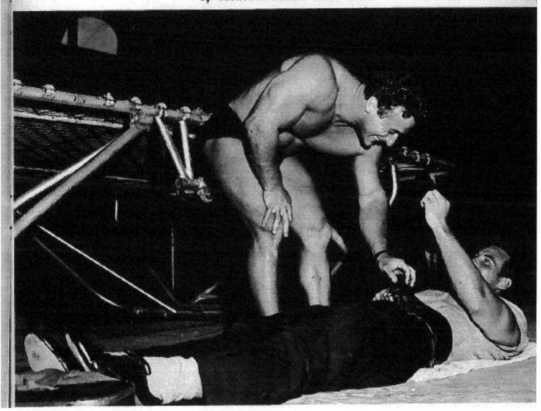

That's STEVE REEVES lying on the floor with a chain secured around his waist... and that's GEORGE EIFERMAN who's preparing to lift Steve by his teeth! These long-time friends frequently practice this difficult strongman feat!

★ As most of you **Muscle Builder** readers know, I have been traveling in the interest of our great sport, bodybuilding, for almost more years than I'd like to count. I've clocked well over 700,000 miles, just by automobile alone! Add to that the many cities I've visited by plane and train and you'll see that I'm well-traveled.

When you get about that much and meet so many great physique stars, advanced bodybuilders, and those whose careers are just now beginning, you collect a lot of memories... some amusing, some a bit sad... but always interesting. Just a few days ago when Publisher Joe Weider was in Southern California to check up on our Weider West Coast office, we were shooting the breeze one afternoon, and I happened to tell Joe a couple

61

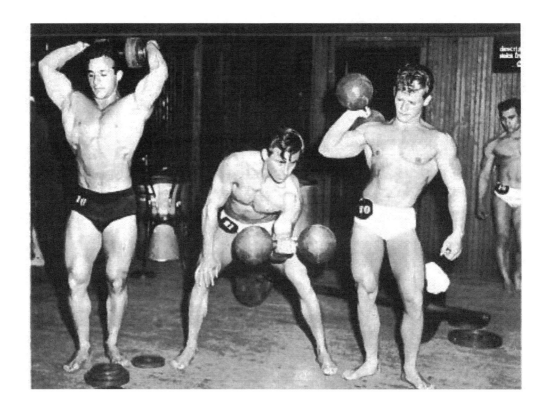

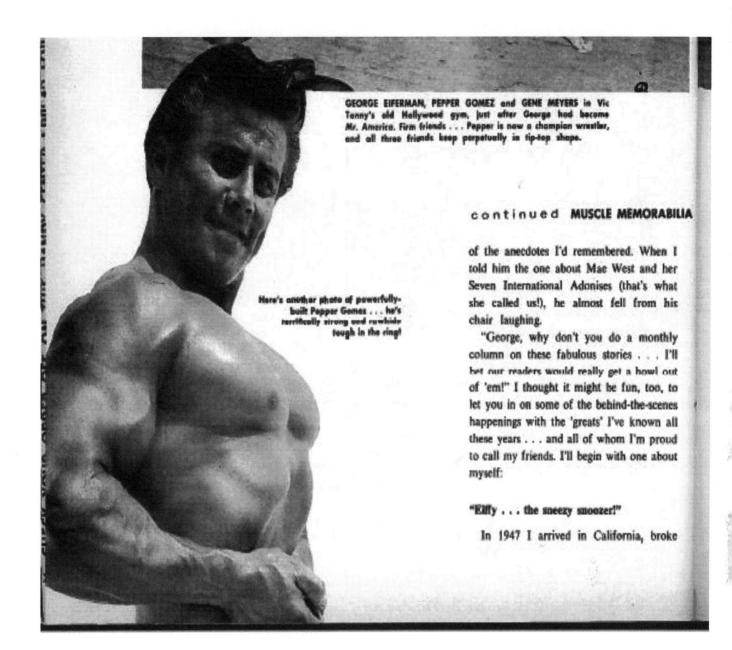

GEORGE EIFERMAN, PEPPER GOMEZ and GENE MEYERS in Vic Tanny's old Hollywood gym, just after George had become Mr. America. Firm friends . . . Pepper is now a champion wrestler, and all three friends keep perpetually in tip-top shape.

Here's another photo of powerfully-built Pepper Gomez . . . he's terrifically strong and rawhide tough in the ring!

continued MUSCLE MEMORABILIA

of the anecdotes I'd remembered. When I told him the one about Mae West and her Seven International Adonises (that's what she called us!), he almost fell from his chair laughing.

"George, why don't you do a monthly column on these fabulous stories . . . I'll bet our readers would really get a howl out of 'em!" I thought it might be fun, too, to let you in on some of the behind-the-scenes happenings with the 'greats' I've known all these years . . . and all of whom I'm proud to call my friends. I'll begin with one about myself:

"Eiffy . . . the sneezy snoozer!"

In 1947 I arrived in California, broke

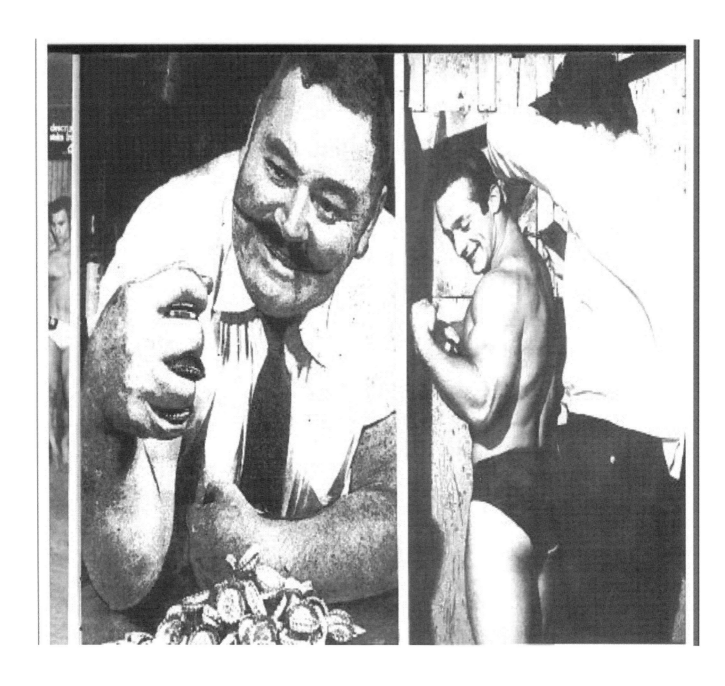

The one and only Mac Batchelor Demonstrates the fabulous beer cap bending feat described in the article (left), and Look who's giving Eiffy a haircut... none other than Steve Reeves. As George would say "But he wouldn't have so much to cut these days... I'm growing a high forehead!"

and jobless, and was given a place to sleep in Vic Tanny's old gym... by none other than the great Vic himself. A trampoline was my bed ...if you can imagine such a thing! Whether there was some material in the trampoline I was allergic to, I don't know... but I do know that something made me sneeze... and when Eiffy sneezes it's like a marathon... I keep it up for reps, about 16 sneezes per set.

Well, if you don't even try hard to visualize it you can still see what a sight I was sneezing away on that old trampoline. "Oh ... he flew through the air with the greatest of ease... the daring young man on the sneezy trapeze!"

You should have seen Vic's face as I bounced up   (Continued on page 101)

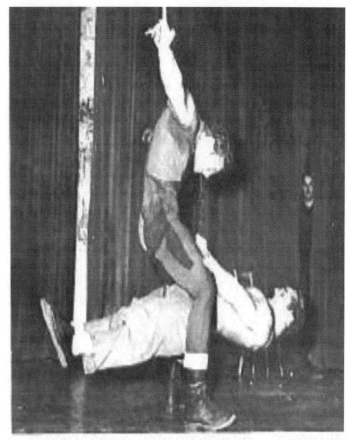

Now it's Steve's turn to lift George with his teeth... and it surely must be good for the teeth, for Steve has 32 absolutely perfect, dazzling white, cavity-free molars!

MUSCLE MEMORABILIA

(Continued from page 63)

and down ... he tried so hard to contain his laughter he actually turned purple! There were two other noted bodybuilders of that time who are now very successful professional wrestlers ... you know them as

"Pepper Gomez and Gene Meyers."

Every morning, as certain as dawn breaking, Gene and Pepper would come bouncing down the gym stairs for their three-hour workout. They'd roust me from my bouncing bed and get me to train with them. Having had a very complete workout all night long on that darned trampoline I really was reluctant to lift even a tiny dumbbell. But I did, anyway. I recall that Gene was the only man I've ever seen who could curl his bodyweight with dumbbells. It was almost unbelievable to see this 170-pound athlete take two 85-pound dumbbells and quick-curl them. It was easy to understand why Gene was Los Angeles City Gymnastic Ring Champion, for his arm strength was — and still is — phenomenal.

"Mac Batchelor"

One day Vic Tanny invited Steve Reeves, Floyd Page, Vic's brother, Armand, and me to visit Mac Batchelor, world champion wrist wrestler. The five of us entered Mac's tavern and from behind the bar in his big white apron, Mac welcomed us. After extending the greetings — and a seidel o' suds — Mac got down to business of what he is most famous for ... beer-cap bending.

Mac showed us the incredible strength of his fingers by placing four bottle caps between his fingers and applying pressure so that he bent each cap. We were astounded! Imagine being a cow that Mac milked!

One by one, each of us wrist-wrestled Mac, and were promptly defeated. Floyd Page in a suit does not look as strong and rugged as he really is, and a man at that bar singled out Floyd and challenged him to wrist-wrestle. They sat down at a table and locked arms. Floyd turned the man and the table over in one motion! The fellow promptly left and we all had a good hearty laugh.

"Mae West ... a wag with the wigs!"

The Mae West show was breaking all records in the major nightclubs across the country. One of Mae's "Seven International Adonises" was Zabo Koszewski, who has won more best abdominals awards than any other man in the world.

Although Zabo is tops in the muscle department, he doesn't have exactly 20-20 vision and had to wear glasses. Since, obviously, it would have appeared a bit odd for an almost nude muscleman to appear on stage with spectacles, Mae had Zabo get some contact lenses fitted. Fine ... Zabo didn't mind at all. But one night, unfortunately, when we were playing the famed Ciro's in Hollywood, Zabo somehow misplaced them. When the cue came for all the athletes to march out onto the stage, Zabo walked ... and walked ... right off the stage into the orchestra pit.

"Hot damn!" laughed Mae. "This is better than real show, let's put it into the act!"

Another pretty funny thing that happened while I was with the show was when Mae noticed that some of us were growing bald ... let's say that we were

101

developing awfully high foreheads.

She therefore went to great expense and had hairpieces (wigs) made for Zabo, Joe Mauri and me. I disliked wearing mine and put it on one night very low over my forehead, giving a werewolf effect, and also looking like an idiot! When I came out on stage at my cue, Mae couldn't help laugh and cancelled the wigs thereafter!

"The days of wine and roses!"

One hot summer day Armand Tanny, Joe Gold and Bob McCune, after months of preparation and hard work, sadly said farewell to all of us at Muscle Beach. They were leaving for the Pacific fishing waters in their newly-bought surplus Navy landing craft. They were going to make a fortune in the fishing industry.

Two weeks went by with no word from them and we all began to wonder what was wrong. We considered contacting the Coast Guard, fearing that they had been swallowed by the heavy seas. Then, suddenly on the scene appeared Joe, Armand and Bob . . . suntanned and rested and with the biggest grins you ever saw! They never got past Catalina Island with its wine, women and song! What they caught wasn't a load of fish, but a lot of fun!

ever go back to Atlantic City I'm going to look for Bill's head again . . . I hope he finally came out of the water!

"Steve Reeves . . . and his secret diary!"

Steve Reeves kept a secret notebook on his training. Being his best friend for many years he showed it to me one day. He was a real pioneer on the concentration-sets system which Joe Weider later organized and taught to the rest of us.

When Steve and I trained hard we'd try to work out in the morning. Our breakfast consisted of concentrated frozen orange juice mixed with two egg yolks in a blender. This was light and easily digested and gave us quick energy. Today we'd use the same formula plus Weider Hi-Protein. Very few people knew of Steve's great strength. In fact, many think it isn't strong at all!

Yet I've personally seen him clean an Olympic barbell weighing over 200 pounds **while on his knees!** At an exhibition at Woodbury College he lifted me (205 pounds at the time!) with his teeth. Steve has the most perfect teeth you can imagine . . . all his own and not a cavity in them!

Steve believed that if one walked slightly pigeon-toed he would get a better calf development. His favorite Curl was the dumbbell Incline Bench Curl.

"Catch that man!"

Busy Joe Weider was out on the coast recently, organizing his new Muscle Beach office. Bobby Vernon, the West Coast manager, and I had to get some important matters settled with Joe, but it was time for Joe's workout and nothing can make him postpone that.

So we all headed for the sands where Joe stripped down to his trunks to squeeze in his daily run along the beach. "Great for the calves!" said Joe. He invited us along. So all of us in our street clothes and shoes were about ten feet behind Joe, huffing and puffing away to keep up with him! Suddenly two strangers joined us in the rear. One yelled to me, "Say . . . what did that guy up there do? We'll help you catch him!" He misjudged the whole scene and thought we were after someone. It gave us all a good laugh and a chance to catch our breath, too.

"Tommy, the incredible!"

While visiting our local YMCA some years ago, some athletes told me of a young boy who could lift over 300 pounds overhead. One hears of many Paul Bunyans and everyone knows someone who lifts prodigious weights, so I paid little heed to this.

"On the boardwalk at Atlantic City!"

Going back through the 1950's and remembering funny things, I recall that one day I was on the boardwalk in Atlantic City, and I noticed a head bobbing in the water twenty yards away. The man looked familiar to me. Sure enough it was Bill O'Brien of Fritsche's Gym ... a former **Mr. Philadelphia.** During the conversation only his head showed. I wondered and waited for him to walk out of the water onto the beach so we could talk further. He wouldn't budge. Finally I had to go. I found out later from his wife who was sitting on the sand, that Bill wasn't in good shape and didn't want someone in the iron game to see him without his 'mukkles'. If I

He never wanted to work his trapezius muscles so he did his forward dumbbell raises on the incline bench also.

I noticed that Steve always worked his neck from front to back and sides. I asked him why and he replied, "You have to keep it balanced, and to get a column-like neck you must give equal resistance to each part of the neck ... front back, left and right sides." Steve preferred hand resistance or a neck strap rather than the wrestler's bridge. So did Alan Stephan.

Alan Stephan who had one of the greatest lat spreads of all time explained to me that a wide chin or the lat pulley broadens the shoulders fastest. He used to do over 6 sets of chins when the lat pulley wasn't available ... averaging 10 reps per set.

While taking my workout in the weightlifting room, a handsome Oriental boy approached the heavy train wheels we called our Olympic set, and in a flash lifted it overhead! I swore off carrot juice as I saw a world champion being born. We drove down to Ed Yarick's big show in Oakland and Tommy was the sensation of the California meet. Tommy who? Kono, of course ... who today is the greatest championship lifter in the world ... in character as well as in lifting ability.

* * *

Hope you've enjoyed rambling along with me through my muscle memory lane and will join me next month for more of same!

—MB

Here is a nice cover shot of Pepper Gomez on Muscle Builder;

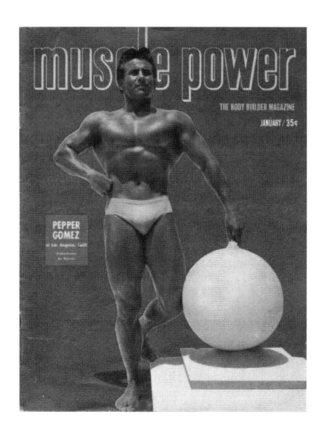

Previous to this one, he was a Strength & Health cover guy;

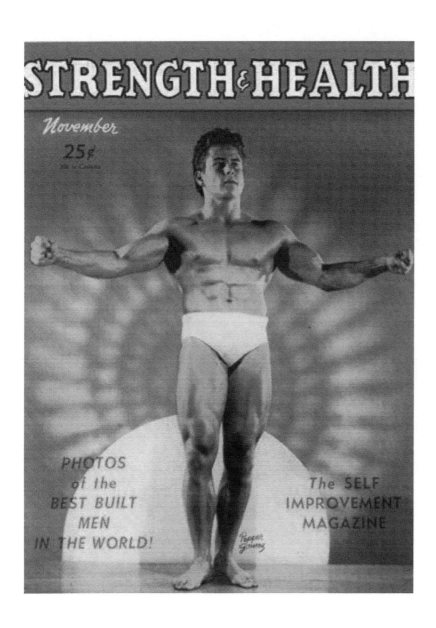

Here's one of Gene Meyers, who was mentioned above in Eiferman's article;

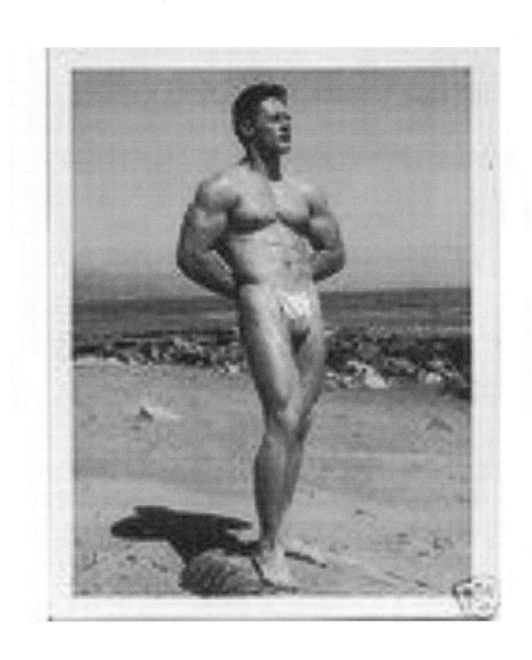

Another of the greats that trained at Tanny's in its early days is this guy:

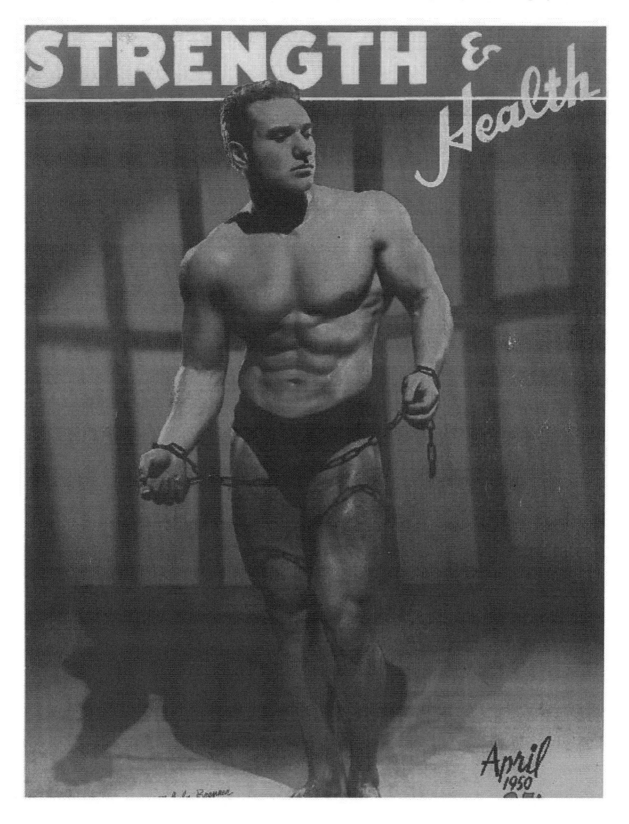

THE MAN ON THE COVER

By GEORGE EIFERMAN

I COULD hardly believe it. This giant of muscular perfection was only 20 years of age and already possessed the strength of an ox. One was amazed and surprised when he watched Malcolm training because he always did some unusual exercises and strength feats every time he trained.

I first met Malcolm Brenner when he came down to Tanny's Gym. The very first

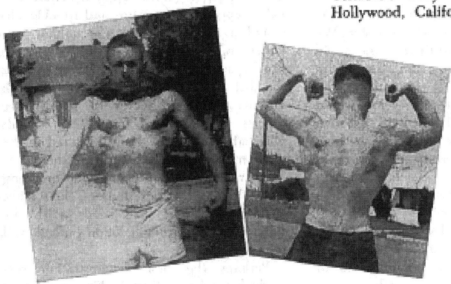

These snapshots, though not very clear, show MALCOLM BRENNER, our cover man, after one year of barbell training. He was already building the framework that was later to make him one of the best built men in the world.

bodybuilding with great enthusiasm. Shortly after, with only a few weeks of earnest training, he entered the "Mr. California," "Mr. America" and several other contests where he impressed everyone so much with his fine muscular development that he placed high among the top men in each event. He won numerous awards for his fine back and deep chest.

Brenner is currently training at Tony Terlazzo's body building gymnasium in Hollywood, California under the training supervision of Tony Terlazzo himself, that great little world champion, Olympic champion, and thirteen times national champion for whom Malcolm has the greatest admiration. For his money Tony Terlazzo is tops as a lifting champion and rates him among the best as a physique man as well. Malcolm admires him so because Terlazzo is almost twice his age, still retains his great lifting skill and thing I noticed was his remarkable sense of humor. He seemed to have all the boys in the gym laughing. Later when I was introduced to him he kept making funny remarks which made me laugh in spite of my trying to be serious. He is ever making people laugh with his funny antics and humor. He is a fine fellow to have around when the weights feel heavy and one needs a lift in his training. He livens up your spirit.

Here is a little history about this new Hercules so you will know more about him, being somewhat of a newcomer to these pages. He was born in the big town where there isn't "one living baseball umpire"—Brooklyn, N. Y. He came to California when he was only four years old so is almost a native of this sunny state. Malcolm started weight training when he was 15 years of age at a bodyweight of 123 pounds, a full fledged featherweight. His training was often interrupted but he thrived in spite of it. While in the army during the last world conflict he never followed a steady routine of training but did the best he could in way of exercise under the circumstances. The army officials were impressed with his commanding appearance and felt he would make an ideal M. P. guarding Japanese war criminals, which post he served commendably.

When Malcolm was discharged his bodyweight was already up to 180 pounds and he was already making plans to begin strength while his physique continues to improve at an age when most men have acquired a bulging belly. Terlazzo has Malcolm on a strict lifting program as he feels this young giant can become a fine lifter if he applies himself. Already he has made wonderful progress and in a matter of a few months Malcolm should do some amazing lifting. In the Odd Lifts cham-

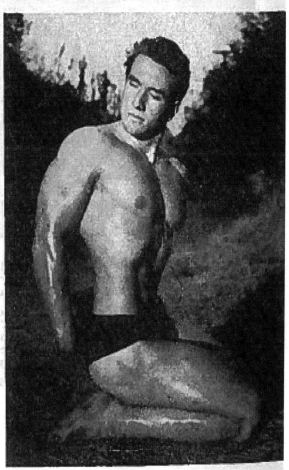

After his stint in the Army, MAL looked like this—very impressive. We first featured him in S. & H. in 1945.

—Malcolm Brenner... Coming Champion

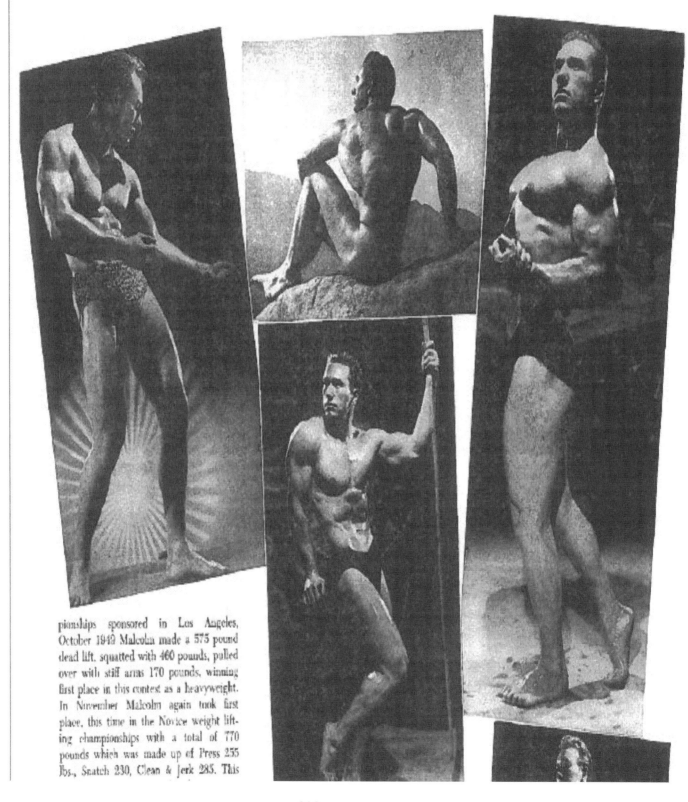

pionships sponsored in Los Angeles, October 1949 Malcolm made a 575 pound dead lift, squatted with 460 pounds, pulled over with stiff arms 170 pounds, winning first place in this contest as a heavyweight. In November Malcolm again took first place, this time in the Novice weight lifting championships with a total of 770 pounds which was made up of Press 255 lbs., Snatch 230, Clean & Jerk 285. This was the highest total ever lifted in a novice meet here in California. He only had about five weeks of training for this contest which proves he is capable of much more in the future.

I heard recently that Malcolm is now pressing 285 pounds regularly at Tony Terlazzo's gym where admirers often gather to watch Terlazzo and his boys go through their training. Malcolm himself told me he is focussing his aim on the next Nationals and hopes he can participate in this annual event. If he continues to improve on all his lifts, all of us who know him feel sure he will make a fine total. Naturally we wish him luck in this field and hope one day he will win the championship.

Another ambition Malcolm has is the ability to draw. He has extraordinary talent along these lines and some day he might make this his life's work. At present

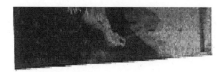
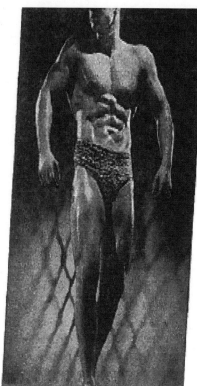

MALCOLM BRENNER *of Los Angeles as he is today. (Photos by Athletic Model Guild of Los Angeles).*

he is attending an Art school here in Los Angeles. Many times I have seen his amusing and clever cartoons decorating the bulletin boards of different gymnasiums. This gives many of us a hearty laugh.

Malcolm Brenner is six feet one and one half inches tall and now weighs 230 pounds. He has 53 inch chest (51 Normal) and an 18½ inch arm measured "cold." His other measurements are also impressive: a 28 inch thigh, 15 inch forearm and a 16½ calf. This 20 year old coming champion has a lot of "stuff" and (*Continued on Page 31*)

The Man on the Cover
(*Continued from Page 9*)

will be heard of much more in the future both in physique contests and in lifting championships. As a matter of fact last summer he was given the title of "Mr. Muscle Beach." The judges selected him from a large number of entries.

Among his more recent accomplishments are: a one hand dead lift of 550 pounds, and 650 pounds with the aid of a handkerchief. He does ten repetitions with 410 pounds in his workouts. In the Prone Press on bench his record is 380 pounds. In the under-hand Clean & Press he has done 275 pounds. In the presence of Tony Terlazzo he did a perfect Crucifix with 75 pound dumbell in each hand. His record in the one hand military press is 145 pounds. Seated he has pressed 260 pounds from behind the neck. He curls 185 pounds and can Snatch the 135 pounds of the York Olympic barbell by holding the plates rather than the bar. All these lifts have been done in the presence of well known lifters and physique men such as Terlazzo, Armand Tanny, Buford MacFatridge, Bob McCune and others. Says Malcolm, "My greatest ambition is to be 'Mr. America' and also a weight lifting champion."

This gent was another well-known bodybuilder that spent some time training at Tanny's;

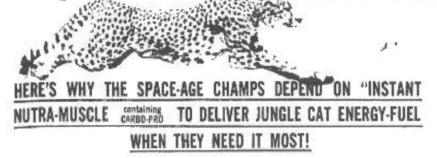
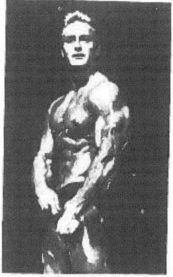

Bill McArdle

Here is something penned by Vic himself, writing for Strength & Health;

Here is a brief summary of Clancy Ross' training program from the **April 1949** issue of Strength & Health in an article by **Vic Tanny**. Quotations are from the article:

1. Squats 4x10
2. Leg Presses 2x 20
3. Calf exercise 4x30
4. Prone Press 3x10
5. Incline Presses 3x10
6. Pushups between boxes 3x10
7. Upright Rowing 3x10
8. Side deltoid raise 3x10
9. Bar curl 3x10
10. Bent over dumbbell curl 3x10
11. Triceps exercise 3x10
12. Overhead wall pulley 3x10
13. Five foot wall pulley 3x10
14. Lat stretches 3x10
15. Sit-ups 100 reps
16. Side bends 50 reps
17. Leg raises 50 reps

"You will notice that in this program Clancy does 10 reps on each set of squats, 20 reps on each set of leg presses. 30 reps on each set of calf work. 10 reps on all chest exercises. 10 reps on all sets of shoulder work. 10 reps on all arm work and 10 reps on all "lat" work. 100 reps in sit-up and 50 reps on both side bends and leg raises. This program takes Clancy about two hours of steady work *with* a training partner. The buddy system of training is an excellent method and one that most men adopt sooner or later. It makes both parties work harder and more conscientiously. I've advocated this system in my gym for many years, and with excellent results. Try to pick a partner who is consistent and a hard worker. If you team up with a playboy you might wind up doing one arm curls at the nearest bar instead of your regular exercises."

Here is an article by Vic about training at his gym that showed up in the February, 1949 issue of Strength & Health; the 1st 2 pages were separated into 2 pages each and blown up for easier reading. Please read down the first column of the 1st 2 pages as if they were one page, and then do the same for the following 2 pages. You'll see how the text flows.

TRAINING AT

I HAVE been asked by both Bob Hoffman and John Grimek to write a series of articles on training. It is with a certain amount of misgivings that I am starting on these articles because making arbitrary statements on what is the right way and what is the wrong way to train is at best a risky business. I say risky because no two people react to a given program in the same manner. The best I can do when I do not know the training history of the victim is to give a series of programs that tend to generalize rather than specialize. I'll try not to be too technical because if you are anything like myself you will become bored by five sets using the same amount of repetitions and weight.

Many question the feasibility of more than three times per week. Personally I have found that in my gym the pupils who work out five and sometimes six times per week seem to make the greatest gains. They don't at first but as the body becomes adjusted to the increased work the gains seem to be greater. Once you start working more than three per week you will find it easier to get started on your workout. Sometimes the rest day feels so good that a person gets the feeling he'd like to prolong the rest. If he does then his conscience bothers him and he finally becomes unhappy.

I would suggest that you follow this program for two months. I feel that two months is a satisfactory period of time in which you can derive the best results from a program of this type.

In checking on your gains during this two months period it is best to take both cold and hot measurements. By that, I mean before any working out, for a cold measurement and during a workout for a warm or blownup measurement. You should also take six or eight snapshots before and after the two month period. Make your before and after poses identical and your lighting conditions as identical as possible.

You will very likely hit a plateau somewhere about the fifth or sixth week when you seem to be retrogressing instead of progressing. Do not become discouraged or think you are doing the wrong exercises. It is best to keep on and do your best until this slow streak dissipates itself, which it will inevitably do. I sometimes recommend to my pupils that they cut their repetitions from 10 down to six repetitions and use heavier weights. They can do this for a week or ten days and then go back to the regular number of repetitions. They seem to break out of the slump and become stronger for having followed this procedure.

The necessary equipment is an important factor in your training. It will be time and money saved in the long run. In the preceding program it is necessary to have an inclined bench, a flat bench, a leg pressing machine, and a pulley for your latissimus work, and of course enough weight in barbells and dumbells to get a decent workout. Don't fool yourselves about this equipment problem, fellows; the more equipment you get, or can get, the better you can train.

In my gym I usually measure the fellows after a two month session on a program such as that above and make a

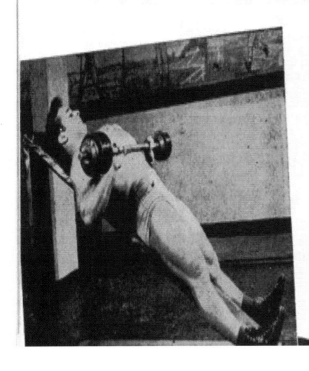

technicalities long before you learn anything. So with this thought in mind I'll give a program that you might try as a starter.

1. Prone press on inclined bench with dumbells (elbows wide) 3 sets of 10 repetitions.
2. Leg raises on flat bench. 2 sets of 10 to 15 repetitions.
3. Pull in on 45 degree angle latissimus pulley. 3 sets of 10 repetitions.
4. Curl, squat, and press with dumbells. 3 sets of 6 repetitions.
5. Leg press (preferably on leg press machine). 3 sets 10 repetitions.
6. Curl on inclined bench. 3 sets 10 repetitions.
7. Lateral raises on flat bench with dumbells. 3 sets 10 repetitions.
8. Upright rowing motion with barbell (grip bar in middle, hands together, overhand grip).

This can be followed from three to five times per week. If you have a lot of energy and don't feel tired the day after a workout you might be able to work this program five times per week. If three sets don't seem to extend you enough, work the program from three to

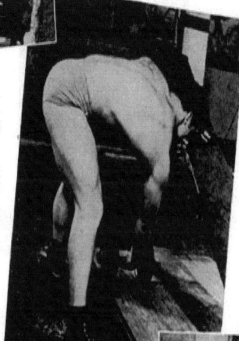

Top to Bottom: GEORGE EIFERMAN, "Mr. America" *performing supine press on inclined board. One hand curl while leaning and the wide press with dumbells on inclined board. All photos by Cecil Charles of W. Los Angeles.*

new program to suit their individual needs. Since each one responds differently to the same program each pupil's second program is different and made out to improve the muscle groups that failed to respond satisfactorily to the first program.

A pupil who makes uniform and average gains might possibly get a program such as the following:

1. Press behind neck. 3 sets 10 repetitions.
2. Situps 1 set of from 15 to 25 repetitions.
3. Bent arm pullover and press on flat bench. 3 sets of 8 repetitions.

Page 24

TANNY'S

By VIC TANNY

4. Upright dips on high parallels (using a hip belt for added weight). 3 sets of 10 repetitions.

5. Hack exercise. 3 sets of from 10 to 15 repetitions.

6. Alternate curl and press with dumbells. 3 sets of 8 repetitions.

7. Prone press on flat bench with dumbells. 3 sets 10 repetitions.

8. Lateral raises on wide pulleys. 3 sets 10 repetitions.

9. Optional ex. Toe raises using hip belt 5 to 10 minutes (or) One arm pull in on latissimus machine or pulley. 3 sets of 10 repetitions with each arm.

By the Hack ex. we mean holding the barbell tightly against the buttocks and doing squats with heels raised on a board or object 2 inches thick.

As I mentioned before we can get much better results by working with the individual and understanding his weaknesses, living habits, occupation etc. When we know all these things it is much easier to give him a program that will bring him the ultimate in gains.

I think the most important factor involved in your training is your degree of consistency. You must be consistent above all. I cannot emphasize this point too much. All of us have a tendency to slough off or find excuses why we shouldn't train today. Use the positive approach and try to think of reasons why you should train.

and started. You almost always get your best workout on the days you don't feel much like training.

Some fellows suspend their training when going through a period of emotional upset. This I believe is a big mistake. If they keep up with their training, they will find that they can relieve the emotional strain and avoid many illnesses that follow extended emotional strain. A bridegroom will often quit training to apply himself more diligently to the task of proving that two can live as cheaply as one, and other such malapropisms. Those newlyweds who do this are making a mistake because most men can make their best gains when married. They usually adopt better living habits and live a lot more scheduled and orderly life. That prowling around looking for excitement and more beer every night when a man is single, has an enervating effect upon him and retards his progress to a great extent.

That great strongman and weightlifter of ten years ago, Frank Jares, gained 30 pounds in bodyweight and a hundred pounds on his total in the first three months of his married life due to his improved and regular habits. The point I'm trying to put across is that a man should not let marriage interfere with his workouts but should use it

start weight training. I have found that the fellows who rave the most about how wonderful weight training is, and how wonderful they feel, and what phenomenal gains they are making, are the ones who give up first. Take a somewhat cynical approach or rather a more level headed approach and you will last a lot longer. I hate to say this but the grumblers usually do better than the idealists, because they expect nothing and are pleasantly surprised when they find they are getting results. The idealist will look at a Grimek or a Stanczyk and be sorely disappointed when he finds that after 3 weeks of intensive training that he is not quite as good as these stout lads.

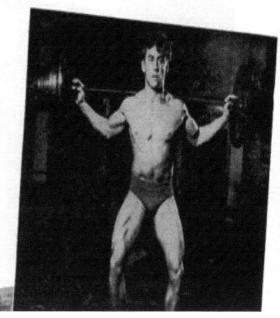

My pupils often come to the gym and say they cannot train today for this reason or that. When the reason is analyzed it is usually found to be a mere fabrication or at best a poor and flimsy reason for missing a workout. I usually advise them to take a five minute workout. Once they get warmed up and started they usually get in an excellent, full workout. Half the battle is getting warmed up as a stepping stone to greater gains and improved life. Get your wife interested in working out and you won't run into difficulties when you want to go to the gym for a workout.

Don't get over anxious when you first

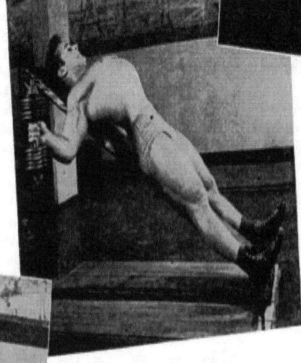

Top to bottom: PEPPER GOMEZ doing a 400 Lb. Deep Knee Bend. EIFERMAN performing the "Flying Exercise" (Bent Arm Lateral Raises) and the Stiff Leg Dead Lift.

Use a little introspection on why you wish to train. A fellow usually is not conscious of the real reason why he wants to look like superman. They usually start out by telling me that they don't want a huge build, or muscles, they just want to feel good. I doubt this is the real reason for most of them who say that, because they usually feel good anyway. They are the same ones who after a couple of months put up a kick because they are not getting a 16 in. arm fast enough and their chest isn't quite 50 etc., etc. If you can understand the real reason or reasons why you want to train you can set a more sensible goal and approach it from a sane viewpoint. I prefer to believe that personal vanity and the wish to impress some starry eyed little "mouse" is the great motivating factor in a fellow wanting to

(*Continued on Page 40*)

Page 25

"one-hand-stand"... the one-hand-planche ... pressing up from the "planche" into a handstand ... the most difficult stunt in all handbalancing.

The above mentioned chapters are only a few of the many in the new York Handbalancing Courses. These new methods teach you right in your own room! You learn quickly, correctly and safely.

ENROLL NOW

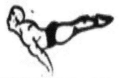

The complete York Handbalancing Courses are priced at $5.00. Send this coupon.

....

YORK HANDBALANCING
P. O. Box 1484,
York, Penna.

Dear Sirs:
I would like to enroll at once in the new YORK HANDBALANCING COURSES. I am enclosing $5.00. Please send me the complete courses at once.

My name ....
Address ....
City .... State ....

....

Page 40

Training at Tanny's

(Continued from Page 25)

work out. I can be wrong of course but I have come to this conclusion after much personal and not necessarily scientific observation. The wish to get strong and beat up on someone who did you dirt on some occasion is sometimes a factor but the desire for revenge is soon forgotten and a better reason is soon substituted or the desire to workout slows down. Some men are accelerated by the idea they have always been physically inferior and here is an opportunity to show their superiority. This theory holds some water but I think that is soon lost in the shuffle otherwise all those fellows who are thin and run down would train religiously and as you know not many of them do. If they did we would all be millionaires. (I mean the gym owners.)

Good food is a most important factor in your progress. There are thousands of diets you can follow, some good, and some bad. Some fellows go overboard and become strict vegetarians. This is fine but I am inclined to think that the young should eat some meat, especially vital organs such as kidney, liver, brains, etc. These meats should be cooked medium rare. Animal protein is more easily assimilated than other types of protein and they are very necessary in muscle building. Vegetarianism is a good thing for older people who do not do much manual labor.

The fellows at muscle beach try to watch the quality of their food intake and seem to thrive splendidly. They eat as much fresh fruits and vegetables as possible and short cook their cooking vegetables with little or no water. Meats are usually broiled rare. Buttermilk and yogurt and brewers yeast in the bulk, as well as a satisfactory amount of vitamin A each day, make up the diet of these health seekers. You do not necessarily have to go overboard on diets but nevertheless you should not take the lazy man's out and say "I eat anything," because just anything isn't always the right thing.

I have often been asked how much smoking and drinking should be done when in training. Naturally I advise against smoking and drinking of alcoholic beverages. Some fellows don't seem to be able to bring themselves to a stop on either of these habits, so once again we have to take the common sense view and ask that they limit themselves to five or less cigarettes a day. It keeps the trainee from becoming too unhappy and he very often quits smoking altogether after a few weeks, without any noticeable mental strain. It is of course better to stop smoking altogether if you find it doesn't make you too unhappy to stop abruptly. People do stop abruptly you know, and feel better almost immediately.

As far as drinking is concerned the less the better. The small nip each day doesn't work too well with most people because most people feel that one good nip deserves another so with this happy little thought in mind they go around and around with Mr. Gigglewater. The end product is cataclysmic. So we must approach the problem from this angle, namely, to have just a bottle or two of beer every other weekend and if you should slip off the deep end by mistake you will at least have a week or two to recuperate. Meanwhile don't miss workouts. The best solution is to stop altogether. (Not the workouts, Buster—the drinking.)

HERCULES *Barbell Bargains*

For those who desire to enjoy the many benefits of weight training, who do not wish to invest as much in a barbell set as the price of the York Deluxe or York Aristocrat sets we offer the York Hercules barbell sets. They are good, strong, durable outfits which compare favorably with the sets which are being offered for sale by other companies. Economies have been made in their manufacture which make it possible to offer these truly wonderful prices, prices which, considering the quality and durability of the Hercules sets make them the Best Barbell Bargain in America today. Consider these low priced sets.

100 lb. Hercules Weight Training Combination. Includes 4 each of 1¼, 2½, 5 and 7½ pound Hercules plates, 5 foot polished steel bar with extra heavy duty inside and outside collars, weight 25 pounds. Pair of solid steel, 14 inch, dumbell-swingbells with heavy duty collars and revolving hand grips. 3 books of training courses, barbell, dumbell and swingbell training. With this set in addition to the barbell you can make up a pair of 37½ pound dumbells or a 52½ pound swingbell. Very moderately priced at..................$14.95

150 lb. Hercules Weight Training Combination. Same as the 100 pound combination with the addition of 2-25 pound plates..................$21.95

200 Lb. Hercules Weight Training Combination. Same as the 100 pound combination with the addition of 4-25 pound plates. We recommend the 200 pound set for better and faster results are obtained when you train with heavier weights. This set is suitable for a strong man..................$28.95

With the combinations described on this page you will have the pleasure and physical benefit of training with barbells, dumbells and swingbells, these permit the practice of scores of good result producing exercises.

Order from

YORK BARBELL CO., YORK, "MUSCLETOWN," PA.

YORK *Aristocrat* 30lb. DUMBELL SET

You saw Vic referencing a guy named Frank Jares, yet another Pro wrestler, who spent some time training at the Dungeon;

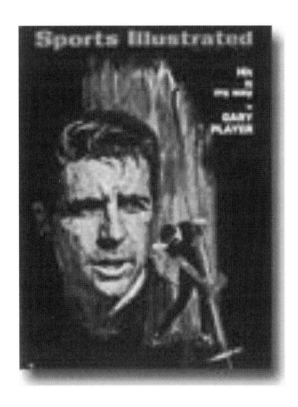

March 21, 1966

My Father the Thing

A son's fond reminiscence of his dad's colorful career as a professional wrestler (left, bleeding) and of a summer spent with Frank Jares on the road, where Joe learned there are some real dangers involved, too Joe Jares

Not that it helped me much in childhood frays, but I was the only kid on my block who could boast, with absolutely no fear of contradiction, "My father can lick your father." Frank August Jares Sr. was a professional wrestler, the nastiest, meanest, basest, most arrogant, cheatingest, blood thirstiest eye-gouger around. No rule, referee or sense of fair play ever hampered his style. In short, the sort of man a boy could look up to. In his prime Pop was just a shade under 6 feet tall and weighed 230 pounds, with short brown hair, a neck like a steel pillar, big biceps and ears much more like cauliflowers than rose petals. Most people can fold their ears in half, but Pop's seem to be made of solid gristle and will not bend more than half an inch. He had, and still has rather thick lips and prominent cheekbones, a Slavic countenance that would fit perfectly in a Warsaw union meeting or the Notre Dame line. His wrestling stage name was **Brother Frank, the Mormon Mauler** from Provo, Utah, but really he was just Frankie Jares from north-side Pittsburgh, the son of a Bohemian butcher from Czechoslovakia and a U.S.-born mother, also Bohemian. He never heard English spoken until he went out on the streets to play with the other kids. At age 12 he had both upper arms decorated with tattoos, and at 14 he was out of school and driving a truck. Naturally, he grew up to be a tough guy, but sometimes a gentle tough guy. He spanked me only twice in my life. Even though he traveled a lot, I thought I knew him, but I actually did not know him well at all until I spent one summer with him in Tennessee and Alabama—the summer of 1956. Pop was Southern Junior Heavyweight wrestling champion, operating out of Nashville (the senior champ, I figured, had to be King Kong, but I never met him). I finished my freshman year at USC in June and flew from Los Angeles to Nashville to join Pop, Mom and Frankie Jr., who were living in a nice trailer park alongside some *Grand Ole Opry* stars and other assorted footloose folk. It was my job to accompany the old man on the southern wrestling circuit—usually Birmingham on Monday, Nashville on Tuesday, Kingsport, on Wednesday, Thursday to Bristol, Friday to Knoxville and Saturday in Chattanooga. After the matches in Chattanooga, we would drive all night back to Nashville, stopping once on the way at a mountain café' for sausage sandwiches and ice-cold milk. Sunday was rest time at the trailer park swimming pool. Back on the road Monday. "I don't know a single damn highway number," Pop said, "but I can take you to the back door of any arena in the United States by the shortest route." He told me I was a bodyguard, a ridiculous idea (the only thing I guarded was his precious 1956 Studebaker Golden Hawk, a favorite target of his enemies after the matches). On his brawny arms he had that faded green artwork—a flag, an anchor, a star, a sailor girl, an Indian maiden, a Kewpie doll and so on. The only tattoo that would have fitted on one of my arms was a skinny snake, and not even that if the snake were coiled. Pop often said I had arms like garden hoses and a neck like a stack of dimes. He could see better out of his one good eye than I could with my glasses. But we entertained each other, I by listening and he by telling tales of his travels, his brawls, his riots and his bloody third-fall finishes. For instance, somewhere between Nashville and Blytheville, Ark., he told me about Hawaii. There he had not been Brother Frank, but **the Golden Terror,** mysterious scourge of the mat. Yellow mask, black sleeveless shirt and, according to irate fans, yellow streak down back.

By pulling hair, illegally using the ropes and just generally ignoring the Boy Scout Code, he prevented any good-guy opponent, or "baby face" in the lingo of the trade, from ripping off his cover. Actually, he had such an intricate way of fastening the hood that it would have taken the Pacific Fleet to unmask him. And if it had happened, nobody would have known him anyway. Well, hardly anybody. In his free time Pop wore his own face as he lifted weights and wrestled at the YMCA with various Islanders, including one Harold Sakata (later to become Tosh Togo, the evil Jap ring villain, and, still later, Odd job in the movie *Gold finger*). "You know," said one of his friends after a workout, "you're such a good wrestler you should go down and challenge the Golden Terror." Pop felt a little like Clark Kent, and somehow no one connected the giveaway tattoos. Of course, there had been other aliases. Pro wrestling is a world of unrelated brothers and Italian noblemen from The Bronx. Every Indian is a chief, every Englishman a lord, every German a Nazi. Pop was once Furious Frank Jaris. And Frank Dusek of the roughhouse Nebraska Dusek clan. And Frank Schnabel, brother of that despicable duo, Hans and Fritz. **One of his finest guises was The Thing**. He used a horrible orange-red dye on the hair on his head and on a new crop of whiskers. He fixed up a wooden suitcase with THE THING printed on it in spangles and a hidden button that could be pressed to bring forth a sound similar to an aroused rattlesnake. He flew to Chicago to make his fortune and was granted an athletic commission license in the name of M. T. Bochs. He strolled the sidewalks of such towns as Gary, Ind. and Racine, Wis. in top hat, elegant topcoat, vest, striped pants and spats—and that fluorescent hair. Decent citizens who had seen his matches would curse him. "That's just what you are," said one little old lady, "a dirty, dirty thing." Pop smiled politely and said, "Why, thank you." As long as little old ladies had no hatpins he was polite to them. But he made no fortune and eventually went back to being the plain old Mormon Mauler. Between southern whistle stops that summer of 1956, as the souped-up Studebaker cruised along at 60 mph and we tried to hit rural mailboxes with empty Dr. Pepper bottles, Pop often talked about wrestling fans, as testy a group as you can find this side of a Brazilian soccer stadium. One time in Pico Rivera, Calif., Pop told me, he was walking to the dressing room between bleachers, and a man 12 feet above him reached down to hit him, slipped, fell to the concrete floor and broke his own neck. At various times in the ring Pop had been hit by whiskey bottles, lighted cigarettes and paper clips shot with rubber bands. During a match against Vincent Lopez (not "Lopez speaking") in Redding, Calif., Pop pulled himself under the ropes while flat on his back, a sneaky trick to get the referee to make the baby face let go of his ankle. A ringsider stood up and slashed Pop's forehead with a beer-can opener. The wound took 17 stitches to repair. He also had been stabbed with a knife, cut with a broken mirror and punctured with fingernail files. In Bremerton, Wash., Pop treated kindly, fair-dealing giant Primo Camera with something less than minimal courtesy. As he ran the gantlet on his perilous journey to the dressing room, an indignant woman threw a lighted book of matches that hit his sweaty body with a painful sizzle. He stopped to analyze the woman's ancestry (even Pop could not hit a lady), but between them stepped a belligerent man who said, "That's my wife." Pop slugged him and yelled, "Then teach her better manners." The arena erupted into a riot, and dear old Dad had to stay under police guard in the dressing room half the night. The fans were really stirred up one night in Bridgeport, Conn., he said. They completely misunderstood Pop's gentle nature and were intent on dismembering him. "I know my crowds," he said. "If you don't have the experience, you get killed. You have to jump right into the middle of the milling mob, never go in the opposite direction. A silent crowd is much more vicious. That silent 'heat,' that's the vicious crowd. The punchers and scratchers are much less dangerous. They wind up hitting each other most of the time." Well, this night in Bridgeport,

Pop was in the middle, all right, and not enjoying it, but he happily sighted a policeman battling his way through the mob. The cop finally made it to Pop's side and then unhesitatingly bashed him over the head with a billy club. At the Wilmington (Calif.) Bowl in the mid-'40s Pop and his original partner, **Brother Jonathan** (who was really from Utah), won a tag-team match and were chased around the building by an angry pack of sailors intent on seeing justice done. The Brothers made it into the dressing room finally, but one sailor made it inside before they got the door locked. Another wrestler held the sailor and said, "Here he is, Frank." Pop walked toward him with fist cocked, and the poor man collapsed in a faint. Then there was South Gate, Calif. For 32 straight weeks, Pop recalled, he and Wee Willie Davis took on and defeated all comers, each week with some nefarious tactic. Their favorite ploy was to have Willie, a huge man, slowly back up into his own corner so Pop, standing outside the ropes, could reach through his legs and yank the opponent's legs out from under him. There were 27 sellouts in those wild 32 weeks. After a while the South Gate police refused to respond to any more riot calls, so Promoter Frank Pasquale had to hire his own guards. One night after the South Gate chaos Pop was driving through East Los Angeles when he was forced off the road by four men in a jalopy. They were going to teach Brother Frank some manners. They got him as he was halfway out the driver-side door and beat and stomped him until he got away by rolling under the car. Pop was so furious he went out and bought a pistol, stashing it in his glove compartment for the right moment. Nothing happened the next week, although he and Wee Willie were as wicked in victory as ever. But two weeks later the quartet forced his car over at almost exactly the same spot. Pop leaped out of the car brandishing the pistol like Jesse James (not the Houston wrestler Jesse James, but the outlaw). Three of the attackers jumped back into their car and sped away, with Pop emptying the pistol into their trunk. The fourth was so scared he fled across a field, leaving one of his shoes in the middle of the street. Pop twisted the shoe into a useless hunk of leather and ended his gun-slinging career the next day by tossing the weapon into the sea. At Long Beach's civic auditorium, he told me, a drunken fan once climbed up on the ring apron and hit him behind the neck. Pop shoved him off, as a man would shoo a fly. A woman sitting at ringside claimed the man landed on her, and she sued the arena, Pop and everybody else in sight. She lost the suit (because, luckily, the match had been kinescoped and the jury could see for itself what happened), but it still cost Pop more than $500 in legal fees. After the trial a man in the courtroom, the very same one who had climbed onto the apron, walked up and apologized. He did not offer to pay Pop's lawyer. Of course, antagonizing the customers was the whole idea, Pop explained, so you had to expect a little jab from a fingernail file once in a while. On those long rides between little towns he told me about "finishes," building up the "heat" to just the right temperature until the arena seemed ready to explode, then ending the match in some super-duper, slam-bang manner guaranteed to bring all the people back the following week for a sequel. There was this time down in Panama, where he was known as Hermano Frank, a holy man from Utah with seven wives. He wanted to be a heel, as usual, but the Panamanians loved everything he did and he gradually became, much to his chagrin, a baby face (just imagine The Joker helping Batman catch crooks). He taught a husky sailor, Strangler Olson, how to "work" (throw fake punches, apply harmless step-over toeholds, etc.) and play the villain's role. For the big finish Strangler was to throw Pop out of the ring and be disqualified, thereby setting up a juicy return match. To make it look better, Pop had a razor blade carefully secreted in the waistband of his trunks. During the inevitable confusion at ringside he was supposed to cut himself just slightly on the forehead. It would not hurt any more than running a fingernail over the skin, but it would look as bad as a battle wound.

However, Pop could not find the blade and used the next handiest thing, a bottle cap lying nearby. He stood up with a face full of gore, and the fans went berserk, attacking poor Olson like maniacs. "The crowd was beating the poor guy to death," said Pop. "I figured I had to save his life. So I started screaming, 'Let me at him! I'll kill him! Let me at him!' The mob parted and allowed me to get to him. I pretended to beat him right into the dressing room and the door slammed safely behind us." Some finishes were more goofy than bloody. In San Bernardino, Calif., Pop and a cohort were wrestling the Dirty Duseks in an all-heel main event. A moth landed in the center of the ring, so he put up his hand and stopped the match with silent-movie pantomime. Very slowly he leaned over and tried to pick up the delicate little moth and, naturally, it fluttered up and away. In awe he looked up and watched its flight. Then boom, that dirty Emil Dusek sprang from his corner, socked Pop on his inviting chin, knocked him cold and won the bout. That summer in the South had its share of crazy adventures, too. Pop had been on his way to Charlotte, N.C. and was supposed to stop off in Tennessee just to help out the local bookers for a couple of weeks. The couple of weeks stretched into nearly two years. He quickly won the Southern Junior Heavyweight belt from Sonny Myers in Birmingham in 1955 and from several other guys in several other cities. It was such a big territory that nice little "bits" could be reused in practically every town. Pop kept the big, fancy belt in the trunk of his car and wore it into the ring for big matches. Baby faces loved to grab it away and chase Pop around the ring bludgeoning him with it. He won a big trophy in Memphis, then promptly broke it over the Mighty Atlas' head. The belt stood up under the punishment, though, and made a dazzling prop. Pop was wrestling Spider Galento in Chattanooga one night, and it was sort of a contest between them to see who the crowd hated the most. In such instances the people usually pick a favorite, and he is forced into being honorable and decent. Galento entered the ring first and by a series of struts and poses had the fans despising him immediately. So Pop came into the ring and showed off his ill-gotten belt. Still, the crowd obviously hated Spider more. So Dad shouted up to the Negro section, way up in the back, that he was tired of their being deprived and he was going to give them a close look at his belt. He did just that, delaying the start of the match 14 minutes as he slowly wandered among them. By the time he got back in the ring the whites hated him as much as if he had sung *The Battle Hymn of the Republic* over the loudspeaker. New Good-Guy Galento proceeded to please the white portion of the crowd by punishing Brother Frank with good, honest holds. In a few minutes even the Negroes were back hating my evil father. At one point Galento had Pop by the throat and, in the time-honored wrestler's pantomime, asked the Negro gallery if he should hit him. "*Yes*," they screamed. Then he asked the lower balcony. "Yes," they screamed. Then the ring-siders. "Yes," they screamed, in a frenzy of anticipation for the delicious moment. But when he asked the vendor selling Cokes at ringside, Pop came alive and did the slugging himself. "What the hell," muttered Spider during the next quiet headlock, "can't you wait until I get my heat?" The riots in Knoxville, Pop's most lucrative payoff town, sometimes started as he *entered* the ring, depending, of course, on how vile he had been to the hero last week. He usually needed a riot-squad escort to make it back to the dressing room after the matches. I remember once we had to sit there until 1 a.m. as the mob milled around outside, all the time Pop worrying about his Studebaker. We finally walked out a side exit and encountered a large, hostile crowd. Pop just picked out the guy with the loudest mouth and invited (invited?) him to shut up. Then we calmly climbed in the car and drove off. At least he was calm. We always hated to go to Gadsden, Ala. The people were nasty, the arena was a junk pile and there were no showers.

The wrestlers had to take spit baths in the men's room, treatment even Class D baseball players do not get. Pop was champion and thus had a $50 guarantee, but the other boys usually had to settle for the $15 to $20 minimum. I was kept pretty busy. First I counted the house (you could do that in the weed patch towns) to make sure the promoter did not pull anything on the old man at payoff time. I had to guard the men's room door while he was cleaning up and then run out and guard the Studebaker. After an unruly main event in Gadsden near summer's end, he was leaving the ring amid flying insults and flying chairs. Two or three teen-agers were giving him a particularly bad time, and he looked over at the dressing room door and saw me peeking out, enjoying the rhubarb from a safe distance. He beckoned me out. He, a former weight lifter who had pressed 270 pounds, snatched 260 and clean and jerked 330, was calling out his arms-like-garden-hoses son to protect the family honor. Reluctantly I went, wondering why the hell I had not been born to a hod carrier. I challenged the leading heckler to come down from the stands and fight me—which should have been an easy assignment for him, but a peace officer burst out of the crowd just then and grabbed my arm, apparently thinking I was causing the hassle. Pop grabbed my other garden hose and dragged both me and the sputtering officer into the dressing room. It took an hour's argument, a phone call from the head booker in Nashville and some phony flattery to keep the Jareses out of the Gadsden jailhouse. And when we got to the car, the aerial had been bent in half (it was not as tough as my father's ears). We never went back to Gadsden, but I'll always remember that night as the most exciting since **Gorgeous George** gave me a gold-plated "Georgie" bobby pin and swore me into his fan club. The best melee of all was in lovely Kingsport, jewel of northeast Tennessee. I was in the heel's dressing room (heels always seemed to be the funniest storytellers) when someone stuck his head in the door and said, "Riot!" The dressing rooms were on either side of an unused stage, and when we ran to the curtains we saw Pop fighting his way to the far doors with the aid of a couple of cops. The crowd was in a nasty mood—which was typical. Three or four of us sprinted the long way around the side hallway to the front doors, but by the time we got there Pop had realized he was going in the wrong direction and had started back through the howling mob to the stage. We raced back down the side hallway, bounded up the steps and saw that the policemen were busy knocking fire-breathing fans off the stage. Brother Frank was lying face down on the floor of the stage, not moving a muscle, as what seemed like the entire population of northeast Tennessee tried to reach him for one last swing or kick. Finally the cops quieted the crowd, which must have thought the old man was dead or dying. The curtains were drawn, and I waited for the wail of an ambulance, for surely Pop was in need of medical aid. But the sly possum suddenly jumped to his feet, not a mark on him, and strode into the dressing room with a sinister grin on his face, basking in the hatred of the fans and confident that next week there would be a packed house. How many people showed up or what foul deeds Pop perpetrated I don't know, because I returned that week to college for my sophomore year, which turned out to be awfully dull somehow.

Chapter 4   Gold's Gym

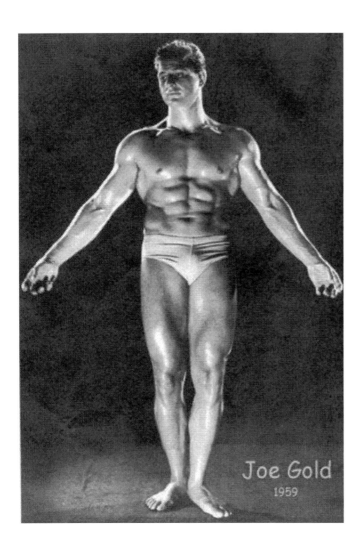

We can't talk about Gold's Gym without first talking about the man who built it, Joe Gold;

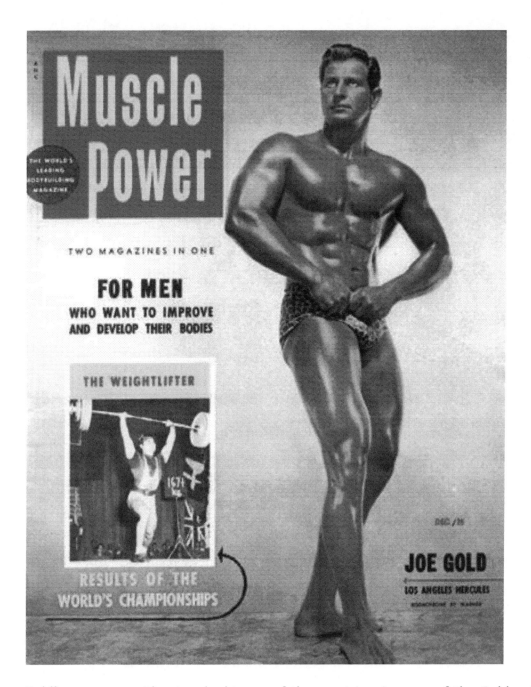

Gold's gym was without a doubt one of the most iconic gyms of the Golden Era. This next section is an excerpt from my previous book "**Forgotten Secrets of the Culver City Westside Barbell club revealed**" Gold's gym showed up quite a bit in that book, as it was one of several places that the original Westside guys trained at, and happens to be the place where my friend Joe DiMarco met Bill West before that club became what it later would be. There are lots of ties between the men who trained with West & friends and the original Gold's gym, as well as the other Golden Era gyms.

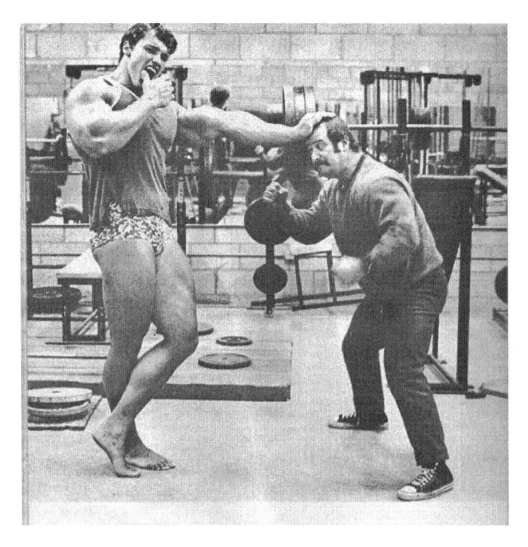

2 icons at Gold's, clowning around as usual.

Here are some tidbits from a couple of "Muscle Rags" of the era;

Gossip from Muscle Beach

By Dick Tyler
Mr. America Magazine, August 1965

Here's big news to all the BIG men reading this column. Well-known California muscle man, Joe Gold will soon e opening a gym at 1006 Pacific Ave. in Venice. For those of you who know, Venice is just a stone's throw from famed Muscle Beach. Joe, who owns some real estate hereabouts, is building the gym from the ground up. Nothing "made over" for Joe. Now this is going to be a gym for men. No fancy rugs or chrome - just plain old-fashioned weights and the greatest apparatus you ever saw. How's this for dumbbells? The gym will have two complete sets of dumbbells going from 10 lbs. to 80lbs. in five pound jumps. From there they'll go to 150 lbs. by tens. Already Joe is having equipment made to order for the specialists. Joe is a Weider man and you can bet your bottom dollar that this is going to be a hot bed of training for Southern California strong men. Co-managing will be ole Zabo Koszewski himself. How can they miss? Those of you not already here in "Sunsville" better make Gold's gym a tourist attraction.

The Famous GOLD'S GYM - Where the Champions Train

By Our Roving Reporter
Al Antuck
Ironman vol 34 no 4
May 1975

Why are some restaurants and other establishments the "in" places to go? What is the aura of a place that makes it "the" place ? Bigness or expensive decor certainly do not make any place "in" automatically. In fact, bigness or costly trimmings might turn many people off, making those establishments Chapter 11 cases very quickly. Many businesses thrive because of good management; some businesses thrive in spite of poor management. What is the charisma of an establishment that attracts regardless of its management, size or decor? Whatever it is, Gold's Gym on Pacific Avenue, one block from the beach in Venice, California has it. Gold's attracts many of the top California physique stars -- Schwarzenegger, Zane, Draper, Columbu, Bill Grant, Birdsong, to name a few. Gold's is definitely not a plush gym ala Jack LaLanne's, and it is not a big gym as most gyms go. Gold's appears to be the size of a medium-sized store. From the street you can look inside and see a floor crowded with barbells, benches, and other equipment. You can see members -- many of whom you will quickly recognize -- working out. Gold's is a bodybuilders' gym. Here you won't find business men types who work out just to stay in shape. Most members are bodybuilders who work hard to gain bulk, density and symmetry, and they work hard with minimum time for kibitzing or goofing-off. The lockers and showers are on the ground floor in the rear of the building. On the second floor above the locker area is the manager's office where you might find Ken Waller, who not only trains here but also manages Gold's Gym.

Gold's Gym is a nice place to visit, and you may want to work out there.

GYM DANDY

The Gold's Story

By Don Ross
Muscular Development

The California Gold Rush of the mid-19th century brought thousands of settlers to the West Coast. But it has been gold of an entirely different sort that has brought top strength athletes flocking westward for the past 20 years: the world's first internationally recognized gym chain, Gold's. The flagship of the more than 300 Gold's Gyms worldwide is found in Venice, California. Here famous athletes and celebrities commingle with the dedicated bodybuilding locals. Just two decades ago no businessman in his right mind would have invested a penny in a hardcore workout facility lacking a sauna, Jacuzzi, spa, pool, or racquetball court. Now, as many of the chromed and gleaming health clubs go out of business, Gold's continues to grow in membership and recognition the world over. Fitness buffs today are more interested in a no-frills approach to serious results. To better understand the story of Gold's we need to go back nearly a quarter century. Joe Gold had already been a competitive bodybuilder, movie stuntman, and co-star of the famous "Mae West Show" of the 1950's when he opened a small training space in Venice. Joe kept up with the evolving strides in new equipment and techniques and made sure they were a part of Gold's Gym. Before long, the word had spread. Bodybuilders began leaving their gyms for Gold's. Muscle magazines jostled for the opportunity of making Gold's a backdrop for their photo shoots. By the late 1960's, bodybuilding champions from around the world came to train where the action was, to combine their knowledge and techniques in a new atmosphere of "training community." Gold's had become the Mecca of bodybuilding. One of the early members who greatly influenced the Gold's physique fraternity was a young Austrian named Arnold Schwarzenegger. Since Arnold's early days at Gold's, scores of international champions have made the Mecca their training ground. In 1970 Joe Gold sold the gym to Bud Danitz and Dave Sachs. Yet the change of hands did nothing to diminish Gold's tradition and following, and the gym went on to attract world attention when, in 1975, it was featured in the film *Pumping Iron*. The movie made stars out of Arnold Schwarzenegger and Lou Ferrigno, and expanded world awareness of both Gold's and the sport of bodybuilding. Gold's has undergone several changes and face-lifts over the years. Dave Sachs sold his share in the company to partner Bud Danitz. Then in 1977, the gym was bought by former bodybuilder and fitness expert, Ken Sprague. Meanwhile, business continued to boom. Several prestigious contests were hosted by Gold's Gym, starting in 1977 with the Mr. America. In subsequent years, Gold's was the arena for several national Men's, Women's and Mixed Pairs competitions. Gold's led the way in promoting the recognition of women in the sport by co-hosting the first national woman's championship. It seemed that no changing of hands could hurt the reputation of the facility, but it didn't *help*, either - until 1979, when bodybuilding great and Mr. World titleholder Pete Grymkowski, along with Mr. Empire State Tim Kimber, and architect Ed Connors bought the facility for $100,000.

These three men combined their marketing know-how and noticeable changes began to take place. Their plan for Gold's Gym came from a dream that went far beyond simply expanding the original facility. Their dream was to popularize the image and benefits of hardcore gym training in the minds of the businessperson, housewife, actor, athlete, and other non-competitive, but health-conscious people. Once this reputation for state-of-the-art training techniques and equipment was established on a public level, they moved on to a larger audience - the world. In June, 1980, Ed Connors became the first Gold's Gym licensee by opening Gold's in San Francisco. Today, over 310 Gold's Gym licensees operate gyms all over the world. As the United States became more aware of their diets, Gold's saw the opportunity to expand into nutritional supplements for the purpose of energy, muscle recuperation and overall health. After interviewing athletes on their expectations and needs, after four years of research, including human clinical studies, Grymkowski, Kimber and Connor launched Gold's into the forefront of a new frontier, pharmaceuticals, with its own formulas for vitamins and minerals, called Pro-Line. A whole new technological horizon opened up in the field of physical fitness and Gold's owners seized it with both hands. They developed a computerized program to analyze individual nutrition and fitness, which was sold not only through the gym, but through sporting goods and health food stores throughout the country. A line of sportswear was designed bearing the Gold's logo, picked up by major department stores and sold to athletes of every stripe, who carried off designer name with the alacrity produced by an alligator only a decade before. The ball was rolling and there was no sign where Gold's mania would stop. Today there stands in Venice, California Gold's Bodybuilding Hall of Fame. The original gym had become a regular stop for tourist "weekend warriors" to train alongside Mr. and Ms Olympias. The driving concept of Gold's had always been that there was no stereotypical muscle man, that working out should be open to people from every walk of life: not like some jet-set nightspot, all manners of weight trainers flocked to perform the reps beside such personalities as Lyle Alzado, Kareem Abdul-Jabbar, Mych Thompson, Ken Norton, Reggie Jackson, Charlie Sheen, Richard Dreyfus, Judge Reinhold, Carrie Fisher, Linda Rondstadt, Jodie Foster, Michael Landon, Carl Weathers, David Lee Roth, Janet Jackson, Jermaine Jackson, Hulk Hogan, 700 pound bench presser Ted Arcidi, and the world's strongest woman, Jan Harrol. From a gym where the locals use to sweat and grunt is now spawned a Motion Picture & Television Division! Single-handedly, in its own name, Gold's was creating an industry where none had existed. In film, television, radio and print media, through film shoots in the gym, guest posing and seminars, Gold's promoted male and female bodybuilders and gained the sport international "showbiz" exposure. The Gold's phenomenon is the embodiment of the American Dream. Today, in the small gym from which it all began, the Mecca has turned into the Mega-gym. Vacationing athletes work out side by side with locals in the expanded three rooms, on everything from free weights to Keiser air pressure machines; competitors visit the private posing room where they rehearse their routines to music in front of multi-angled mirrors; and soon the gym will add a fourth room, for boxing, martial arts and wresting.[1] In many ways, Gold's was responsible for putting bodybuilding on the global map and thankfully, it's not Kansas anymore, Toto.

Don Ross is a former Pro Mr. America and the author of Muscle Blasting.

Gold's Gym Tug of war team featuring Steve Merjanian

Please forgive some redundancy if you have already read my "Forgotten Secrets of the Culver City Westside Barbell club revealed", as these following pictures were also in that book. For those who have not seen the Culver City book, I think these pictures will be a treat.

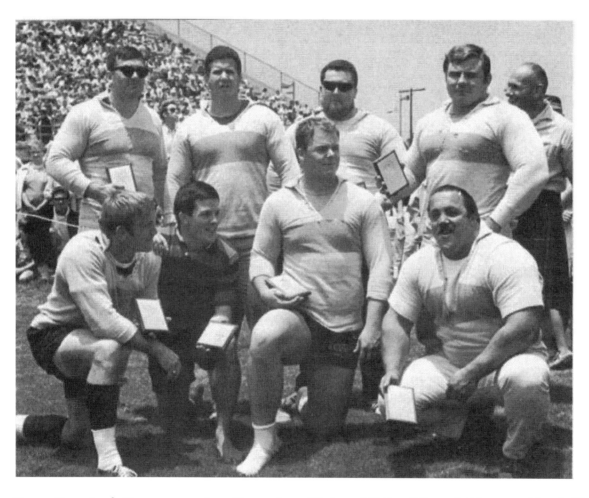

Tom Cas, Jack Summers, Joe Kanaster, Richard "The Moos" Mooos, Hank "The Tank" Breaker at 300 lbs!, Dick Fulmer and John Roehr and of course Steve Merjanian

The 1968 Gold's Gym Tug of war team known as the Gold Ropers, at the Southern California Highland Games

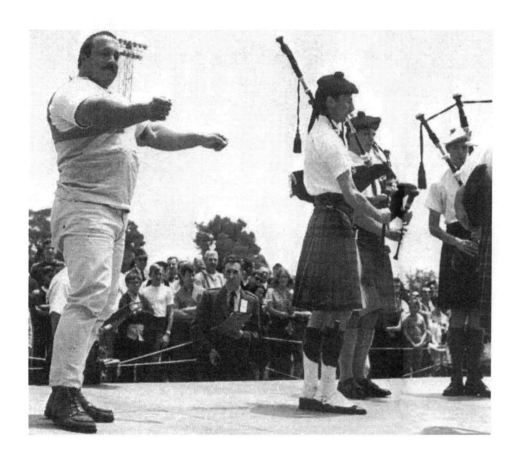

Steve hamming it up

In the Picture below, you can see the team in action

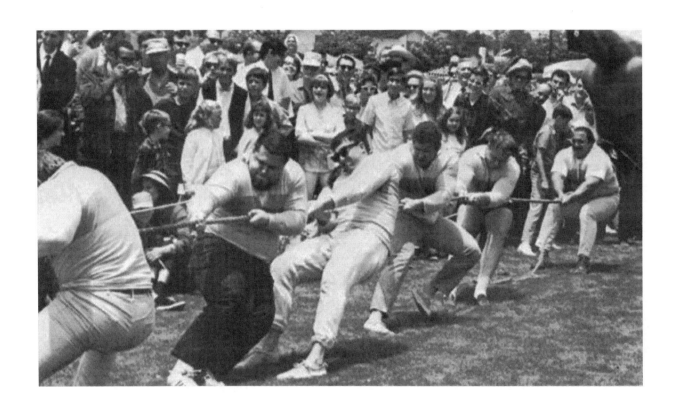

And below we see the team getting their awards

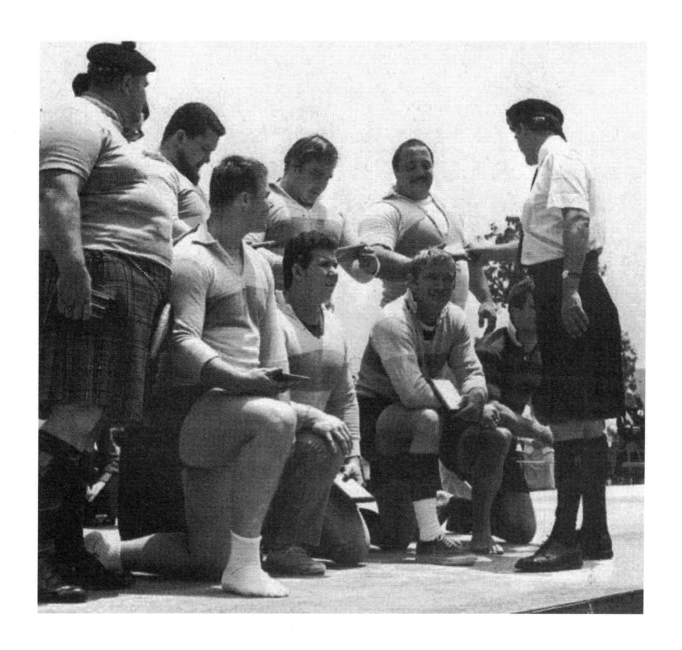

The next picture shows Steve signing his autograph on a woman fan's arm

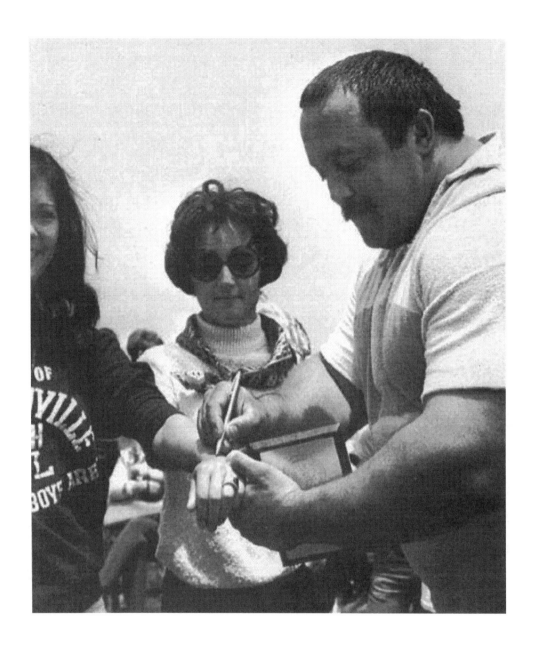

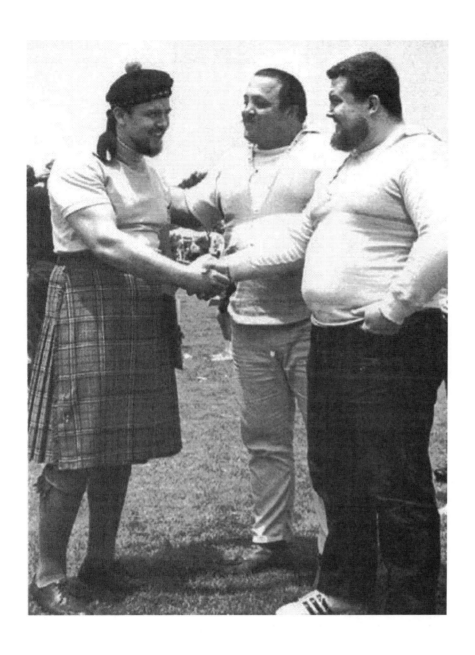

And A Hearty Handshake

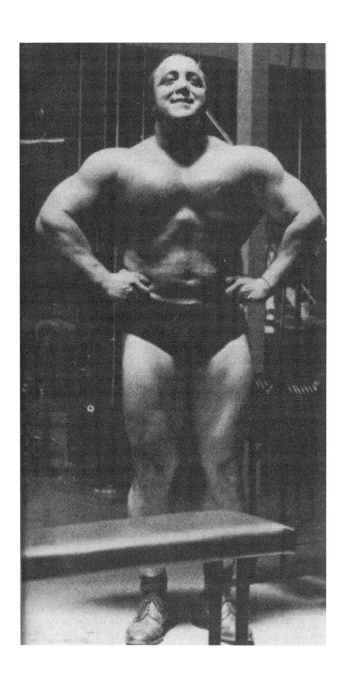

Big Steve

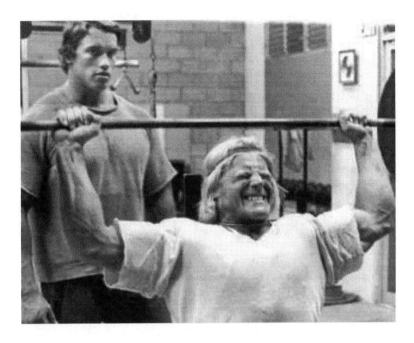

The tell-tale cinderblock wall of Joe Gold's original gym in Southern California provides the back-drop for 2 icons of the Golden Era.

The following excerpt is from Dick Tyler's Book (with captions by Draper),

Excerpted from
West Coast Bodybuilding Scene

It all began so quietly. The men started to assemble in the cool of the evening. The sun set over the horizon of the Pacific and the soft blue of the evening was beginning to accept the blackness of night. An ocean breeze drifted across the sands of the beach and wound through the crooked little streets of the city. The lights in the homes and apartments flicked on as the windows of the hippies' pads glowed with crazy hues of blue or red bulbs and the sounds of hard rock music fought those of Lawrence Welk. It was night in the city of Venice. Still they came. First there was Zane. He quietly nodded to Zabo, who was sitting behind the desk, and went upstairs to the dressing room. Soon Franco and the current Mr. Belgium, Serge Jacobs, arrived. Draper was next, followed by Eddie Giuliani and Mike Katz.

After a few minutes, Don Peters came in and within seconds, Arnold arrived. Gold's Gym was now busting with championship lumps. Already at work was Ken Waller, who is one of the most massive bodybuilders of all time. The cannon was loaded and was ready to explode. All this concentration of bodybuilders was for the sole purpose of getting ready for the big contests in New York. With the exception of Waller, all the others were IFBB bodybuilders and were stomping like mad bulls for the tension of the big event. Already Zane and Jacobs were working abs. This would last for as long as an hour and a half without rest. Arnold and Draper went over to the squat rack in the corner. They started loading the bar, which was already bent from the tons of weight it had been forced to carry over the years. Katz took some dumbbells from the rack and started blasting away at his delts. Columbu was on the calf machine lifting a stack of weights that rack and started blasting away at his delts. Columbu was on the calf machine lifting a stack of weights that was almost taller than he, while Don Peters was warming up with some light presses. What made the whole scene a little scary was the almost unearthly quiet that seemed to descend. Everyone was concentrating on what they were doing. This was serious business and there would be no useless rapping this night. I looked over at Arnold, who was heavily clothed in a sweat suit. The stains of sweat began to show under the arms and around the chest. Dave slapped more plates on the bar. Now it was his turn. Again and again he went down to the full squat position, only to fight to stand. Arnold leaned forward with each rep and counted them out. When it seemed Dave would burst if he made one more effort, the Oak would lean even closer to the Bomber and say, "You can do it, Dave. You can do it." Then as if in some kind of hypnotic state the mighty Draper thighs would ram out another rep. "Do another one, Dave," said Arnold softly, another rep done. Then it was Arnold's turn and he worked until his thighs looked like they would split his pants. There was no resting between the supersets, and then both Dave and Arnold started doing sissy squat moves on the hack machine. All that could be heard was the clank of Olympic plates and an occasional yell of encouragement. "Dick," said Arnold finally, "I think my thighs are going to come off my leg. They feel so heavy with blood. Tonight we are doing torture routine number two." "Torture routine?" I asked. "Ya. On Monday its torture routine number one. That's the heavy day. On Wednesday it's torture routine number two, when we combine the heavy with the supersets, and on Friday we do nothing but supersets for the legs. On Tuesday, Thursday and Saturday, it's the same thing for the upper body." "Why do you call them torture routines?" Arnold looked at me with baleful eyes under his brow, now dripping with sweat. "What else would you call a routine that makes your whole body scream for relief; that makes you want to vomit or pass out from exhaustion?" I nodded. "Torture." "It's your turn," said Dave as he got off the leg curl machine. By this time Mike Katz was doing presses behind the neck. He was seated on a back-supported bench and ramming out reps that forced him to grind his teeth until I thought I saw the enamel crack. Zane and Jacobs were still doing sit-ups. I got seasick just watching them. "Do another set," I heard the familiar voice of Arnold roar from across the gym. For a moment I thought he was urging Dave on. Instead it was aimed at Don Peters on the preacher bench. Don was standing in a pool of sweat. I could see his muscles twitch involuntarily. "You want to kill me or something?" he asked. "If that's what it takes for you to win the Mr. America this year, yes." He couldn't have made it much plainer than that. "Okay, but I have to take a rest first." "No," said Arnold as he turned back to the calf machine for another set, "you wait too long." Don shook his head in disbelief and went back to another set of curls. By this time the whole place was chugging away like a steam engine. I've never seen anything like it. There were more shouts of "Go, go, go!" I got up on the stairs that lead to the dressing rooms. From the balcony I could see the entire gym.

Everyone was now dripping with sweat. Great pools of it seemed to surround each apparatus. The smell was getting pretty musty. The yelling was increasing with the clanking of the plates. Nostrils were flared, eyes were wide and staring, teeth were grinding, blood vessels looked like they would burst and steam was almost seeping from the floor. For a moment it reminded me of Dante's inferno. No money on earth could make men toil in a hell like this, but they were doing it all for just the glory of a few minutes on a posing dais. After the workout Peters and I walked toward his car. "You come here every night?" I asked. "Yes," said Don, "but it's worth every long mile. I found myself getting in a rut. I had it pretty soft. I had a whole house to train in with a pool outside and soft music on the stereo. It was pretty great if I was training to win the Mr. Pismo Beach title, but not for the Mr. America. In order to have the kind of muscle that wins the big titles, you have to suffer. It's not suffering laying by a pool and listening to the stereo playing Doris Day or Johnny Mathis. No one ever won a title with those two as training partners." As I was driving home I began to think back on my bodybuilding past. I began to wonder if I could have ever won a physique title. Maybe, I thought, if I had really tried. I turned on the car radio. It was Doris Day. No, I guess its best I stuck to writing.

author's note

Incidentally, I have purchased & read this book, and it was well worth the investment. You can order it directly from Dave Draper's site;

http://www.davedraper.com/west-coast-bodybuilding-scene.html

One of my favorite forums is this one;

http://forum.iron-age-classic-bodybuilding.com/index.php?board=24.0

One of many sub-threads on this Forum is the one about the filming of "Pumping Iron" that took place at Gold's. Here is a comment by an owner of one of the later Gold's Gyms;

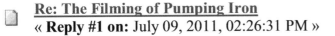

Re: The Filming of Pumping Iron
« **Reply #1 on:** July 09, 2011, 02:26:31 PM »

Right from the top, none of the training scenes at Gold's were "staged" for the camera. What you see on the film was a fair representation of Gold's at that time---except that we turned down the music so as not to interfere w/ the sound recording. The cameraman crept around the gym, Butler and the sound man in tow, catching the guys train as best he could.

The training intensity was real, not manufactured. [Nobody cared much about adherence to fixed routine of sets, reps or exercises---intensity was all (How else can you explain Corney keeling over from a set of squats?). Exercises were selected ad lib among training partners, as long the exercise fit the body-part trained that day.]

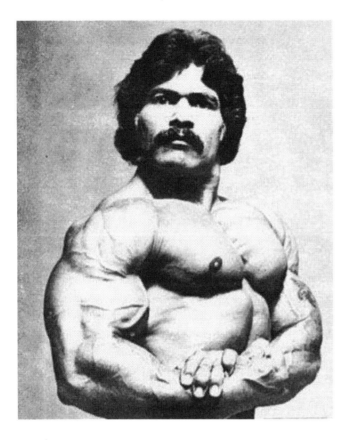

Ed Corney

Cameras need light; that was especially the case before the advent of high speed film. Before the first day of filming, studio electricians mounted high intensity lights on the gym ceiling. That allowed for spontaneous filming; the film crew could walk into the gym any day, day or night, and be lit to film w/ the flip of a switch, often catching the guys in action mid-routine. There were huge electrical cables on the floor to feed the overhead lights, but they were stepped over w/ a little bitching. The whole deal lasted about three weeks. Those of you that have the book and the film might notice the change to the front windows of the gym that preceded the filming. The covered windows permitted interior filming from any angle---no need to worry about filming into the sun. For you technical guys, filming was done w/ a 16mm handheld Arriflex. A little aside, in Los Angeles---and perhaps nationally---Vince's and Pearls were as well known or better known than Gold's at that time; at least very near that time. My understanding was that Butler's original idea was to film at Pearl's and Vince's as well as Gold's. But lights couldn't be installed in either Vince's or Pearl's since both had low ceilings; hence, Gold's was by default the primary location---particularly since the "owner" offered free use of Gold's for the filming. And it certainly didn't hurt that Arnold, Franco, Waller, et al trained every day at Gold's. I don't remember a complaint from any of the members that the film crew was an undue interference---I suspect the guys fancied the possibility of inclusion in the film. After all is said and done, bodybuilders are drawn to cameras. The icing on the cake was that Arnold supported the film---that pulled the other guys into line. [Butler had (correctly) convinced Arnold that Pumping Iron would be a great promotional vehicle for Arnold.]

Pumping Iron is an icon. Unfortunately for Butler, the film did not make money, but we should all congratulate him for a job well done---and putting The Oak on the path to major mainstream success.

Ken Sprague
Gold's Gym Owner

In another interesting thread from the forum, the inevitable question, much like that posed about the Dungeon earlier;

 Strongest bodybuilders at Golds?
« **on:** October 09, 2011, 08:31:25 AM »

Ken, during your tenure as owner, who were the strongest bodybuilders at Gold's?

Report to moderator   Logged

Ken Sprague
Gold's Gym Owner
Olympia Level
★★★★
★
Offline

Gender: ♂
Posts: 1454

Make Muscle, Not War!

 Re: Strongest bodybuilders at Golds?
« **Reply #1 on:** October 10, 2011, 03:43:57 PM »

Intenseman,
I've thought about your question for a couple of days. The problem in answering it stems from the fact that Gold's was a bodybuilding gym in the true sense---pure strength displays were few and far between.

Of course, Franco was strong. But as I've noted before, I don't think he would have ever been a champion power lifter. He did bench over 400# (shirtless)---the joke was that he only had to move the bar 10" because of a wide grip and short arms. And was a good dead lifter---the best in the gym.

Waller was strong w/out any lifts that would be considered exceptional as a heavyweight, but could probably generate more power than all but a few because he was also quick.

Kal came along a little later and as I recall could bench ~500#---but he was light in the pull and squat.

The following is a Muscle Builder "Gossip "column excerpt from the same column that had the picture with Bill West donning a necktie and Arny looking at him with a disapproving face. I told this story as Joe DiMarco recollected it being told to him from George Frenn, who was a key part of the story;

I've heard it said that truth is more exciting than fiction. Over a period of years I've sometimes had cause to doubt that saying, but an incident which recently occurred at Gold's Gym makes me wonder. It all happened one night not long ago when the gym was packed with its usual muscle denizens. One of the boys really digs the incline bench and had worked his way up to quite a sizable poundage. He was able to get the poundage up rapidly because he would bring the bar to the chest with incredible force. He wouldn't just let the bar drop to the chest. He'd literally *pull* the weight to himself until he could almost bend the Olympic bar from the force. I suppose he felt that it was some kind of a super bounce. He was warned by almost everyone that what he was doing to get the weight up might cause him a great deal of trouble as the weights got heavier. He wouldn't listen and continued pulling the bar into his chest with great force. Then it happened. He finished a set and got up to walk away. Suddenly he began to sway. Before anyone could help he tumbled to the floor as if he'd been pole-axed. His head hit the cement floor like a piece of lead shot. In fact it literally bounced. People ran over to help him up. He didn't move. His eyes were closed and his lips parted. Something was wrong—seriously wrong. George Frenn, the great track and power champion elbowed his way through the crowd that had gathered.

"What's wrong?" he asked.

By this time the young lifter's mouth was turning blue.

"He's not breathing," Frenn said as he lept forward and started to give mouth-to-mouth resuscitation. Thus began the battle to save a human life. George worked until the sweat was pouring from his brow. Still he didn't respond as his face started to turn blue. George started to pound on his chest hoping to stimulate any heart action that might have ceased

"Breathe, breathe!" he yelled frantically.

The young lifter's face was turning ranker by the second. In desperation Frenn lifted the man in his arms and started squeezing him around the chest to force his lungs to work. At last there was a gasp for air and a man's life was probably saved because of the efforts of George Frenn who wouldn't let death win. The young man was taken unconscious to the hospital. The following week he came back to the gym. Everyone seemed astonished to see him walking around.

"How do you feel?" someone asked.

"Fine. Why shouldn't I?"

"Don't you remember what happened?"

"Yeah, I heard I got a little faint."

"A little faint! Man, you nearly cashed in your chips and went to that great gym in the sky!"

"Are you kidding?" said the young lifter.

Everyone just stared as he loaded up the bar and prepared to do his inclined presses.

Here is a recent article posted in the popular Men's Journal magazine:

In the 1970s, a new breed of American man emerged from the weight rooms of <u>Gold's Gym in Venice Beach</u>. Led by Arnold Schwarzenegger, a clique of world-class bodybuilders — muscle-bound, steroid-fueled, bronzed like suntanned gods — pumped iron, chased girls, and changed the world's exercise culture forever.

By Paul Solotaroff

Robby Robinson, a wedge of black marble, arrived in Venice Beach in 1975 with one oversize suitcase and seven dollars. That was every dime he had after quitting his job and selling everything of value but the trophies he'd won at bodybuilding shows in the Jim Crow South. He'd left behind a wife, three small children, and a certain localized fame as the best-ever body in the state of Florida, fronting 20-inch biceps, a 28-inch waist, and 205 pounds of peaked, freak muscle on his hourglass, 5-foot-8 frame. But if your dream back then was to make the cover of *Muscle Builder* and storm the palace of giants in your sport, there was one thing to do and one place to do it: Join Gold's Gym in Venice Beach. With the ocean at its back, the sun through its skylights, and the biggest men on Earth trooping in by the dozen to bench 450 before breakfast, Gold's was Camelot-by-the-shore. You felt its pull in your hypertrophied heart, deep in the belly of that reckless muscle. Robinson, born and raised in the swamps of Tallahassee by an illiterate mother and a bootlegging father who later abandoned his 14 children, had a deep and perfectly rational terror of whites. Driving to shows in Mississippi and Georgia, he had seen the signs posted on rural light poles: niggers, don't get caught here come sundown. But it was a letter from a white man that had brought him to Venice: a written invitation from no less than Joe Weider, the publisher of *Muscle Builder*, to come out and join his stable of champion bodies living and training large in Los Angeles. Robinson got off the plane expecting to be met by Weider, or if not by him then by Arnold Schwarzenegger, Weider's Austrian prince, who'd won the title of Mr. Olympia five times running. Neither showed up, though, and after standing around for hours, Robinson tossed the suitcase over his shoulder and walked nine miles to Venice in platform heels. He found a place to crash at a fellow bodybuilder's and showed up at Gold's one morning that spring, gawking through the window, dumbstruck. "I couldn't bring myself to train. I was so in awe. All my idols in one room! Arnold and Denny Gable, Bob Birdsong and Franco Columbu; these beasts working out with no shirts or shoes and a crowd of people watching from the street." The gym manager, Ken Waller (a Mr. America and Mr. Universe), saw Robinson hulking by the door. "You," he growled. "You wanna train here? Fine: Come lift what we lift." He pointed to a pair of humongous dumbbells, 150-pounders with tapered grips. "Get down on that bench and give me 10," he said. "Otherwise, get the #$%* out and stay out."

Robinson, who'd built himself in backwoods gyms, had never seen dumbbells half so big. Somehow he got them onto his thighs, then, trembling, winched his back down on the bench. Each rep was a carnival of toil and pain, the weights teetering as they went up and ticked back down, the fibers of his mid-pecs shrieking. "I've no idea how I did that set," says Robinson, now 65 and still wondrously carved, his traps and triceps bulking through a linen shirt, his waistline waspish as ever. "But the adrenaline going through me then, that drive to be one of them — it was like a double shot of steroids and B-12." He fought the 10th rep up, screaming and twisting, then dropped the weights on the concrete floor. "You're in," grunted Waller. "You're one of us. Now go and give me a dead lift of 700."

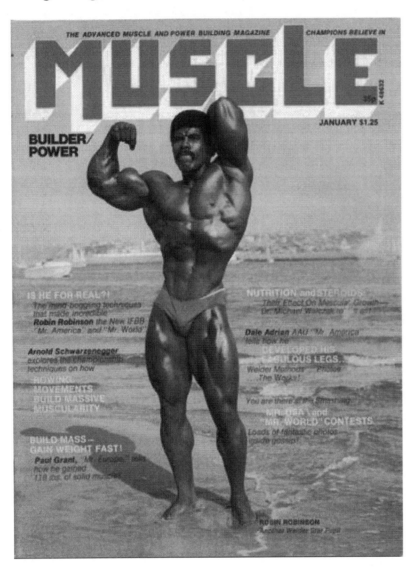

One of Robbie's early cover shots

Muscle, in all its meanings, is such a deeply American trope that it feels like part of our national narrative. We've made strength the flag of our exceptionalism and believe, however vainly, that our might will prevail in any test of wills against our foes. We've even found a way to monetize muscle, building an industrial complex of health clubs and home gyms and their hugely lucrative sideline: nutritional supplements. Thirty years ago, men stopped at a bar for a cold one after work; now those bars are Bally's and Crunches, and the person sweating beside you is as likely to be a woman as the guy who used to buy the second round. Most of them aren't there to build contest-quality mass or prepare for strongman shows; they go in pursuit of fitness, which is strength by another name — muscle fit for stock traders and internet geeks. But if you were born anytime after the release of *Conan the Barbarian* in 1982, it may shock you to learn that as late as the 1970s, Americans were repelled by the sight of brawn. "I'd go to the beach, and they'd give me the wolf whistle, guys on a blanket wanting to fight," says Eddie Giuliani, the 1974 Mr. America (short division) and one of the early legends at Gold's. "Nobody liked guys with the lumps back then. They thought we were all morons and fairies." George Butler, co director of *Pumping Iron* — the landmark documentary that made a rock star of Schwarzenegger and almost single-handedly changed America's view of well-built men — says, "I always liked to walk behind Arnold in the street so I could check out people's reactions as we passed. They'd point at him and sneer: 'God, look at that #@$% freak. What a clown.'"

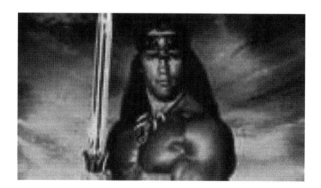

Gold's Gym didn't blow that bias away the day it opened for business in 1965. But in less than a decade, it became the Athens of muscle, the cradle of a full-blown body culture and the place where the gods of iron inspired millions. Everything we have now, from moonshot-hitting shortstops to film stars busting out of their bandoliers, began in that no-frills bunker by the beach. **Joe Gold**, the ornery seaman who built the place and has since been largely forgotten, had a lot of timely help from other people, not least of them Butler, whose charismatic film spread the Gospel of Huge to a scrawny nation. None of that would have happened, though, without Gold's vision. He made a space where titans congregated.

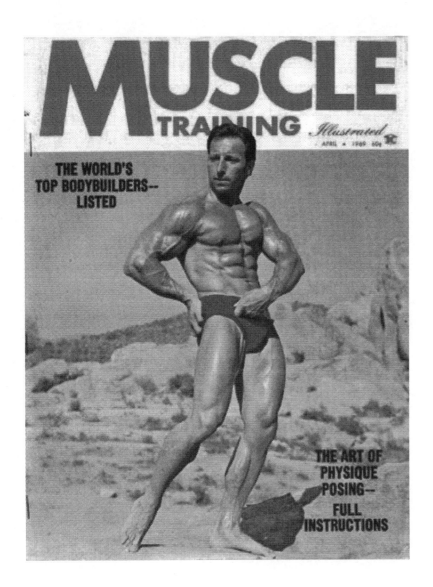

Eddie Giuliani

Gyms in the 1960s were scarce and vile, most of them unfit to train a dog. When Gold's opened its doors on **Pacific Avenue in Venice**, there were only three other clubs serving 7 million people in Los Angeles, and one of them, **the Dungeon**, was so unsavory that even powerlifters left their wallets at home. There was next to no money in the major competitions — Mr. Olympia, the top show at the time, paid $1,000 to the winner (Phil Heath, the 2011 winner, earned $600,000) — and the stars of this firmament worked knuckle-dragging jobs just to earn enough to train. (Schwarzenegger and Franco Columbu, a future Mr. Olympia, took bricklaying gigs; Lou Ferrigno carried caskets at a mortuary in Brooklyn and lived with his parents well into his 20s.) Bodybuilding was beached on the far shores of pop culture, poking along, barely in the muscle magazines, which existed to sell barbells to skinny teens. "They had smallish circulations," says Wayne DeMilia, a masterful promoter who raised the sport's profile in the 1980s by turning tournaments into sex-bomb pageants. "Weider earned off his products, the equipment, and protein powders." DeMilia, who left the sport in 2004 after Weider sold the business, by then a media empire, for $350 million, adds, "If you were one of his boys, he'd give you free ad space to hawk your own mail-order crap. That's how Arnold made his first money, selling exercise booklets to kids." **Gold's Gym was a money pit from the day it opened until Joe Gold sold it in 1970**; it seemed Gold went out of his way to avoid making a buck. He'd built a two-story bulwark of concrete blocks that had all the amenities of a morgue — a place exclusively for hardcore lifters, many of them friends of his from boyhood. The gym was big for its day, 30 feet wide and 100 deep, and consisted of a single, large, double-height space, unlike the rabbit-hutch layouts of other gyms. Up a narrow staircase was a smallish loft where members could change and shower after workouts or dose themselves with the first, crude anabolics — typically, Dianabol tablets and Decadurabolin shots, a combo that grew muscle but also compromised heart walls (as these men would come to regret in middle age). The gym's windows were sealed, there was no sign on the facade, and Gold usually kept the front door locked, lest any casual lifters happen by. "You'd go in the back door, which was always propped open — that way we'd get the breeze from the ocean," says **Ric Drasin**, a pro wrestling legend in the 1970s and '80s who joined Gold's Gym in 1969. "You could park back there, but most of the guys walked. They could barely afford rent, let alone gas."

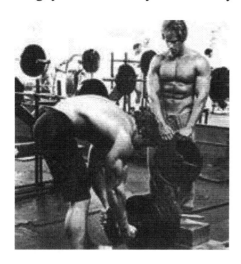

Ric Drasin with Arny

Gold fitted the place out with equipment he'd forged himself in the shop behind his house: signature dumbbells with tapered grips that snugged perfectly in your palm and reinforced benches with closely set stalks that you could push against for leverage in heavy sets. He'd also had the foresight, or dumb luck, to install a bank of skylights in the roof, and the flood of natural light brought photographers down in droves to shoot the half-clad bodybuilders. "There was no heat or A/C, and you could really freeze your ass there in the winter," says Drasin. "We'd go to Joe and bitch, and he'd say, 'So put some damn clothes on,' because guys would train in tiny posing trunks." Gold had no patience for complainers; he made gladiators, not big-armed girls. The son of a Jewish junkman, he'd grown up in the working-class slums of L.A., and he had learned to fight his battles when the Polish toughs hassled him after school. In high school, he began hanging around the Muscle Beach Weight Pen, where the giants of the day posed for boardwalk crowds that grew to the tens of thousands on weekends. Gold got big there and formed lifelong friendships, and though he was gone for long chunks of the next two decades — to the South Pacific in World War II, where he was injured by a torpedo strike, and to South America with the Merchant Marines until he quit sailing in the early 1960s — his heart was firmly docked off Muscle Beach. When the authorities shut the Pen down in 1959, declaring it a magnet for "low morality" (read: big bodies, small swimsuits, horny tourists), Gold's friends scattered to dives like the Dungeon and a new, bare-bones weight pit on Venice Beach. Gold built his gym to bring those beasts home, and charged them the sweetheart rate of $40 a year. "If you didn't have the cash, though — and a lot of them didn't — Joe would let you slide," says Drasin. "Hell, at some point or another, he supported half those guys. Paid 'em to show up and do nothing." The great ones enrolled, and the grotesques did too — the split seemed to run about 50-50. Among the former was **Dave Draper**, the surf-tanned Mr. America whose presence on Weider's magazine covers was a clarion call to bodybuilders, and mighty **Steve Merjanian**, an Armenian strongman who benched 500 pounds for fun. Then there were the wackjobs whose fixed compulsions would have gotten them ousted from other gyms. They included Bob Schott, who'd leave between sets and punch the walls outside until he bled; a huge German named Yogi, garbed head to toe in SWAT gear, who boasted of blowing more than 100 Marines a day in the park behind Camp Pendleton; and Bugsy, who dressed like a Chicago gangster and drank a fifth of vodka while he trained. "So many nuts there," says Drasin. "Then Arnold got famous and was on the cover of every mag. That was when the real fun started."

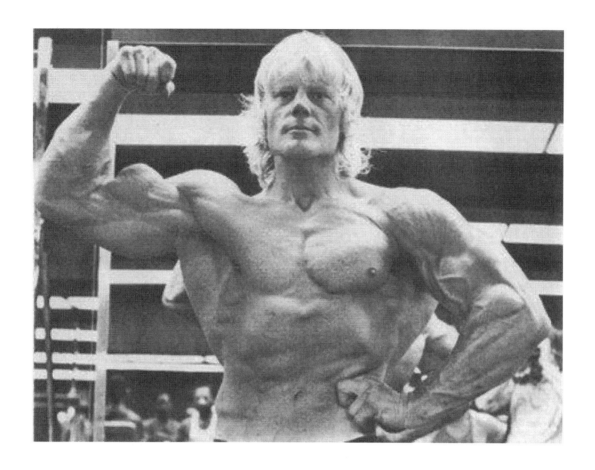

A ripped Draper

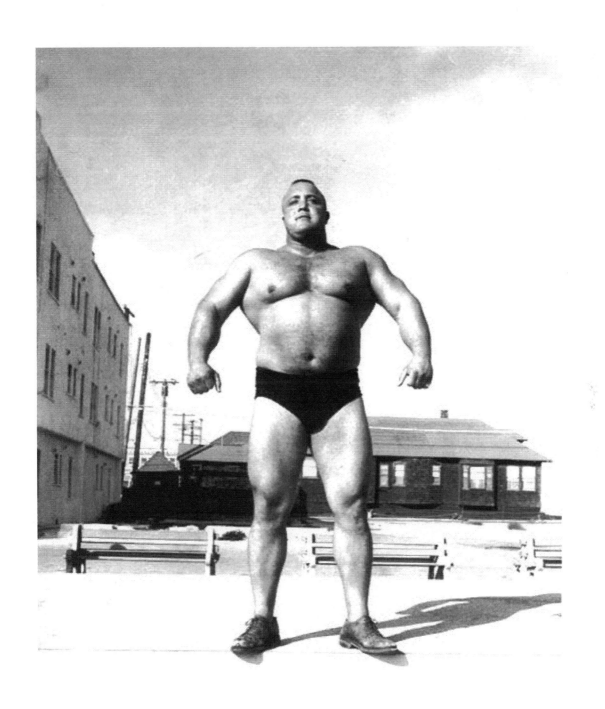

Steve Merjanian

http://www.musclebeach.net/smonica.html

A clip from the Gold's current site:

http://www.goldsgym.com/golds/press-room/press-news/mens-fitness-magazine-muscle-paradise

Men's Fitness Magazine looks back at Muscle Beach and the golden age of Bodybuilding in Venice, California.

04.02.2007

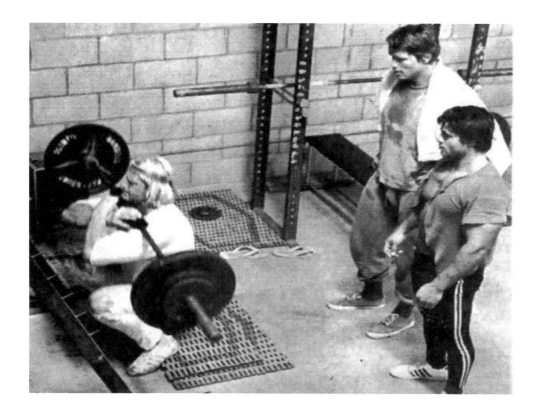

Here is a hard-core trio if there ever was one… hitting it hard at Gold's

If there's a heaven for guys who lift weights, it would have to be a re-creation of the original Muscle Beach of the '40s and '50s, and the bodybuilding scene in Venice, Calif., circa 1970. For a span of about 40 years, everything a guy could enjoy about the fit lifestyle was at his fingertips in Southern California. You could pump iron in a hardcore gym with your buddies all morning and chase girls on the beach all afternoon. You'd go to a restaurant, get a seven-egg omelet for a dollar, and then glance over at the next table and see Steve Reeves or Arnold Schwarzenegger looking back at you. And maybe one day, while you were showing off on the parallel bars on the beach or making a human pyramid with nine other guys, a director would stroll by and ask if you wanted to be in a movie. Of course, a place this perfect couldn't last. But the legacy of the eras survives, and it has transcended the bounds of Los Angeles County and the bodybuilders themselves. Their "good time" has become our everyday routine. Whether we're conscious of it or not, every time we touch a dumbbell, cut a carb from our diet, or strike a pose for our girlfriends, we're emulating an age in which a bunch of so-called muscle heads laid the foundation for modern fitness. And all they were trying to do was have fun in the sun.

The Cradle of Muscle

While the exact origins of Muscle Beach are in dispute, numerous sources credit one woman with starting it all. Kate Giroux, a local physical-education teacher, convinced the city of Santa Monica in the mid-1930s to supply the public with a tumbling mat (though some argue it was just a strip of carpet) and some gymnastics equipment, such as a pommel horse and rings. The gear was set up on 200 square yards of sand just south of Santa Monica pier. "During the Depression, the only recreation for people was the beach," says Bill Howard, a former bodybuilding champion and resident. "It was free." Naturally, local athletes particularly gymnasts and acrobats, at first took notice and began using the equipment to practice their flips and tumbles in the open air, while also escaping their economic blues for a time. Regular folks began to crowd around to watch the stunts, and as the site grew in popularity, city officials supported it, ultimately installing proper weight-training equipment and a platform for stunt shows.

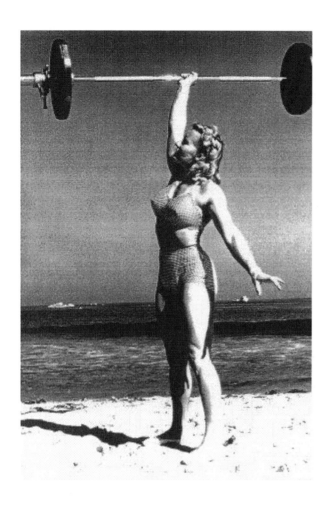

"Pudgy" Stockton

Around this time, Muscle Beach found its first hero, another woman, named Abbye "Pudgy" Stockton. Despite her nickname, Stockton was regarded as 118 pounds of perfect feminine proportions; muscular and strong (she once clean and jerked 135 pounds) yet lean and soft enough to make any man drool. Stockton provided perhaps the earliest evidence that lifting weights didn't have to make women bulky or masculine but could instead give them tremendous strength and athleticism. She and her future husband, Les, were early celebrities on the beach, taking part in weightlifting contests and acrobatics displays that included hand balancing, throwing people into the air and catching them, and stacking 10 or more men toward the sky, one on top of the other. Witness the events just once, people say and it was impossible not to want to get behind the weights and see what you could do, too. During this time, in the midst of World War II, word of the physical and cultural anomaly taking place in Southern California began to spread across the globe. GIs on leave in Santa Monica would get an eyeful and relay pictures and stories to people they met overseas. After the war, there was a buzz practically everywhere people exercised about "this place in California where people run around with their bodies hanging out," says Howard. Though at the time weight training and bodybuilding were considered strange pursuits adopted mostly by narcissists and insecure men, the message most were getting was that on Muscle Beach, no such rebuke existed.

By the mid-40s, everyone who trained, including bodybuilders, circus performers, and movie stunt people, was doing it in Santa Monica. From that motley melting pot, a unique and wonderful camaraderie grew. The performers and contestants at the Muscle Beach shows (presented free of charge) made no money for their efforts, participating instead for the love of sport and for fun. Though they played to audiences of several thousand on a weekly basis, the muscle folk themselves remained a relatively niche group of around 50 members, and they exchanged health and nutrition ideas as well as gut-wrenching workouts. "People would ask us, 'What can I do to get another inch on my arm?' or "How can I get started with exercise?'" says Howard. "We were on the covers of muscle magazines that went around the world, so anybody who was interested in fitness was there." It wasn't long before nearby Hollywood came calling, snatching up champion lifters and bodybuilding pioneers such as **Reg Lewis and Steve Reeves**, and casting them as leads in the popular "sword-and-sandal" epics of the 1950s and early '60s. And suddenly, the men lifting weights on the beach became celebrities. "It would be like you going into the gym and running into someone famous," recalls Howard, but it wasn't a big deal for us. These were the people who were around you every day, and you could train with them."

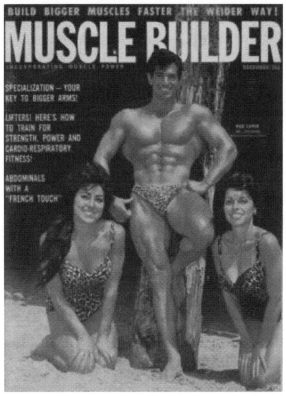

Reg with his wife and a friend

And so things continued... until one day in 1959, when Muscle Beach lost its innocence forever. A scandal erupted in which several bodybuilders were accused of raping underage girls. A week or so later, bulldozers arrived in the middle of the night and leveled everything. The particulars of the case are still highly controversial. "It's not on any police records," says Howard. "Many think the city squashed it." Rumors abound: Some believe the incident was actually statutory rape between only one man and one girl; others say there were more pressing reasons for cleaning out space on the beach (such as to create parking for the city's growing population). Since then, the conspiracy theory has only grown especially since the charges against the accused were eventually dropped.

But most people agree in the end that city leaders believed Muscle Beach had begun to attract a bad element and had to be closed. Though one era had come to an end, weight trainers would not be out of a home for long. The seeds of bodybuilding culture had been sown in Santa Monica, but they would grow to huge proportions just two miles south in Venice.

Bodybuilding's New Mecca

By the early '60s, some of the original Muscle Beach training equipment got the chance to resurface in a new facility in Venice. **Nicknamed the Dungeon**, the gym was a far cry from its old beachfront. Located in a basement that got no sunlight and offered only heavy weights, the locale became a refuge for hardcore bodybuilders and a harbinger of modern fitness's transition from acrobatics to pure muscle. As such, it made the ideal training ground for many famous bodybuilders to get their start, including muscle-magazine icon Dave Draper. The camaraderie lived on as well. The Dungeon had no official owner, and everyone who trained there contributed a few dollars for rent. "It would be a horror story for anybody today," says Draper, winner of several titles, including Mr. Universe, "because the equipment was so dilapidated. But it was wonderful to work under those circumstances. You had to improvise. You didn't know anything better, because this was all you had." While the Muscle Beach lifters worked to regain their footing, other gyms began to pop up as well, all hoping to satisfy a new generation's taste for iron. One such place was **Vince Gironda's Valley gym in the San Fernando**. Of all the training gurus of the day, Gironda remains one of the most respected, as so many of his theories about exercise and nutrition have been proven true. He knew that ab exercises didn't automatically trim the waistline and that fat intake supported testosterone. "Vince helped me win titles when I was in my 40s," says Bill Howard, who took home the Mr. America title in 1974. "He was more into the aesthetic look of muscle," he says. It was this change in thinking and training a move from functional athletic skill to the idea of transforming muscle into art that ultimately gave rise to the bodybuilding of today. Just around the corner, the most famous and enduring training center of its time was getting its start. **Gold's Gym opened in 1965**. Founded by Joe Gold, a bodybuilder who had done a stint in Mae West's traveling male revue, Gold's offered a unique blend of the romance and glamour that the original Muscle Beach personified and the intense bodybuilding training that made the Dungeon and Gironda's gym such productive places to work out. **"The gym was a cinder-block building with nothing on the walls and a concrete floor," says Ric Drasin, a bodybuilder and professional wrestler who frequented Gold's, later designing its legendary muscleman logo.** At about 2,000 square feet, the gym contained some very bare-bones equipment, including homemade barbells and dumbbells enough for about 50 guys at a time to work out with. "It was also just a few blocks from the beach," says Joe Weider, fitness-magazine magnate and mentor to many bodybuilders of the day, "so all the champions gravitated to it." After an intense workout, the men could walk to Venice Beach and work on their tans or show off their pumps to gawking onlookers. It wasn't long before Dave Draper and most of the future cast of *Pumping Iron* (including a 245-pound, gap-toothed Austrian) were calling Gold's home sometimes quite literally. Since the cash prizes in bodybuilding at that time were paltry at best, Gold allowed a number of homeless bodybuilders to sleep on the gym's shower-room floor and even on the roof. "Joe wasn't looking to make a lot of money," says Draper, recalling that most of Gold's early members weren't even required to pay gym dues. "He was just putting a place together for the guys." Gold's enormous generosity went hand in hand with his ferocious enforcement of gym rules. No music, no dropping weights, and no silly behavior, or you were out (nevertheless, stories of crazed antics remain see "Muscle Memories," at right, for some examples).

The strict atmosphere provided for some balls-to-the-wall workouts, the likes of which set a precedent for how to conduct oneself as a bodybuilder. **"The first thing that came to my mind when I walked in the first time was that I had to train harder," says Lou Ferrigno, who had already captured back-to-back Mr. Universe titles when he arrived in 1976**. "It was all blood, sweat, and tears in there." More than a construction site for monstrous physiques, Gold's also served as a cultural meeting ground. Whether bodybuilders arrived seeking greater motivation, the fellowship of training around icons such as Schwarzenegger, or a chance to test their resolve against that of other determined champions, men flocked to Gold's from around the world. "And they would be accepted right off the bat," says Drasin. "If you were from another country, that was even better. It was a melting pot of ideas, and everyone got along." For these reasons, the gym came to be called **the Mecca of bodybuilding.**

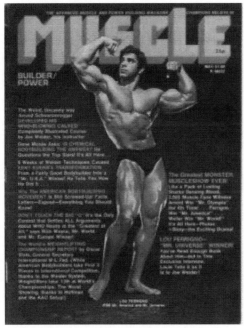
Big Lou

Muscle Media

Although Gold's reputation was solid, it took Joe Weider (and his magazines *Muscle Builder* and *Muscle Power* forefathers of our own *Men's Fitness*) to cement the gym's legendary status. In an age when bodybuilding was reviled by the media, Weider celebrated it, distributing information on the sport to newsstands around the world. "I believed that men who worked out and were strong were comparable to the ancient Greeks," says Weider, who sold his magazine empire in 2002 and recently co-authored the book *Brothers of Iron*. "The Greeks did feats of strength, and our bodybuilders would more or less do the same with their workouts. I wanted to carry on the Greek tradition building the perfect body." By photographing bodybuilders in loincloths and sandals against the backdrop of California's ocean and canyons, Weider created a heroic, cinematic, and indelible image of the pumped-up male body and he sold it with great success. Arnold Schwarzenegger saw it in Austria and dedicated his life to looking the same way.

Lou Ferrigno saw it in Brooklyn and did likewise. "That got our attention," says Ferrigno. **"Everyone knew that to be the best, you had to come to California and be a part of Gold's Gym."** Though Weider did much to publicize the benefits of training with weights, he wasn't the first to do so. **Bob Hoff man,** a weightlifter, had been publishing a revolutionary fitness magazine called *Strength and Health* since the mid-1930s. Hoffman's agenda was very different from Weider's. He wanted the world to know that weightlifting (explosive lifts such as the clean and jerk and the snatch, as seen in the Olympics) was the best route to athleticism and power. (Hoffman, like the rest of the planet, believed that bodybuilding was self-indulgent and, worse, nonfunctional.) However, Weider shrewdly observed that bodybuilding training, with its attention to building each muscle group evenly and minimizing body fat would ultimately have broader appeal. "I figured that for every one guy who wanted to lift heavy weights, there were at least 10 guys who wanted a beautiful body," says Weider. "When World War II began, the Army took the weightlifters, and weightlifting competition was dead. That's when bodybuilding really began to rise." Though Hoffman continued to fight Weider and his bodybuilders, his magazine lost momentum. **By the 1960s, Weider's publications ruled the muscle media**. Fitness aficionados no longer cared if you could lift 500 pounds but it was particularly important that you *looked* like you could. The magazines' focus on aesthetic body development buried the more attainable athletic look and functionality that ruled the day at Muscle Beach. Back then, physique contests were only one part of the festivities, and they usually included some exhibition of strength and flexibility in addition to muscle posing. Now bodybuilders would only be required to flex onstage. The quest for gargantuan size and sharper definition led to the popularity of then-legal anabolic steroids, and the overall health of the participants became more questionable. "I was a natural bodybuilder for 15 years," says Bill Howard. "But then I couldn't get into a contest. We'd lie and say to each other that we weren't using steroids, but then we'd look at each other in the gym and think, "That son of a bitch is, so I'm going to, too!""

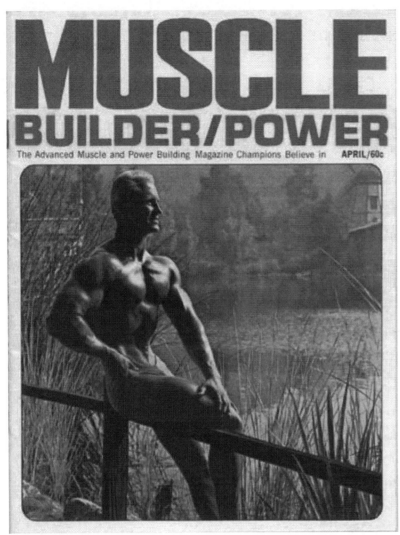

Bill Howard

The Golden Age

Muscle historians and fans refer to the 1960s and '70s as the golden age of bodybuilding. It was the era of Arnold, bodybuilding's all-time most charismatic and visible champion, and *Pumping Iron*, the docudrama that introduced muscle mass to the masses. The physiques were awe inspiring yet conceivably attainable, and as with Muscle Beach before it, men trained to be part of a brotherhood not for a purse. But mostly it was a helluva fun time to be alive.

Muscle Beach had a resurrection of sorts in the Venice Beach "pit," a small, city-run club overlooking the Pacific where bodybuilders could train outdoors again. While the serious training was still done a few blocks away at Gold's, the pit allowed the bodybuilders to show off for crowds and work on their suntans. "They would save one for the sun," says Howard. "After their main workout, they'd go out and do a little extra work at the pit, showboat a little, and have fun with the public." The lifters particularly enjoyed attention from the ladies. "We didn't really need pickup lines," says Ferrigno.

"The women felt an instant attraction it was like having a bear for a boyfriend. They felt protected and safe with us." Though L.A. today is notorious for its gridlock traffic, that wasn't so in the 1970s. "It was easy to get around," says Drasin, and even beachfront property wasn't out of a young man's price range. "I paid $225 a month for two bedrooms, two baths, and a sundeck," he recalls. "That's probably $2,000 today." Bodybuilding food wasn't hard to come by, either. The men had their fill at places like Zucky's Deli and German's, "where you could get a seven-egg omelet with ham and cheese for a buck," says Drasin. Afterward, they would drive to the House of Pies for dessert. And if you think they needed a lot of cardio to burn it off, think again. "We used to get lean by using higher repetitions and a strict diet," says Howard. "If you were doing eight to 10 reps normally, you switched to 14 to 18 to get lean and hard."

Muscle Goes Mainstream

Ultimately, the golden age outgrew itself. The fame that *Pumping Iron*, the Weider magazines, and Arnold Schwarzenegger brought to the area led to a mass influx of would-be bodybuilders and businessmen looking to capitalize on the craze. "All the guys who had made bodybuilding what it was had gotten older and moved on," says Drasin. "New personalities began coming in. The training changed and there were more steroids. And there started to be other places to train, too. It wasn't only in California anymore." But the more bodybuilding and fitness spanned the globe, the more people became nostalgic for their Muscle Beach and Venice origins. Today, these gyms and beaches are viewed by competitive bodybuilders and fitness enthusiasts alike as sacred ground, giving "the Mecca of bodybuilding" a more literal meaning. **In 1991, Howard finally saw his beloved Muscle Beach restored when the city of Venice allowed him to refurbish and reopen the weight pit under the official name of "Muscle Beach." He now hosts contests and shows there that are akin to what he first saw 50 years ago in Santa Monica.** Weight training today is bigger than ever, and it's the No. 1 fitness activity among regular folks. Nutritional-supplement sales are a multibillion-dollar industry, and diet books sell millions. "Every diet you see whether it's the Zone or anything else's all the same," says Drasin. "Everything is a bodybuilder diet.

It's all about high protein and low carbs to build muscle and lose fat." Even Gold's Gym has worldwide appeal, with gyms in 26 countries and a membership that numbers more than three million. Ferrigno, who still trains in Venice, has come to grips with the expansion while also carrying the torch of yesteryear. "Nowadays, we have actors and rock stars and regular people working out here," he says. "But everybody respects the bodybuilders because this is our home. We got here first."

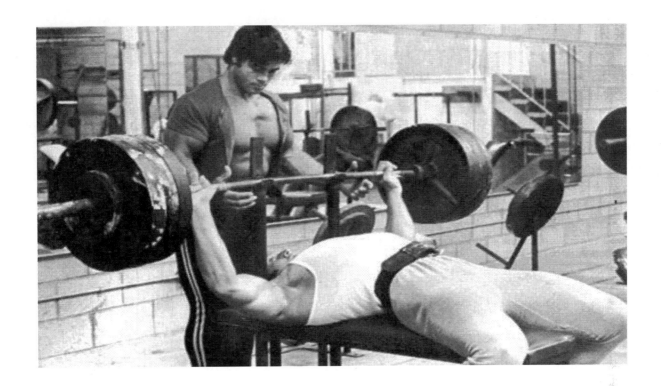

Franco spotting Mike Katz at Gold's.

The following piece about Ed Corney shows Ed training under the watchful eye of the "Master Blaster", Weider himself at Gold's

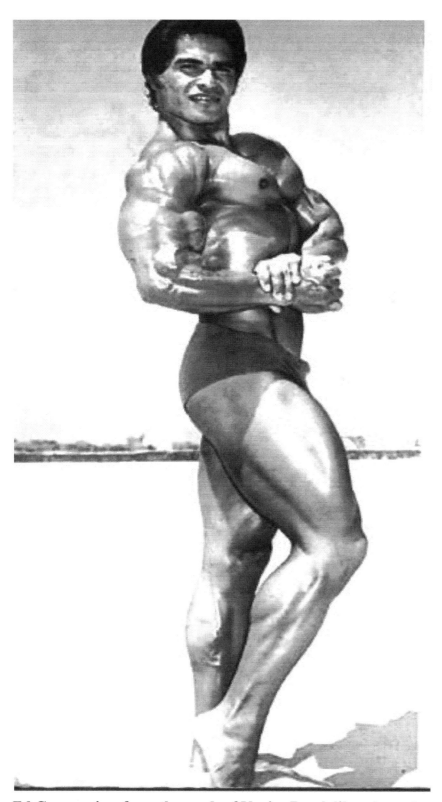
Ed Corney rises from the sands of Venice Beach like a legendary Greek god. His outstanding muscularity and flawless symmetry have catapulted him into the international physique spotlight

ED CORNEY
THE INCREDIBLE HAWAIIAN TRANSPLANT

by Dick Tyler

I remember some jerk in a gym say once that all physique contests were the same. "You see one you've seen them all," he said in a matter of fact way as he put down the two pound dumbbell he was using and shuffled his fat, hairy body with the skinny arms and legs into the shower.

It always intrigues me the way some people will so in a muscle gym to "get in shape" and suddenly become authorities on everything in bodybuilding. By this particular goof's reasoning, all books are the same so all we have to do is read one and we've read them all.

That's the great thing about bodybuilding—the contestants are as individual in their personalities as they are in their physiques. Sure, you can always find someone who reminds you of this or that person but in the last analysis, Larry Scott is Larry Scott and Arnold Schwarzenegger is Arnold Schwarzenegger. The only similarity is that their last names begin with the letter "S"

You'd never guess it but I love going to physique contests. Bodybuilders are the wildest bunch of dedicated hard-nosed, single-purposed men you ever wanted to know. There's never a dull moment either in the audience or backstage. If you've never been to a physique contest—just try

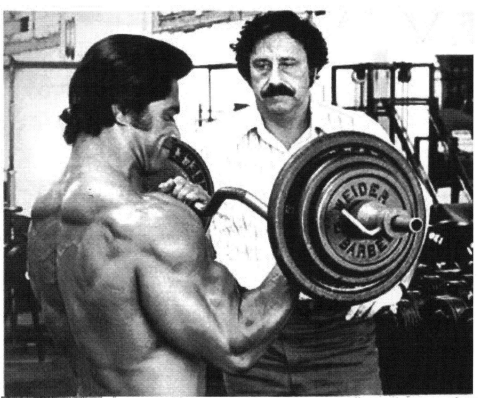

Scrutiny time Joe "The Master" Weider stands over Ed during a session at Gold's. Now that Joe is on the West Coast he can personally supervise more and more rising stars. Careful supervision and application of Weider training methods are essential if Ed is to continue to improve.

it and see.

A couple of years ago, I went to an AAU show in downtown Los Angeles. I used to enjoy waiting to see what new men would make their appearance in a local meet. No matter how great the present champs are there is always someone climbing up the ladder to become tomorrow's hero. As the house lights darkened a hush fell over the audience and the contest began. There were the usual oldtimers who picked up fringe trophies year after year and there was a sprinkling of new boys to make the show entertaining, then they announced the name of Ed Corney.

On to the pedestal jumped a sun-bronzed athlete who made everyone sit up. It wasn't that his arms were so large or that his abs were so well defined or that his legs were so well balanced. What made most of the audience so impressed was that he had so many good things placed in just the right places. To put the icing on the cake, he was able to display in the most artisitic posing routine I had seen in years. Often a bodybuilder will think that a posing routine is great if it is weird. I've seen them get into all kinds of contorted positions and twirl around like a ballet dancer in an effort to dazzle you with movements and obscure the vacuum left by the muscles they don't have. This wasn't the case with Corney. He had the ammunition and he knew how to deliver it. Of all the men that appeared in that contest that evening--he was the one

I remember. I couldn't tell you who won the event, but I sure remembered Ed Corney.

Ed was one of those late starters. He didn't begin serious weight training until he was 25 years old and he didn't enter his first physique contest until almost 10 years after that. Fortunately he's made up for lost time. Ed is the kind of person who takes his time in deciding a course of action but when he does decide, he

An expression of dedication. The road to success has been paved by hours of grueling work and Ed Corney has been more than willing to give 110% each and every workout. Note the superb frontal deltoid separation as he strains through one final rep.

18

clamps on and rides to the end of the line.

Born and raised in Hawaii, he eventually moved to Northern California. It was here that he met Millard Williamson and the course of his life was changed Williamson is one of the best physique men in that part of the country. It's little wonder that Ed was astounded when he first saw him One of Corney's favorite sports is volleyball. It also happens to be the favorite of Williamson. After a game they played was over Ed introduced himself to the man he had been playing against just a few minutes before

"I've never seen muscle like yours." said Ed "Did you get it from training with weights?"

"That's right." replied Williamson. "Weights are the fastest and most complete way of developing muscle ever devised."

"I always thought that weights would slow you down, but you're one of the best volleyball players I've ever seen."

Williamson looked astonished. "Weights don't slow you down. In fact, proper weight training and nutrition only tend to make you faster and better coordinated."

Corney couldn't argue with what he had seen with his own eyes

In the days that followed Ed kept thinking how he too would like to have muscles like Williamson. Why couldn't he? After all he had the proper amount of arms and legs What was to keep him from building them the way he wanted to? With this idea in mind Ed became a man of great physical purpose. Under the tutelage of Williamson, Ed's great natural potential began to assert itself. For years it began to assert itself. In fact, it asserted itself so much that people began to wonder why this physical phenomenon didn't enter any shows

Ed always responded that he wanted to train only for health and appearance and not for the cups he could win. Still his naturally competitive spirit kept digging on his biceps and urging him to get in there and try the waters of bodybuilding competition

The right moment seemed to arrive. The year was 1967 and they were holding the Mr. Fremont contest in the Central California area. The pressure mounted. Ten years of it and at last Ed Corney entered his first event. He won the title handily

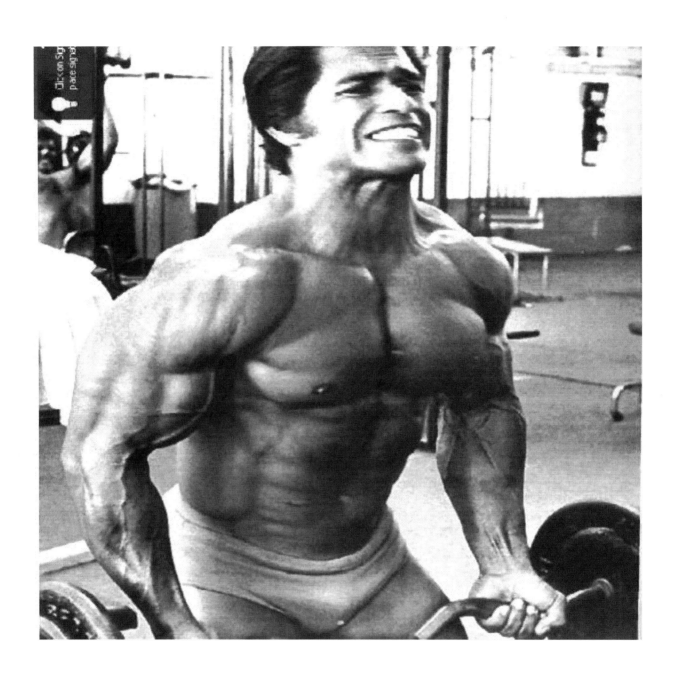

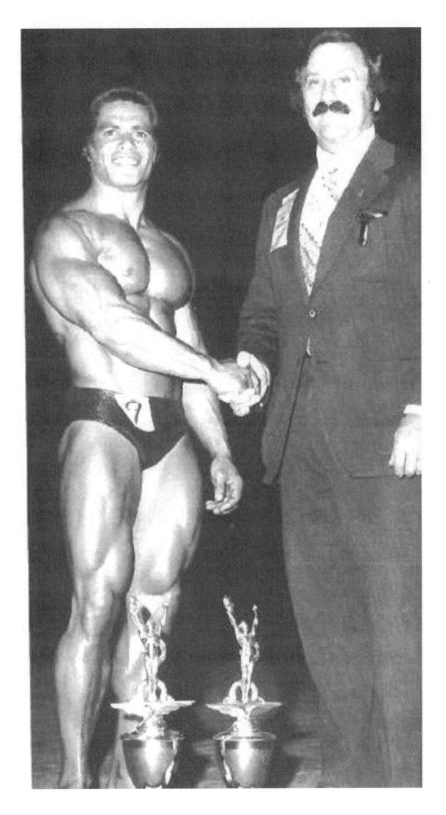

And here is where the hours in the gym pay off Joe Weider proudly congratulates Ed on becoming the latest in a long and noble line of Mr USA after Ed's victory last fall in New York A fitting tribute to the methods and the man

OK, let's finish up the section on Gold's with this little gem;

Mr. America Magazine, Vol 2, No 4, Page 10, July 1959

Modest to a fault, retiring, self-effacing Joe Gold has been little known in the bodybuilding world. Here is a true champion who can inspire the man of 35 as well as the teen-ager to build a physique of incomparable excellence. It is with the thought of revealing to you one of the best-built but least-known physiques starts that we ask you to meet

JOE GOLD

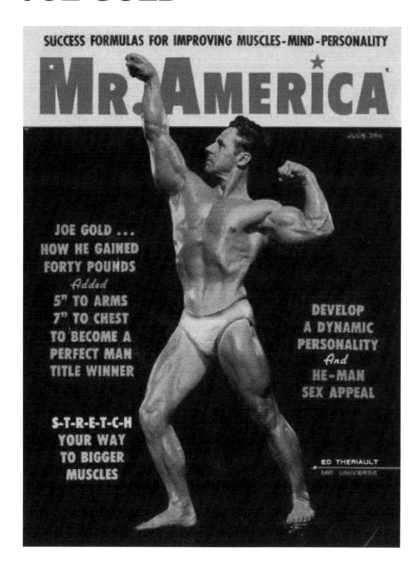

America's Undiscovered Physique Champion

by Joe Weider, Trainer of The Champions

One of the greatest of present-day bodybuilders is virtually unknown to the muscle world at large. In an era when the white spotlight of publicity is turned on far lesser champions Joe Gold remains unique. He **avoids** publicity, **shuns** physique contests . . . and you'll never find him spreading his lats on Muscle Beach! It is because he is so modest and retiring that little is known of this stellar bodybuilder. I first saw Joe Gold when he was appearing with the famous Mae West show in New York. I had gone one night to get some up-to-date stories of Dick Dubois, Armand Tanny and George Eiferman who were also members of her troupe. And as I sat in the audience enjoying the show I was stunned by the physique of a man whom I remembered vaguely from earlier pictures, but who would certainly be indelibly etched in my mind from that moment on. Later I went backstage to greet my other friends who in turn introduced me to Joe. "Great Scott, man . . . where have **you** been all this time?" I enthused. "Oh, I've been around," was the shy and diffident answer. "You certainly can't have been around very much or I would have heard of you before now." I exclaimed. "Oh, I've never gone in for physique contests and muscle shows . . . as a matter of fact, this is the first time I've ever done show work like this. I guess that's why no one knows very much about me." "But Joe, think what an inspiration you could be for the countless thousands of men who are thirty-five and over who think they're too old to train. At your age you are the **proof positive** that weight-training can keep **any** man's body in **peak condition**, perfectly-**functioning**, wonderfully **flexible** and muscularly **coordinated** far into later life. "I feel that I **personally** mustn't let the opportunity pass to tell your story and to show the bodybuilding world how magnificently you are developed and how superbly you keep that development in tip-top shape." Okay, if you think I'll be of help," Joe agreed. And so here is the story of America's **undiscovered** physique champion. When Joe Gold started barbell training he stood five feet eight inches tall and weighted a miserable 135 pounds. Because of his under-par physical condition he was always shy, lacked self-confidence . . . was afraid of meeting people. He was the skinniest kid on the block. Because he lived in a very rough neighborhood he was continually being drawn into fights and brawls by those who glorified in bullying the underdog. Too many beatings caused Joe to retreat into himself . . . to avoid others whenever he could and live in a little world of his own imagination. But like so many other young lads . . . like so many of our Weider champions, Joe had the wisdom to realize that this state of affairs couldn't go on forever. He reasoned that he had the same God-given right to a happy, healthy life as anyone else . . . and he further reasoned that the only way he could achieve that happier life was to develop his body the best he could. How to go about it? That was the question. About this time, as though in answer to a prayer, Joe Gold met famous Harold Zinkin - one of the most outstanding of West Coast bodybuilders - who inspired him to take up weight-training. At Harold's suggestion, Joe joined the East Los Angeles Barbell Club and began a bright new adventure in living the bodybuilder's way of life! Under Harold Zinkin's expert guidance, Joe made rapid progress right from the start. To Joe it seemed as if his muscles had lain fallow for years just waiting to be stimulated. Every day saw amazing progress as his muscles just "soaked-up" exercise like sponges. His gains were so rapid; his muscles grew so full and shapely, that in just six months he had slapped 30 pounds of solid muscle on his young frame. Then he took up wrestling and boxing to better defend himself. Needless to say the neighborhood "bully beatings" soon stopped, once the hoodlums had a taste of the Gold strong right arm.

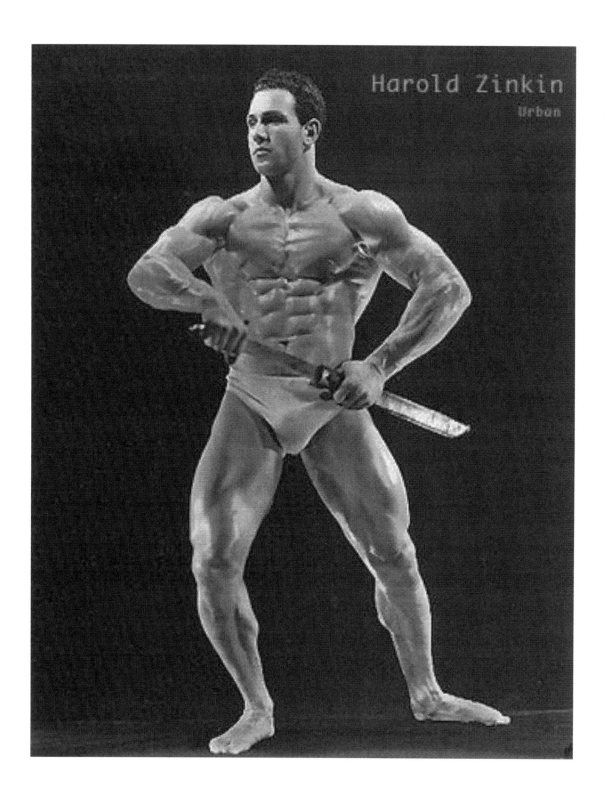

The taste of his first victories was sweet indeed to Joe Gold . . . but was nothing to compare with the new lease on life that barbell training had given him. And the lessons he learned in the care and development of his body have remained with Joe throughout the 35 years of his life. Today, he gives the same scrupulous attention to every detail of his workouts . . . the same complete concentration . . . the same directed purpose with which he began twenty years before.

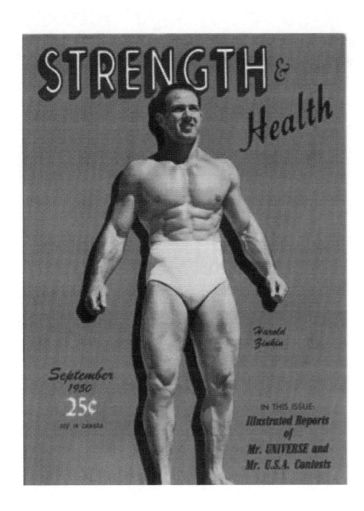

Here is another shot of Zinkin, gracing the cover of Strength & Health. Zinkin co-authored a book about Muscle beach;

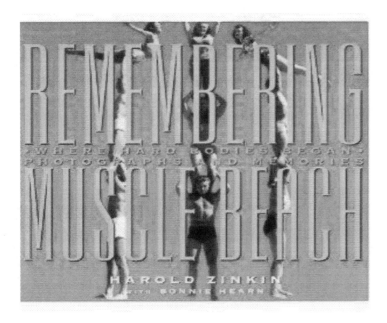

Joe does not **spare** his muscles . . . he works 'em **hard**. He's no "keep fit-er", no "wand drill-er". He doesn't go in for light calisthenics and the "business men's" exercises that are recommended by some for the 35-plus individual. Every workout is a **tussle** with the **muscle!** Today, the Gold physique racks up some impressive measurements . . . like these: Height, 5'10" . . . Weight, 190 . . . Chest (normal) 49" . . . Waist 32" . . . Thigh, 25" . . . Calves, 16" . . . Upper-arms, 17 1/2" and forearms, 13 1/2". In exercising his body, Joe Gold uses many of the famous Weider Principles, particularly the **Split Routine** method, **Muscle Flushing** technique and Weider **Super-Set Principle**. He especially favors the **Split Routine** method because he feels that he cannot adequately exercise his **entire** body in **one** workout. In splitting his routine, he is able to work each body part fully three times each week. He believes that too many bodybuilders mistakenly attempt a complete body workout each training day, that they tire too soon and therefore permit some muscle group to be unexercised or exercised too half-heartedly.

The exercise photographs show here simply do not do Joe justice. We had only one hour to shot them because he had to catch a plane for the next city where the Mae West show was to appear. But they do give you a general idea of his massiveness and shape.

* Sorry but I don't have the referenced pictures from the article here *

Here is his routine:

MONDAY-WEDNESDAY-FRIDAY
Shoulder-Lats-Arms-Abdominals

SHOULDERS

1. Press Behind Neck. 5 sets, 5 reps - 165 pounds.
2. Compound Lateral Raises (raising dumbbells **forward** and **upward overhead**, returning them **sideways** and **downward**). 5 x 5 - 45-pound dumbbells.

Joe works out very fast, going very quickly from one exercise to another. Immediately after completing the last set of Compound Lateral Raises, he goes right into his arm exercises.

ARMS

1. Two-dumbbells Curl. 5 sets, 5 reps - 75-pound dumbbells.
2. Dumbbell French Curl. 5 sets, 5 reps - 120-pound dumbbell.
3. Dumbbell Concentration Curl. 5 sets, 10 reps - 50-pound dumbbell.
4. Barbell Triceps Curl. 5 sets, 10 reps - 75-pound dumbbells

Quite an arm program isn't it . . . one of the most effective we've seen. Now, after a pause for recuperation, Joe attacks his back muscles.

BACK

1. Dumbbell Rowing Motion. 5 sets, 10 reps - 100-pound dumbbell.
2. Pulldown on Lat Machine. 5 sets, 10 reps - 170 pounds.
3. Back-of-neck Chins. 5 sets, 6 reps with 50 pounds attached to waist.

ABDOMINALS

1. Leg Raises. 3 sets, 50 reps, sometimes on abdominal board, sometimes on chinning bar - depending on energy reserve.
2. Situps. 3 sets, 50 reps, on high incline abdominal board.

TUESDAY-THURSDAY-SATURDAY
Chest-Legs-Abdominals

CHEST

Joe's chest work is done in **Super-Sets** and comprises two exercises, with one exercise as an alternate. He either uses the Heavy Barbell Bench Press **or** the Heavy Incline Bench Press, **Super-Setted** with Heavy Bent Arm Lateral Raises.

1. Bench Press. 5 sets, 5 reps - 205 pounds.
2. Bent-Arm Lateral Raise. 5 sets, 5 reps - 90 pound dumbbells.

Joe performs 1 set of the Bench Press, **going without pause** into 1 set of the Bent-Arm Lateral Raise . . . continuing set-for-set in this manner until 5 sets of each exercise have been performed. He rests as little as possible between **Super-Sets** to keep the tremendous muscle **pump** this particular **Super-Set** effects.

On Tuesday he uses the Flat Bench Press in the **Super-Set**, on Thursday he substitutes the Incline Bench Press, and so on, alternating workout-for-workout to give the entire pectoral area a thorough workout.

LEGS

1. Squats. 5 sets, 5 reps - 300 pounds.
2. Leg Curls. 5 sets, 9 reps - very heavy weight.
3. Heel Raise (Donkey). 6 sets, 20 reps.
4. Leg Press. 6 sets, 9 reps - heaviest possible weight.

ABDOMINALS

The same abdominal program used on Monday, Wednesday and Friday is performed on Tuesday, Thursday and Saturday. Into all his exercises Joe Gold pours the most intense concentration. he rarely talks to anyone when training, and he watches himself closely in the mirror to see that the muscles under exercise are working in the exact manner they are intended to. Such patience and zeal are frequently encountered among younger bodybuilders, but in a man who as reached the prime of life they are rare indeed. "I believe it is my great zest for exercise, my determination to keep my body youthful, to avert the slouchiness and lack of muscular tone that older men invariable acquire, that make each of my workouts so progressively successful," says Joe. "I believe that any man of thirty-five and upward can do the same if he will allot himself just a couple of hours each day or three days a week to scientific, modern exercise." Certainly Joe Gold is living proof . . . and what he preaches should be heard and heeded by every man who is discovering that truly "time marches on".

Chapter 5   Abe Goldberg's Gym, New York City

The following pages contain a couple of Muscle Builder articles from the '50s, written by Abe Goldberg, who's gym was an east coast rival to the west coast gyms we have been discussing.

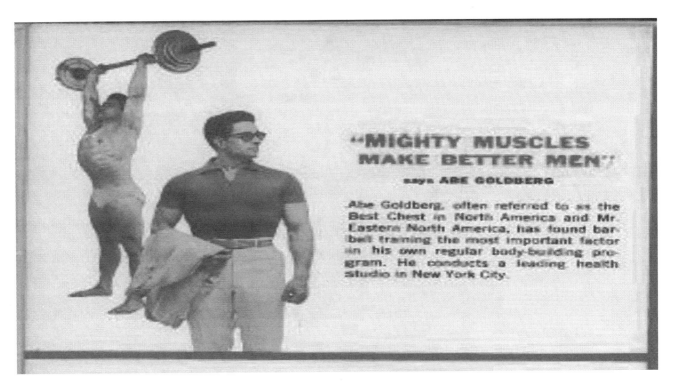

Interestingly, the picture above is from the same Billiard training booklet that featured Bruce Randall earlier on in the book, and in fact, Abe shared the modeling job fairly equally with Bruce in the book.

The picture above was shown right next to this "before" picture of Randall at 400 plus pounds;

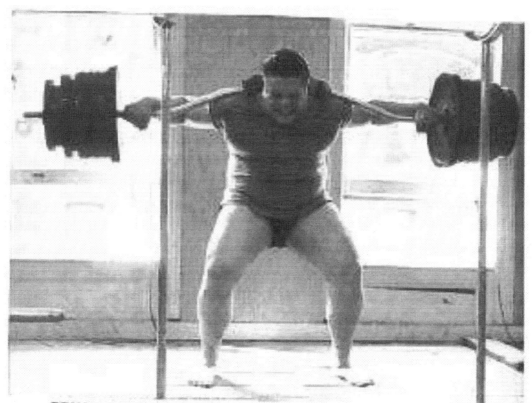

BRUCE RANDALL, AT 401 POUNDS, DOING THE FRONT BEND OR "GOOD MORNING EXERCISE" WITH A 620-LB. WEIGHT.

The following is a page from the booklet featuring Abe as the model;

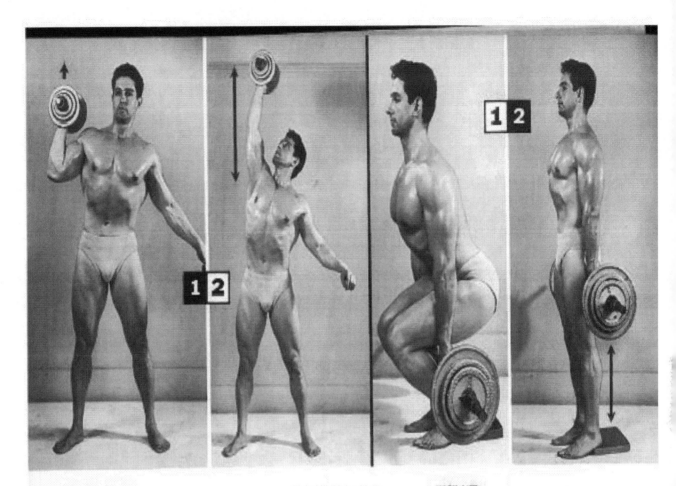

ONE ARM PRESS:

Dumbbell is held at Press Position, and pressed up until arm locks. Lower and repeat.

Recommended: Reps, 3 Sets

HACK LIFT:

Heels on block, in squatting position, grasp barbell, raise to standing position, slowly squat, and repeat.

Recommended: Reps, 4 Sets

ADVANCED EXERCISES

The first Muscle Builder article I have is this one titled

"**Muscle Building is my Business**"

business

BY ABE GOLDBERG
New York City's Foremost Gym Instructor
Gymnasium located at
80 Clinton Street, New York

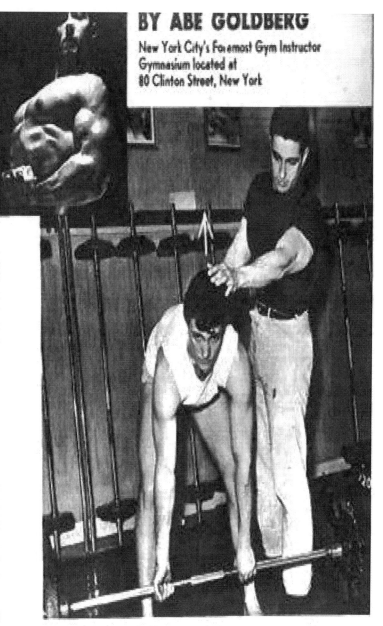

An intimate trip through one of America's most successful bodybuilding gyms where making supermen out of weaklings is an everyday affair.

I DON'T expect to ever retire a millionaire, but already I'm wealthy, richer than most.

I'm not speaking about dollars and cents, but rather of the mental satisfaction of knowing that I have helped thousands to a new, better, healthier and happier life through bodybuilding. Such a true feeling of accomplishment can never be weighed off in terms of money in the bank — it rises above all material wealth.

Often at night, when my last pupil has walked through the doors, out of my gym, I sit back and reflect. Then I am proud *(Continued on page 52)*

Abe takes a personal interest in all pupils. Here he is guiding Joey Rascona in correct performance of the deadlift. —ION.

RAY JIMINEZ

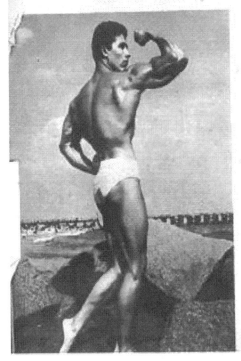

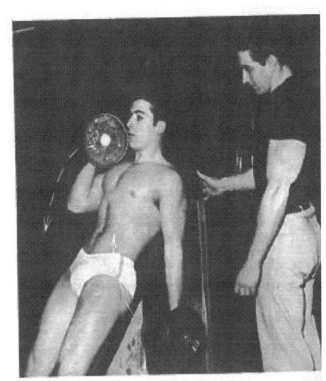

John Alissi performs incline bench curls as Abe watches.

ANOTHER GREAT "V-MAN" CREATION!

the *Hi-Fashion* GAUCHO • • • • • • •

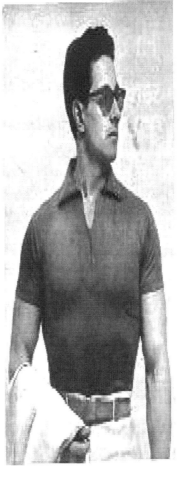

As "cool" as "a breeze in March"
As "smart" as "Paris in N. Y."

THE V-man "Hi-Fashion" is the smartest, coolest gaucho you've ever worn. Made of fine combed cotton... with the "Permathol finish". "Permathol" is the miracle process that guarantees the "Hi-Fashion" against shrinking or stretching out of shape... even after countless washings.

The "Hi-Fashion" gaucho is expertly tailored and designed to meet all the body-builders requirements. It hugs the body like our "V-SHIRT", form fitting and real snug. No bagging or wrinkling like ordinary shirts.

The "Hi-Fashion" comes in beautiful colors: Black, Navy, Powder Blue, and White. The collars are smartly edged in contrasting shades.

BE FIRST! ORDER NOW!

SUPPLY LIMITED

ABE GOLDBERG,
80 Clinton St., New York, N. Y.

Dear Abe,
Please rush me a V-Man Hi-Fashion Gaucho. Enclosed find $3.95 in check or money order.

SIZE: COLOR:
Small (35-38) .... Black ....
Medium (39-42) .... Navy ....
Larger (43-44) .... Pow. Bl. ....
                            White ....

Name ....

---

now that you know how he progressed step by step from his first work-out, you should find following his example easy. I don't feel that Leroy was lucky, or that his present championship arms are the result of any accident. He built them through training, regular hard work, and you can do the same. Just be as determined in your training efforts as he was and you may end up with a pair of arms that rank with the largest in the world. Wishing for them won't get you anywhere. You must work to develop them, the same as Leroy and every champion did. So how about starting to build those 19" upper arms right now!

Muscle Building Is My Business

(Continued from page 24)

that muscle building is my business and I wouldn't change my profession for any other in the world.

Too few people, in my opinion, understand exactly what takes place in a bodybuilding gymnasium. Readers of magazines and even members of gyms usually only see the surface, never digging down into the heart and soul of the business and learning how it affects so many lives for the better.

Making physique champions is only one phase of my work. It is important, of course, for without these stars bodybuilding would lose much of its inspirational attraction. Much of my time is spent in guiding the stars, pupils who have reached the heights of championship acclaim. These are the finished products, the stellar attractions of my trade.

Men like Ray Jiminez, Raul Pacheco, Enrico Tomas, Marvin Eder, Artie Zeller, each is a great champion and each has won fame and glory for himself and bodybuilding. Without proper guidance none would have reached the top. With it, they rank with the best in the world. These men of course realize the importance of proper instruction, and that is why each came to me after training elsewhere, so that they could benefit from the Weider System which is taught in my gym. More than one of these stars was stuck in his training, discouraged with progress, when he joined. I have had the satisfaction of seeing how the Weider System made each a champion and have experienced the Pleasure of knowing that the methods I teach are the greatest in the world.

Still, while these celebrated stars are flexing their powerful muscles in exercise, and other pupils watch them in admiration, hoping some day to achieve an equal degree of physical fame, the daily drama that takes place at my desk remains almost unnoticed, yet it is here that the life blood of bodybuilding is formed.

Day in and day out there is a steady stream of men and boys, of all ages, shapes, and heights who are weak, often sickly, thoroughly discouraged with their way of life, who come into my gym, sit down by my desk and look to me for words of hope that their physical conditions can be improved.

It is with these, the discouraged, often confused beginners in bodybuilder that the professional instructor finds his greatest challenge as well as his biggest opportunity for doing the most good.

The questions these people ask are the same ones any beginner in bodybuilding might. Remaining in them is some remnant of all the old, long disproven fallacies of weight training. The instructor who answers their questions honestly, sensibly, can dispel doubts, convert them to bodybuilding and benefit mankind.

Typical of the type of questions asked me daily, often 10 or 20 times a day by different individuals with monotonous repetition, are: "Won't weight training damage my heart?" "Isn't it true that lifting weights can cause rupture?" "Will I become muscle bound?" "People tell me that training with weights is very hard work, and that once you begin you can never stop or else you'll become fat and flabby!" "Isn't it true that not everyone can build a good body. That some people fail regardless how hard they try?" "Aren't free hand exercises more natural, better for the health than weight training?"

Patiently I listen to their quiries, even though I have long since known by heart just what the questions would be. And one by one I attack the fallacies, pointing out the errors in each.

I tell them the story of Prof. Karpovich, connected with Springfield College, and of the research this learned scientist has done in the physical reaction of weight training. His research covered more than 33,000 cases of weight trainers, men and boys who have been training with weights from only a few months, up to more than 25 years. In this entire group, "not one instance of adverse heart reaction was revealed. In fact, as a whole the group showed a surprising immunity to physical injury and common disease. I show them pictures of John Grimek taken 20 years ago, and let them compare these with those of the present, showing how his physique has actually improved with the years, which certainly would not be possible if he suffered injury to the heart or rupture. Then I speak about my personal friend Barton Horvath who began weight training when he was 16 years of age, weak and skinny, probably in worse physical shape than they. I then tell them the story about his perfect working record, possibly one of the best in the world. Since Barton started to work for his living after leaving school, more than 20 years ago, he has never missed a day on the job due to illness. In this way I impress my visitors with the fact that there is more to bodybuilding than developing muscle. It is an investment in life-time good health which can be used by the individual for success in life.

Next I take out my scrap book of photos and clippings, showing pictures of Roland La Starza, Randy Turpin, famous boxers. Of the great tennis champion Frank Sedgeman, of the decathlon champion, Bob Mathias, of the world's greatest pole vaulter, Rev. Bob Richards, of Lou Thesz, champion wrestler, of Gideon Fortune, discus great, and many, many other stars of the sport world. "What is your purpose of showing these pictures," they ask? My answer—"Just read the publicity clippings now and see where in each there is mention that all these men train with weights to help them in their sports. NOW do you believe that weight training makes a man slow, muscle bound?"

By this time, the prospective pupil is pretty nearly sold. But I don't like to let matters rest there. Now the time has come for me to put in some clinchers. Then, I explain the principle behind weight training. To do this, I generally ask my visitor to step out onto the gym floor. "See that fellow over there? The exercise he is performing is called a two arm curl. It develops the muscles of the upper arms. See the weight he is using? It weighs 15 pounds! This young man has just started, he has been with me only a week. You will have to agree that he doesn't appear to be straining himself. Now, look at that Hercules exercising over there. I point to where Marvin Eder is standing. Look—you can see that he is performing the same exercise, BUT—he is using 200 pounds!"

I continue—"Now, the 15 pounds used by the beginner and the 200 pounds used by that champion are doing each, equal good. The beginner with his weak, underdeveloped muscles benefits from weights which are in direct keeping with his strength and physical condition. Soon he grows stronger, progressing gradually, without strain, until he can use 20, 30, 50 and even 100 pounds in this same exercise. And when he reaches the point where he can use heavier weights, his muscles will have developed so much stronger that he will be able to do the exercise just as easily then as he did with the very light weight as a beginner. In time, if he continues to train, he will develop huge muscles, similar to that man over there who is using 200 pounds. Then, even 200 pounds will be well within his exercise limit and he will be able to use it without strain."

I let this sink in and then continue. "That is the secret behind weight training. It makes absolutely no difference how weak or underdeveloped you presently are. You start training with a poundage that you handle easily. In a few work-outs a difference is noticed and you will be able to add a few pounds to the weight used. And it continues that way, you growing stronger, better developed all the time, and never straining a bit in your training."

I then ask my visitor to step back into my office again where I show him a report which appeared in the American Medical Journal, in which it was agreed that weight training was the fastest method of muscle building known to science.

In answering the question about muscle turning to fat if weight training is stopped, I point to examples of famous champions. Clarence Ross, Leo Stern, Steve Reeves, Alan Stephan, Ed Theriault, and many, many more. "Each one of these men have been bodybuilders for years, 10, 15 years or more. Each one had been a bodybuilder for least several years before the outbreak of world war II. Each spent time in the service, most of them several years or more and they could not continue to work out during that time. Still, not one of them were discharged fat or flabby. The muscle they built with weights stayed with them throughout. Helped them in fact to be better soldiers!"

Finally, in speaking about the natural benefits of weight training as compared with calisthenics, I mention the fact that school children in many countries, including sections of the United States were obliged to follow a weight training program as a means of benefiting their health and physical strength. "If calisthenics were better, you don't believe that these physical educators would dare insist that these children use weights?"

Generally the visitor is sold by this time, but stubbornly, he asks two more questions: —"How do I start and how *long* will it take me to show results?"

"You will start with very light weights, ones well within your limits. You will be required to work-out three times a week. At first, your work-outs will last only 10 or 15 minutes. You will experience a very slight muscular soreness after these first work-outs, but you will not be uncomfortable in an degree. A little muscle soreness is a good sign, for it shows that you are exercising muscles not generally used, encouraging them to grow stronger. Soon, you will not experience soreness any more and will feel so much stronger that you will be anxious to use heavier weights. New and interesting exercises will be added to your program, until you will be spending about 1 hour in the gym, three times a week. Unless you want to be a Mr. America winner, you never have to devote more time than that to your training. You can build a terrific build in that short period of time. Of course, if you want to go further and reach for the very top, you will have to train a bit longer. However, that can be decided by you at that time.

"Now, as to how fast you will show gains. Come out into the gym again, I want you to meet a few of the boys. Here is Tony Palermo. He was very overweight when he began. In three months he lost 50 pounds of fat. You'll agree that is fast! Now, meet Sam Fernandez, who was a skinny wreck when he joined up. Sam gained 40 pounds in 3 months. Say hello to Murray Weissman, he gained 15 pounds in one month, and overcame a severe condition of nervous upset as well. This is Howie Hunter who gained 60 pounds in one year and shake the hand of Bob Murphy, a former boxer who went from 113 pounds to 150 in 6 months. And here is a newcomer, Joe Foltz who put on 18 pounds in the one month he's been here!"

The visitor then leaves, but usually I see him soon again, ready and anxious for his first work-out and to start on the road to physical perfection. Yes, I'm glad that my business is building muscle, for every day, in every way, I can do so much for so many people. I can give them a new start in life, a lift to overcome their discouragement, I even help them in their homes, school work and jobs.

More than one parent has come to see me, extending a grateful hand, telling me how bodybuilding has made better men out of their boys. Wives have told me how much more evened tempered their husbands are, how much more ambitious at work, how bodybuilding has cemented love and security in their home. These are the things, maybe the really important things that so few know about, the glimpses behind the scenes that make me so proud of my career.

Not everything goes smoothly all of the time though. I do have my share of trouble. Like the time an excited mother burst through the gym doors, insisting on seeing her "Johnny" right away. I had a job keeping her from rushing into the locker room where the fellows were changing clothes and I hoped that Johnny would soon come out. He did, and then his mother put her arms around him, kissed him, crying at the same time. It seems as though Johnny hadn't told her where he was spending a lot of his time and when she saw that he wasn't wasting it, getting into trouble, she was overjoyed. She hadn't realized that I was running a gymnasium until she saw her son in a pair of training trunks. Then she sat by my desk, nudging me with excitement, telling me that she guessed Johnny was the strongest, best developed boy of them all!

Another time, one of my most promising rising stars invited me to his afternoon wedding. That evening, he showed up for his work-out as usual. "Being married isn't going to interfere with my work-outs," he bragged. That was six months ago, and I haven't seen him since!

Then there was the case of the fellow who insisted in training in the nude. He had read somewhere that every pore in our bodies breathed, and that for good health it was best to train without clothes. I had one heck of a time convincing him that he could build just as much muscle wearing a pair of training trunks as without them. In fact, only after I threatened to expel him from the gym did he give in. Now, he laughs about it, can't understand how he could have been so extreme.

So there's fun, excitement, drama, in running a gym. It's the greatest business in the world. If you work hard at it, like I do, you end up each day tired out, but in your heart you feel good, because you have done something really fine for your fellow man. And, no matter how busy I am, regardless how much business pressure I may be under, don't you hesitate to drop in to say hello. I've already helped thousands, will be glad to help you in all your bodybuilding problems too. Stop in some day soon at 80 Clinton Street in New York City. I'll be glad to show you around, to assist you in any way that I can!

Here is another article from Abe;

EXERCISE OF THE MONTH
These Exercises Build Champions!

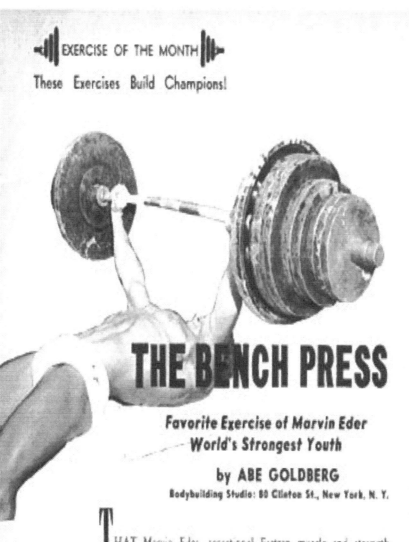

THE BENCH PRESS

Favorite Exercise of Marvin Eder World's Strongest Youth

by ABE GOLDBERG
Bodybuilding Studio: 80 Clinton St., New York, N. Y.

THAT Marvin Eder, sensational Eastern muscle and strength and strength star chose the bench press as his favorite exercise, is no surprise to any bodybuilding authority. For in this lift can be found the key to his determination to become a world beater, to overcome all obstacles and to gain immortality as one of the celebrated GREATS of bodybuilding.

Marvin is not a big man as bench pressers go. Doug Hepburn, Reg Park, John Mac Williams, all outweigh him 30 to 80 pounds in bodyweight. Still he refuses to acknowledge the fact that physically he may not be suited to establish a heavyweight record in the bench press, and he trains as hard on this lift as though his next effort would smash all records.

For the bench press is more to Marvin than just another bodybuilding exercise or strength lift. It is really his silent partner, the one he looks to for encouragement,

(Continued on page 36)

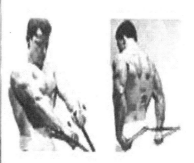

OVERCOME STUBBORN FOREARMS THIS REVOLUTIONARY WAY

AT LAST—This amazing new apparatus smashes stubborn forearm growth! Scientific leverage action reaches deep-lying pronator and supinator forearm muscle masses, forcing them to bulge with power as you twist, bend, rotate and pull against the exercise resistance. Now you can perform ALL varieties of forearm exercise quickly, surely and enjoyably. It adds interesting variety to your workouts, too ... for even the best routine can become monotonous. When this happens, interest lags, workouts lack pep and something NEW is needed to keep enthusiasm high. THIS IS IT! ! Use the Welder Massive Arm "Leverage" Exerciser for MORE training enjoyment. Hold contests ... gain valuable bodybuilding exercise and have fun as well. WE GUARANTEE extra wrist and forearm sinew and muscle growth in one week or you can return exerciser for a refund!

WHAT EXERCISER IS

As shown in illustrations, the exerciser consists of two handgrips, each with a strong coupling

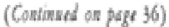

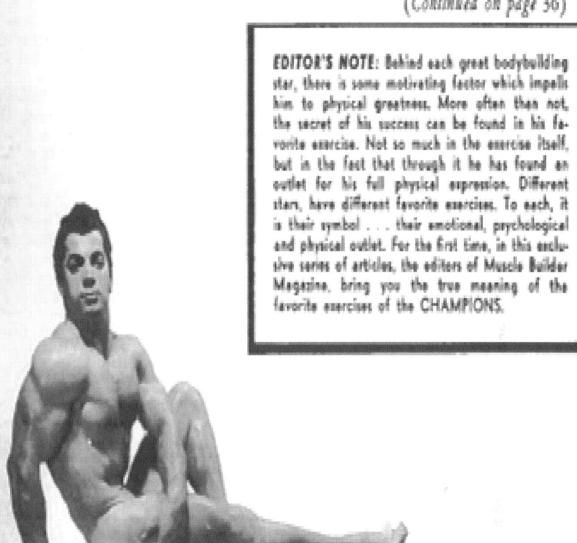

EDITOR'S NOTE: Behind each great bodybuilding star, there is some motivating factor which impells him to physical greatness. More often than not, the secret of his success can be found in his favorite exercise. Not so much in the exercise itself, but in the fact that through it he has found an outlet for his full physical expression. Different stars, have different favorite exercises. To each, it is their symbol . . . their emotional, psychological and physical outlet. For the first time, in this exclusive series of articles, the editors of Muscle Builder Magazine, bring you the true meaning of the favorite exercises of the CHAMPIONS.

help and aproval. Without it he would be just another bodybuilder.

Marvin is a firm believer of psychology in exercise. He feels that the mental and physical must meet in a happy embrace in each exercise session if unusual success is to be had.

However, this was not always so. We can remember Marvin when he was just starting to climb the ladder of physical success, just like any other beginner in bodybuilding. He showed potential then, but it was not until he discovered the bench press that this latent greatness was released and permitted full expression.

At the start, Marvin trained just like any other bodybuilder. He took his work-outs regularly, followed sensible programs and made usual progress.

Then, one day, a group of training partners suggested a contest in the bench press. For Marvin, this was a comparatively new exercise. He had little previous experience with it. Still, he beat everyone else at the gym, making well over 200 pounds his first trial.

To him, from this time on, the bench press became his symbol of success. He began to practice it with real zeal and determination, starting off each work-out session with the exercise. As he improved in the exercise, it was soon possible for him to gauge his strength for his entire work-out by how well he performed on the bench press. When he did well, his entire work-out was a tough, heavy one. When the bench press went poorly, he found that the rest of the work-out was also below par.

In this manner, his psychology of training was developed. With his first exercise he knew exactly how much energy he had to expend in each work-out,—when he could go all out and use limit poundages and when it was more advisable for him to use less.

In this way, Marvin was able to avoid training errors. Even though on occasions he worked out 6 times a week, there was never any danger of him going stale, for the bench press tipped him off. Other times, when he was busy at his job, and could not train regularly, the bench press was his guide as to how hard he could train when time permitted and still not suffer sore muscles as a result.

Marvin has no secret way of performing the bench press. He does it just like other bodybuilders, generally performing 3 or 4 sets a work-out, about 10 repetitions a set. Sometimes he uses the standard grip, other times a very wide one, and still other times a narrow grip.

When he is training for power, he will drop the repetitions down much lower and perform more sets. Other times he will perform a few sets with heavy weights, low repetitions and then wind up his work-out with several sets of higher repetitions with lighter weights.

The secret of his greatness does not lie in HOW he performs the bench press, but in WHAT this exercise means to him . . . the symbol it stands for, the infallible guide to his physical condition he has developed it into.

This is the real story behind the favorite exercise of this great star. From it you can see that to him, the bench press has long ceased to be a movement in which a mass of steel and iron is lifted from the chest to arms length. The exercise lives, as far as he is concerned, just as surely as your own greatest friend and booster lives. It is NOT an inanimate exercise motion, and that is exactly why it has done so much for him. Regardless to what heights the future career of Marvin Eder may rise, he will always have to say . . . "It was the bench press which made me what I am today!"

Other champions have discovered this same key to their greatness in other exercises. Behind each, the story is one which has never been told before. For the fascinating facts, read the future articles in this series of the "Exercises Behind The Champions!"

"If It's Big Arms you're After"

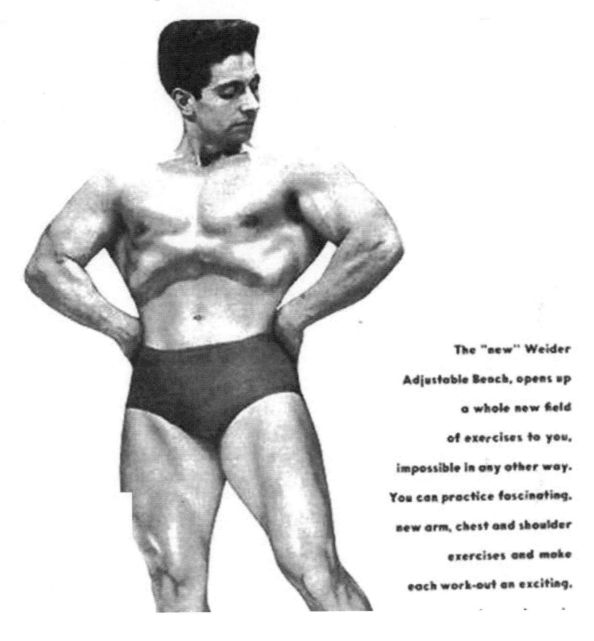

The "new" Weider Adjustable Bench, opens up a whole new field of exercises to you, impossible in any other way. You can practice fascinating, new arm, chest and shoulder exercises and make each work-out an exciting,

Says

ABE GOLDBERG

IT ISN'T the slightest trouble for me to tell you why my bodybuilding studio in New York City is one of the most successful in the Game, successful not from a financial standpoint but as a place where men are made. Please don't think I'm claiming any credit for myself, because in my gym we teach the Weider System, with it's scientific championship principles and up-to-date methods. But in addition to this, there's a piece of apparatus standing in the middle of the exercise room, which I believe has contributed more to the amazing number of outstanding physical specimens produced by my studio, than anything else I can think of ... It's the combination Flat and Incline Exercise bench.

It requires no more than five minutes effort on your part to prove the truth of this statement. Just take any weight training magazine, 25 years old, and compare the bodybuilders in it with those of today. And, in addition to this, if there is a picture of a barbell gym, place it alongside that of a present day studio. Two things will immediately be apparent. The tremendous superiority of the modern bodybuilder over his counterpart of more than two decades ago, and the fact *(Continued on page 46)*

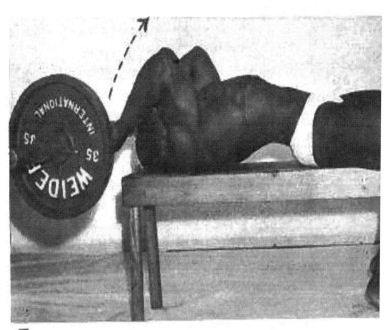

1 *Triceps Press.*

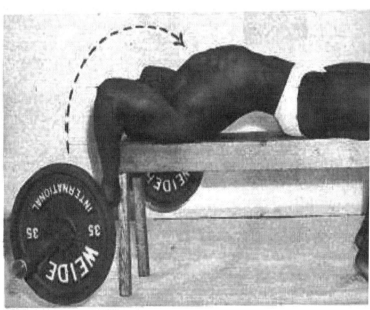

2 *Bent Arm Pullovers.*

If It's Big Arms—Try This

(Continued from page 25)

that in the old style studios, exercise benches which we have always accepted as standard bodybuilding, equipment, are conspicuous by their absence. In the Dark Ages of bodybuilding, the only reason a bench was in a gym, was to sit on between exercises. Today, an exercise bench is used to build arm, chest, and shoulder muscularity and torso form that by any standard is sensational. A gymnasium might just as well have no weights at all, as be without the Flat or Incline bench.

Today's Championship Aspirant demands a heck of a lot more than mere bulk from his exercise routines. He wants a high degree of muscular delineation, strength and, most of all, proportionate development. It is no longer possible for him, as it was for a bodybuilder in the old days, to advance to the top ranks of physique stardom simply because he might possess one outstanding muscle group such as abdominals, arms or chest. Now he realizes that Contest titles are won only by the man whose entire development is pleasingly blended, creating with it's overall appearance an impression of great power, size and definition.

The man whose build gives the impression of masses of muscles plastered on him haphazardly as it were, can no longer gain recognition as an outstanding physical specimen. Instead his place is taken by the bodybuilder whose smoothly flowing musculature conveys a sense of strength and grace, the very physique qualities which exercises performed on the Flat and Incline bench produce swiftly and easily, and which are exemplified in the men who train in my gym, famous stars of the East like Ray Jiminez, Raul Pacheco, Enrico Tomas, Leroy Colbert, Louis Degni and

To show you just what this combination Flat and Incline Bench is capable of, and as an example of what Bench Movements can accomplish for a bodybuilder, I've chosen famous Leroy Colbert, Mr. Eastern America to illustrate this article. Leroy positively states that if it hadn't been for Bench exercises, he'd have never been the first 19 year old boy to build a pair of 19 inch biceps. Exercise Bench routines at the same time have shaped Leroy's upper body in such a manner that the massiveness of his arms in no way detracts from his shoulder and torso development. Training constantly at my gym with other Physique "greats" has taught Leroy that only variety of exercise, plus scientific training principles, can produce outstanding results. These results can be yours . . . right in your own home . . . with the Weider Double Purpose Exercise Bench. Here's your experimental routine. Get to work now, build massive life guard shoulders, tree trunk arms, barrel chest and classical torso. Get the development that will win you contests and fame as a new Bodybuilding star.

EXERCISE 1. *Triceps Press.* Lower the incline Board until the bench is flat and lie on it with a barbell held at arms length above the chest, hands should be 8 to 10 inches apart, palms facing your feet. Lower the bar back of the head by bending the arms at the elbows. When the bar is as low as possible, raise it to commencing position and repeat. In this exercise your upper arms do not move, but are kept still, the elbows pointing straight up. This will pump up all sections of the triceps, increase pressing power.

raising the board and making the necessary adjustment. Clean a pair of dumbbells, and hold them as shown in Illustration 5, sideways to the shoulders with the palms of your hands facing forward. From this position press the dumbbells to arms length, then lower them, pressing down your elbows as far as you can, stretching the muscles across the shoulders. Repeat the exercise. Breathe in as you press dumbbells, out as you lower them. Strengthens shoulder and chest tendons. Widens shoulder structure, packs deltoids and triceps with power.

EXERCISE 6. *Barbell Bench Press.* Lower the incline board so your bench is flat. Lie along it with a barbell held at arms length above the chest, hand spacing two to three inches wider than shoulder width. Lower barbell steadily until it touches the chest, then press it to arms length again and repeat. Don't bounce the bar off the chest, but make the motion steady. Breathe in deeply just before you lower the bar and out as you press it to arms length. Thickens chest, arm and shoulder muscles.

EXERCISE 7. *Incline Bench Alternate Dumbbell Curls.* Alter your flat bench to an incline. Sit on the end, flat portion, and rest your back against the incline. Hold a pair of dumbbells in the hands and allow the arms to hang straight down. Curl the dumbbells up to the shoulders alternately. Don't arch the back off the incline. Don't move the upper arms but keep them pressed against the Board. Don't swing the weights up but make the motion a steady curling on. Pumps up biceps muscle. Prepares muscle for more advanced others.

Why is it that the Combination Exercise Bench does so much for the bodybuilder? Why does it build such a wonderful tie-in of the upper body muscle groups, and in what manner can it be used to gain a torso of classical proportions? First the number of exercises which can be performed on it, either with barbell or dumbbells, is practically without limit. Second, it provides constant change and variety in training. Third there is an economy of energy because of the far reaching effects of the Bench Movements. Fourth because the muscles are worked in groups, in co-ordination, rather than in isolation and it is for this reason that it produces a more proportionate development.

Until recently there were two types of benches in use . . . the Flat bench and the Incline Variety. But with his usual foresight and thoughtfulness, Joe Weider had his designers go to work, and produce a combination flat and incline bench that could be used by any bodybuilder who worked out in his own home. Hitherto, such a piece of equipment was available only to those who trained in large, expensive bodybuilding gymnasiums. Now thanks to Joe, both types of apparatus are ready for use in one neat, compact piece of apparatus, changed from Flat to the Incline bench in less than five seconds.

You'll enjoy using this Combination bench. You'll thrill to the results you obtain, watch with increasing pride the rapid gains you make in development. You'll be able to use heavy bench presses, the kind Ray Jiminez has used to get his chest and arm development. You'll be able to train on the same upper body routine as used by Louis Degni, and you'll progress into such advanced training principles as Super Sets and Isolation routines

EXERCISE 2. *Bent arm pullovers*. Lie on the flat bench with a barbell resting on your chest, hands gripping the bar with shoulder width spacing. Lower the bar behind the head until the plates touch the floor, then pull up and over your face to the chest. Repeat the movement. Keep your buttocks on the bench throughout the exercise. Try not to arch the back too much. Breathe in deeply when lowering the bar, breathe out raising it back to commencing position. Increases size and power of chest and lungs. Develops tapering lats for wedge shaped torso.

EXERCISE 3. *Leg Raises With Iron Boots*. Lie on your back along the Flat Bench, Iron Boots strapped to your feet, buttocks just on the end of the bench, hands gripping the other end for stability. Raise the feet until the thighs are pointing straight up. Lower the feet, keeping the thighs straight, locked at the knees until your legs are level with the bench. Repeat the movement. Burns off excess fat around the lower abdomen. Fines down entire waist line, producing abdominal definition.

EXERCISE 4. *Dumbbell Flying Exercises*. Lie along a flat bench with a pair of dumbbells held at arms length above your chest. Bend the arms a little at the elbows. Keep them in this position throughout the movement. Lower the dumbbells down and out to the sides, until they are a little below level with the shoulders. Raise to commencing position and repeat. Breathe in deeply as you lower the dumbbells. Force out your breath as you raise them again. Don't pause in between repetitions but make the motion of the bells and the breathing continuous. Don't forget to keep your arms bent. Pumps up pectorals. Increases capacity of lungs.

EXERCISE 5. *Incline Bench Dumbbell presses*; alter your bench to incline by movements to follow.

EXERCISE 8. *Seated Alternate Dumbbell Curls*. Sit on the end of the exercise bench a dumbbell held in each hand. Curl the dumbbells up to the shoulders alternately. Palms of the hands face to the front at commencement of the exercise. When the dumbbell touches the shoulder, raise the elbow and pull the upper arm back so it is level with shoulder. Lower weight starting to curl one dumbbell up as you lower the other. Make motion continuous with no pause in between repetitions. Don't allow the body to exert any influence in the curling. Confine the motion to the arms. Works upper section of the biceps. Strengthens entire group.

EXERCISE 9. *Incline Bench Barbell Curls*. Sit on the end of the bench and rest your back against the incline. Barbell rests across the upper thighs and is gripped with a hand-spacing slightly less than shoulder width. From this position curl the bar up to the shoulders, lower and repeat. Don't arch the back away from the incline. Don't allow the upper arms to move. Keep them pressed tight against the body. Lower the barbell down SLOWLY to commencing position and curl it smoothly and steadily to the shoulders. Peak Contraction affect on head of biceps. Increases "split" and "height."

EXERCISE 10. *Incline Bench Peak Contraction Curls*. Stand back of the bench as in illustration 10, arm resting down the incline, a dumbbell held in the hand. From this position, curl the weight up to the shoulder, lower slowly and repeat. Don't move the upper arm off incline. Don't bounce dumbbell off incline to get start to curl. Make movement steady. Exercise arms in turn. Bulks up belly of the biceps. Strengthens tendons and ligaments. Improves starting barbell curl power.

You'll get the best results from all these movements by handling as heavy a weight as possible, starting with a low number of repetitions and gradually increasing them. I personally recommend a start with 6 reps, working up steadily to 12 before you increase the exercise poundage. The first week use one set of each movement. The second week two sets, the third week three sets. Don't go above three sets unless you are training for extra muscular delineation. Three Exercise Bench workouts a week will be sufficient for all but the most advanced bodybuilders. End your training period with squats, legs presses or dead lifts.

It will also be advisable to increase your protein intake. Weider High Protein tablets taken during the workout will keep fatigue poisons down to a minimum and help repair tissue breakdown more quickly. Thus you'll recover more rapidly from the workouts and feel fresher on the day following. Never forget that the old rule "Variety is the spice of life," applies just as strongly to Bodybuilding as it does to living in general. Keep training with the same old program, and you'll reach a sticking point from which it will be extremely difficult to budge. Make use of the Weider Double Purpose Exercise bench and forge steadily ahead to championship form and glory. It's the Choice of the Champions . . . make it *YOUR* choice.

Chapter 6 Bill Pearl's Gym

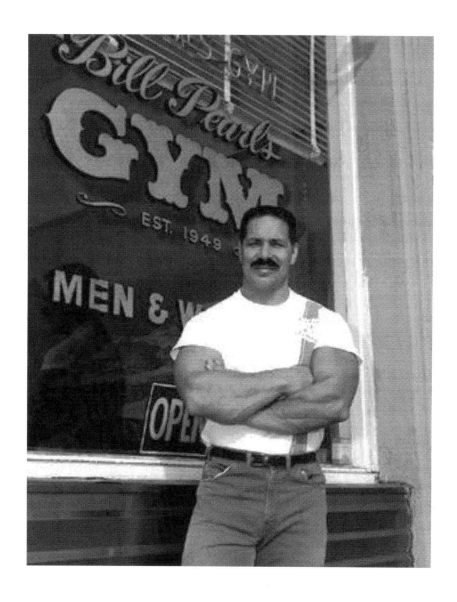

Who is Bill Pearl?

Well, let's see what good old Wikipedia has to say;

William Arnold "Bill" Pearl (born October 31, 1930[1]) is an American former bodybuilder during the 1950s and '60s. He won many titles and awards including winning the Mr. Universe contest five times, and was named "World's Best-Built Man of the Century." He became an expert trainer and author on bodybuilding.

Biography

Pearl was born in Prineville, Oregon. His first major victory was in the 1953 Amateur Mr Universe contest (in which he beat out a then 23-year-old Sean Connery). He actively competed until his retirement in 1971 after winning the Mr. Universe one last time, over superstars Frank Zane, Reg Park and Sergio Oliva. In all, he won the professional Mr Universe 4 times in an 18 year span, which was unprecedented at the time. He was the first professional bodybuilder to author bodybuilding training courses/booklets. He is also the first to pose to music, and was especially noted in performing exhibitions doing an entire posing routine of Eugene Sandow (who is known as the man who invented bodybuilding). Ever the showman, along with his lifelong coach Leo Stern, Pearl would wear a fake mustache, leotards, a fig leaf, and a late-19th century backdrop, all for providing the exact effect of the Sandow era. As if that wasn't enough, Pearl was equally as famous for performing his strongman routine, which included tearing of license plates, bending penny spike nails, and blowing up a hot water bottle. He is the author of the popular exercise book, *Getting Stronger: Weight Training for Men and Women*, which has sold over 350,000 copies in the United States and has been translated into four other languages, including Chinese. His book *Keys To The INNER Universe*, is still to this day considered to be a "must read" for bodybuilders. It contains 1,500 weight-training exercises and weighs five pounds. It is used extensively by professional athletes, trainers and serious bodybuilders and has sold over 60,000 copies.[2] Pearl had his own monthly question-and-answer column called "Pearl of the Universe" in the bodybuilding magazine *MuscleMag International* as well as one in *Muscle Builder* (later *Muscle & Fitness*) magazine, entitled "Wisdom of Pearl" in the 1970s & 1980s. In 2003 with coauthor Kim Shott, Pearl published his autobiography, *Beyond the Universe: The Bill Pearl Story*. Pearl became a vegetarian at age 39 and is the best-known vegetarian bodybuilder. Bill's diet is lacto-ovo vegetarian, which means he eats eggs and dairy products. During the 1980s, Pearl served as a mentor, trainer, and training partner to many of the top professionals that were still competing. One such individual was Mr. Olympia, Chris Dickerson. In 2004, Pearl was awarded the Arnold Schwarzenegger Classic Lifetime Achievement Award for significantly impacting the world of bodybuilding. In 2011 Pearl appeared in the documentary Challenging Impossibility (film) describing when he hosted the 2004 strength exhibition by spiritual teacher and peace advocate Sri Chinmoy. The film was an Official Selection of the 2011 Tribeca Film Festival.[3] Pearl is 5' 9" tall. He currently lives in Phoenix, Oregon.[4]

bodybuilding titles and awards

- 1952 Mr. San Diego, 3rd place (San Diego, California)
- 1952 Mr. Oceanside (Oceanside, California)
- 1953 Mr. Southern California (Los Angeles, California)
- 1953 Mr. California (Los Angeles, California)
- 1953 A.A.U., Mr. America (Indianapolis, Indiana)
- 1953 N.A.B.B.A., Mr. Universe Amateur (London, England)
- 1956 Mr. U.S.A., Professional (Los Angeles, California)
- 1956 N.A.B.B.A., Mr. Universe, Professional, Tall Man's Class (London, England)
- 1961 N.A.B.B.A., Mr. Universe, Professional (London, England)
- 1967 N.A.B.B.A., Mr. Universe, Professional (London, England)
- 1971 N.A.B.B.A., Mr. Universe, Professional (London, England)
- 1974 W.B.B.A., World's Best-Built Man of the Century (New York, New York)
- 1978 Entered into W.B.B.A., Hall of Fame (New York, New York)
- 1978 Elected the I.F.B.B. National Chairman of the Professional Physique Judges Committee (Acapulco, Mexico)
- 1988 Entered into Pioneers of Fitness Hall of Fame
- 1992 Entered into Gold's Gym Hall of Fame
- 1994 Guest of Honor of the Association of Oldetime Barbell & Strongmen 12th Annual Reunion
- 1994 Entered into The Joe Weider Hall of Fame
- 1995 A.A.U. Lifetime Achievement Award
- 1995 Oscar Heidenstam Foundation Hall of Fame
- 1996 American Powerlifters Federation Hall of Fame
- 1997 International Chiropractors Association Sports & Fitness Man of the Year
- 1999 I.F.B.B. Hall of Fame Inductee[6]
- 2000 Spirit of Muscle Beach Award
- 2001 World Gym Lifetime Achievement Award
- 2001 Society of Weight-Training Injury Specialists Lifetime Achievement Award
- 2002 Canadian Fitness Award for 60+ Years of Inspiration to the Industry
- 2002 National Fitness Trade Journal Lifetime Achievement Award
- 2003 Iron Man magazine Peary & Mabel Radar Lifetime Achievement Award
- 2004 Arnold Schwarzenegger Lifetime Achievement Award
- 2006 PDI Night of Champions Lifetime Achievement Award [7][8]

Books

- *Beyond the Universe* – The Bill Pearl Story
- *Getting in Shape*: 32 Workout Programs for Lifelong Fitness
- *Getting Back in Shape*: 32 Workout Programs for Lifelong Fitness
- *Getting Stronger*: Weight Training for Men and Women
- *Getting Stronger*: Weight Training for Men and Women (Revised Edition)
- *Keys to the INNER Universe*

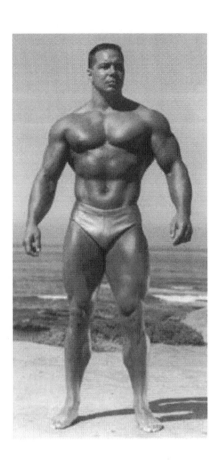

This shot is from Bill's website;

http://www.billpearl.com/career.asp

This excerpt from the website mentions Bill's first gym;

In 1950 Bill entered the U.S. Navy and subsequently had very little time to train until he was eventually stationed in **San Diego, California, and joined Leo Stern's Gym**. This was the turning point for Bill's future. He was now able to receive proper guidance with his training and had the necessary equipment and competition to push him to a higher set of goals. He entered his first physique contest in 1952 and placed third in the annual Mr. San Diego contest. **Come 1953 and Bill Pearl took the physique world by storm. He took the Mr. Oceanside, Mr. Southern California, Mr. California, Mr. America and Mr. Universe titles all in one year.** With his enlistment in the navy finished in early 1954, Bill moved to **Sacramento, California, and opened his first gym with the money he had saved by taking out war bonds the four years he was in the service - a grand total of $2,800.00.**

With the strong determination Bill has for succeeding, the gym was a tremendous success and overnight it was turning out some of the finest physiques the West Coast had ever seen. **At one time he had expanded his gym operation to nine different health clubs scattered throughout Northern California.** This, however, was not BILL. He was not able to get involved with the people on a personal basis. **He therefore eventually cut back to one club and concentrated his efforts on making it the finest in Northern California.** Because of personal problems, Bill sold his health club in Sacramento in 1962 and **moved to Los Angeles, California, and purchased the famous George Redpath Gym.** By this time Bill was in constant demand as a guest poser. He also had a fabulous strength act which included blowing up hot water bottles until they would burst, spike bending, chain breaking, and tearing auto license plates in half with his bare hands. He was also performing such lifting feats as a seated press behind neck with 310 lbs, military pressing 320 lbs, and bench pressing 450 lbs, front squatting 500 lbs and full squatting 605 lbs at a body weight of 218 lbs. He was the most widely traveled Mr. America on record, having made trips around the world performing in nearly every foreign country, giving exhibitions, feats of strength, and lectures on physical fitness. His main theme was always to present himself as a gentleman and a spokesman fitting for the sport of bodybuilding. He appeared before crowds of 25,000 people in India, was the special hose guest of such distinguished men as J. Paul Getty and other top notables. By now the Pearl physique was a legend and he was still improving every year. He continued to set higher and higher standards for the newcomers. **Not only continuing to push himself to higher esteem, Bill still found time to help others reach the top in the physique world by turning out Mr. Americas and Mr. Universes about as fast as he was winning the contests himself.** It was in 1967 when Bill decided to enter the Mr. Universe contest for the last time at the age of 37 and had plans of retiring from competition and devoting his extra time to others he felt would appreciate the limelight more than he. Bill again took Britain by storm and won hands down, taking every first place vote. Most people admitted he was the world's Number One by far. He was in the greatest shape of his life at that time and some of the pictures published of Bill around this time were simply fantastic. Many bodybuilders believed Bill had secrets he was not sharing with the rest of the physique world. **Over the years Bill had long thought of opening a health club that would have universal appeal. His main idea was to separate the businessmen and light trainers for the bodybuilders and heavy powerlifters. This would mean that anyone, regardless of their present physical condition or goals, could use facilities that most appealed to them.** His several years of consulting with North American Rockwell's Aerospace Program as athletic advisor to the Medical Staff, headed by the renowned Harold Morrison, M.D., had made Bill even more aware that proper weight training could improve nearly every person's life style if properly performed. **With this in mind, he sold his gym in Los Angeles and purchased a beautiful modern building in Pasadena, California, that was suitable to his needs. He then proceeded to build one of the finest private health facilities in the United States.**

The website goes on to describe Pearl's big comeback & asserts his philosophy towards steroid use in bodybuilding;

With his contest days over - or so he thought - Bill wanted to stay in excellent health and devote all his time to his family, business, and helping others acquire superb health. THEN CAME THE BOMBSHELL! It was rumored through various physique magazines that Bill was afraid to compete in contests in which other star physiques were entered. He did not take these attacks seriously at first, as he did not think that anyone would expect him at over 40 years of age to do battle with these younger fellows in their twenties. He'd had his share of the limelight. Youth must be served. However, he had not reckoned with the attitude of his old friend and advisor, Leo Stern. These rumors had upset Stern more than it had Pearl. Leo talked to Bill and told him that this would be the ideal way to settle the argument once and for all. Bill was very skeptical because of business pressures and the strain it would put on his wife. Leo kept on insisting that not only could Bill work around the obstacles; he could get into the best shape of his life and beat them all.
So it was the team of Pearl and Stern embarked on what would be the most vital contest in which Bill has ever competed. A lot of these fellows had something going for them that Bill did not and would not have - DRUGS. He absolutely refused to use anabolic steroids in his training methods. He firmly believes that while these drugs have an important place in the world of medicine, they are in no way meant to be used by the man who desires to improve his physique by lifting weights. In fact, this was to be a major factor in Bill's decision to have just one more try and compete against these people. It thus became a quest to prove to the same0minded bodybuilders throughout the world that resorting to the dangerous practice of using drugs is not only unnecessary - it is, in Bill's opinion, "shear madness". With the decision made, Bill, with the help of Leo, began to prepare himself to do battle with the cream of the present-day bodybuilders. It was well publicized early in 1971 that Pearl intended to enter the annual Mr. Universe contest in London. This meant that anyone who wished to compete against him had ample and equal time to prepare himself for the event. Over the course of a year Bill Pearl transformed himself from a great physique to the absolute greatest physique ever! Exercise programs and diets were carefully worked out and from it evolved an absolutely fantastic Pearl that not even his closest friends could believe. On Friday, September 17, the pre-judging was held to determine who would be the amateur and professional Mr. Universe winners for 1971. Great physiques journeyed from all over the world in what would be the most hotly contested Mr. Universe ever. On the afternoon of the next day the famous Victoria Palace was packed to the doors, as usual, for the 23rd annual Mr. Universe contest. The capacity crowd enjoyed a fabulous show, and then waited with baited breath until at last the announcements were about to be made. "Ladies and gentlemen, the 1971 N.A.B.B.A. amateur Mr. Universe Is Ken Waller of the United States." This was a very popular decision and that grand old theater rang to resounding applause. You could almost hear a pin drop when M.C. Cecil Peck went on. **"Ladies and Gentlemen, the 1971 N.A.B.B.A. professional Mr. Universe is... BILL PEARL!"** That huge crowd went wild, cheering what must have been one of the most popular decisions since the contest began in 1948. A hush came over the crowd as Pearl walked toward the microphone to say a few words to his thousands of fans and a little man jumped to his feet and with his finest English accent began to shout at the top of his lungs, "PEARL IS KING."

Returning home from England, after a brief tour of the Continent with his wife and the Sterns, Pearl put himself into virtual isolation from the physique world except for his business. He gave no exhibitions, no appearances, nothing. Being asked why he had taken this attitude, Bill replied, "My main reason for entering the 1971 Mr. Universe contest was to prove a point and I did. The trophy or the title meant very little to me. I wanted it forgotten and over. I actually felt strange onstage and felt I should have been there as a consular or a judge rather than a competitor. It reminded me of an old man trying to act like a kid. I felt I had my day and enough was enough." Bill started competing in bicycle racing in 1972 and purposely dropped his body weight to 185 lbs. Still continuing to weight train daily, he altered his training to fit his new sport. He rode and competed in races until 1975 and then returned to hard training again bringing his body weight back up to 225 pounds and dropped the bike riding to a weekend hobby. With very few photos and articles appearing in the physique magazines, plus the news the Pearl had stopped serious training; he was no longer a threat to the current flock of competitive body builders. Bill was now able to get at the goal he had wanted to attempt for years but could not find the time - getting all the weight training knowledge, material and data he had stored up on paper in hopes of helping others meet their goals in life. Bill's book Keys to The Inner Universe is a part of that goal. After the completion of Keys to The Inner Universe, Bill and his wife Judy moved to Southern Oregon, where they found their ideal haven in a healthful, clean environment, overlooking the beautiful Rogue Valley. The climate and their wonderful neighbors suit them perfectly, while the surrounding hills and the valley provide them with a deep sense of peace and tranquility when they are at home. Bill still gets up regularly at 3:00 a.m. to train six days a week, works on his antique automobiles whenever he has a little spare time, and when he's not doing all that, he is on the road as a consultant for Life Fitness, sharing his expertise in the use of the fabulous Life Circuit exercise system and equipment. His home gym has been updated to include this innovative equipment and he is very enthusiastic about its capabilities for use in sports rehab and exercise. It is used in his gym by everyone who trains there, from neighbor ladies in their seventies, to the biggest, brawniest hulks that come up to challenge him. In short, Bill and Judy have found the best of two worlds through their move to Oregon: peace and tranquility at home, and challenging new opportunities and ways to pass his knowledge and experience of the sport of bodybuilding to others.

Editor's note from above article;

Bill Pearl, 81, is a five-time Mr. Universe and author of the best-selling bodybuilding books, Keys to the Inner Universe, **Getting Stronger**, and Getting in Shape. He has personally coached more major contest winners than anyone else in history. At his own peak as a bodybuilder when he last won the Universe in 1971 at age 41, he weighed 242 pounds at a height of 5'10" and his arms measured 21 inches!

Well, I have some help from the great writings of none other than Dave Draper to add... I love Dave's style, so I think this excerpt from Dave's book will be a nice little addition.

Brother Iron Sister Steel
Book Excerpt: Bill Pearl

Brother Iron, Sister Steel
A Bodybuilder's Book
By Dave Draper

Sequins and Pearls
Excerpt from pages 249-250

It was the weekend before the Mr. America contest in 1965. My training was going well, as far as I could tell. Truth was I didn't yet know how to tell. I looked okay, but compared to what or whom? I was working hard, eating hard, braced with hard discipline and felt hard. **My first months at Muscle Beach were a crash course and I established training methods I would follow forever**; but I learned the essentials quickly and settled into private, unmitigated early-morning workouts. They were silent, undistracted and unrelenting: no compromise and no competition. How sweet it is. Two years of isolated training and I wasn't sure who I had become. I moved with three different training partners at different stages and the reinforcement and friendship were priceless. They knew the Mr. A was on my mind and stood by my side; they were too close, however, to offer the critique and subjective counsel I now sought. Only an outsider could provide an evaluation and dare to place it in my hands. Who could I trust? I needed to know if I was ready for the competition in New York City only eight days away. I also needed a pair of posing trunks. Did I mention—procrastination was one of my specialties, followed by irresponsibility and dimwittedness? Nobody's perfect. If you got on Washington Boulevard and followed it east for five miles you'd find yourself in **East Los Angeles** and standing in front of Bill Pearl's Gym. If you walked in the front door at 6 p.m. you'd find Bill, forearms pouring out of a cut-off sweatshirt, sitting behind a wood desk, chair tilted against the wall. If you arrived at 6 a.m. Bill Pearl was under a bar, bench pressing or squatting some absurd weight for a lot of reps. His training partners would be exuding energy, zeal and perspiration. For my first visit I chose the evening hour after a gentlemanly phone call to assure he would be there. Didn't need to go to East Los Angeles if he wasn't. Bill was the man I could and would trust with the deed of critical analysis; thumbs up or … er … thumbs down.

A legend at thirty-five, Mr. America, Mr. Universe — twice, served in the Navy, **built and owned several gyms over the years,** the man was known for his incredible power and ability to bend coins and tear license plates and phone books in half. "Hi, I'm Dave. Can you tell me if I have muscles? I don't know." "Sure, Dave. Why don't you come here tomorrow morning at six when my huge partners and I can stand you under the skylight and take a good look. Bring your posing trunks."

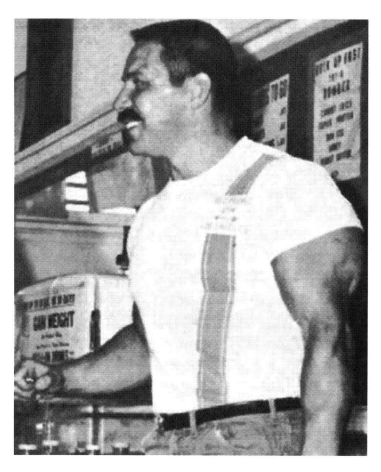

Me and my mouth. How could I say, "Never mind" or "I don't have posing trunks?" There are the tough times, Buster, when you can't go forward and you can't go back and you can't lie. The only thing left was the truth. I was right on time, my big grin and my big gym bag and my big feet. I found the skylight on my own but couldn't find my posing trunks. No problemo, Big D, you can borrow mine. Bill's generosity is also overwhelming. I didn't ask for music. Silence was loud enough. I hit a few shots like Joe Weider, The Master Blaster, had taught me. Joe could pose a molting ostrich and he'd win "the overall" and "most muscular" hands down at any pro show on the globe. The gold metallic trunks offered by Bill fit perfectly and I felt pumped by the end of my routine. The guys were excited and full of suggestions, which further warmed me up and put the disabling self-consciousness to rest. A few more run-throughs with additions and deletions, a change in timing and tempo, posture, facial expression and attitude adjustments and I was a different animal. You can win this thing, Draper. I'm tellin' ya.

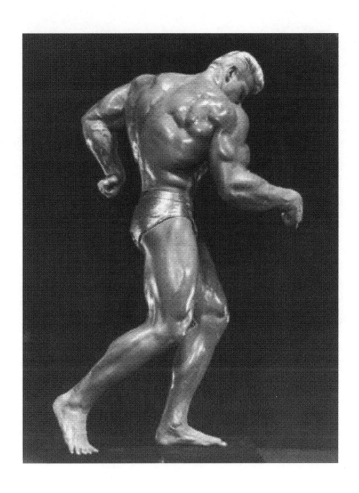

Draper with Pearl's Gold Trunks on

One of the most famous guys that trained at Bill Pearl's place was this giant of the iron game:

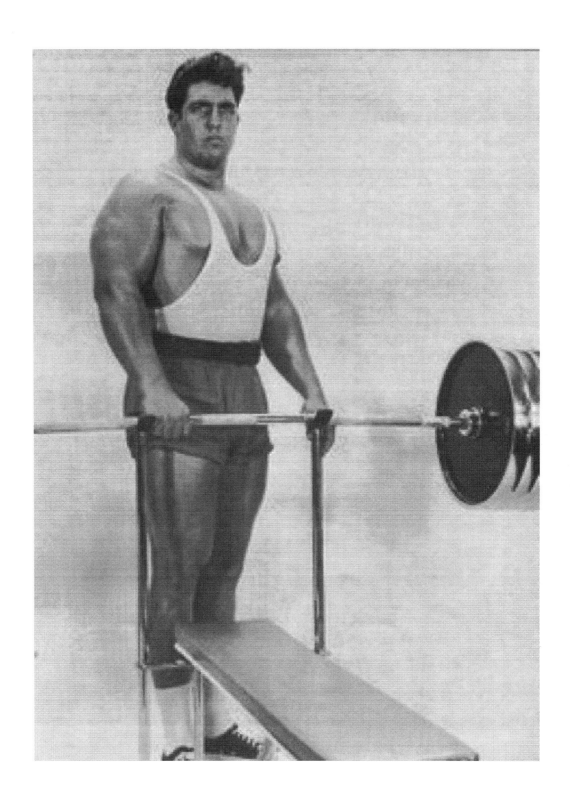

In fact, Casey trained there from his high school days, when it belonged to **George Redpath**, and the gym was known, oddly enough, as Redpath's Gym. Bill Pearl purchased the gym from Redpath.

Some of you probably know that Pat Casey was the first **man in the world to officially bench press 600 pound** (615 on March 25, 1967--without bench shirt, elbow wraps or steroids; he was also the first to officially squat 775 and total 2000).

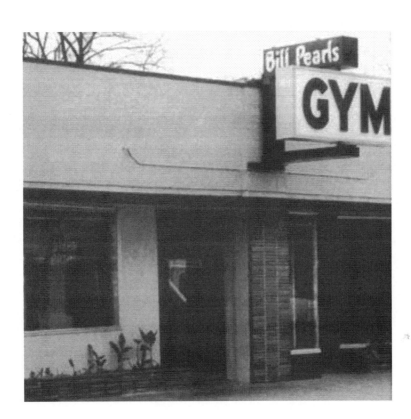

PAT CASEY: King of the Powerlifters

Bruce Wilhelm's booklet on Casey includes a wonderful Foreword by **Bill Pearl**. Casey trained in Pearl's gym for a number of years; lifting such huge poundage that Pearl had to reinforce the benches he used. "I was afraid the benches would not hold the weight," Pearl writes. "**He would do chest exercises with 220lb dumbbells in each hand.** There was a corner of the gym where Pat stored his weights for special lifts. **Nobody touched Pat's weights and nobody other than Pat wanted to touch his weights.**" Significantly, Pearl writes in another part of the Foreword: "He has long legs, long arms, and a short torso. This is the opposite of people like Paul Anderson and Doug Hepburn who were built for strength. Pat over came this handicap through his methods of training and positive attitude." That's what Bruce Wilhelm's booklet is about; he calls it "a training manual/booklet on Pat Casey." It includes interesting information on Casey's background, along with a question and answer session with Pat, and his actual workout and contest poundage—and classic photos of Pat. It's not Shakespeare by any means, but it's an interesting read for anyone interested in strength and Powerlifting. Four decades ago, **Pat Casey became the first man to bench press 600 pounds** - a number that still stands as **a remarkable achievement for anyone who benches raw, as Pat did.** Although Pat was best known for his otherworldly bench presses, he was also the top superheavyweight powerlifter of his day, not a one-lift specialist, as **he was also the first man to officially squat 800 pounds and the first man to officially total 2000 pounds.** Besides his official powerlifts, Pat will always be remembered for his prodigious training lifts, such as walking to the dumbbell rack, picking up a pair of 210-pound dumbbells, walking back to the incline bench, getting the dumbbells into position unassisted, doing his reps, and then lowering and returning the dumbbells to the rack without any help. We are not be lucky enough to still have Pat's company, but wherever heavy metal is hoisted, Pat's spirit will live. Pat was amazing. He has benched 210lb dumbbells, done a weighted dip with 380 extra pounds... amazing strength legend all around.

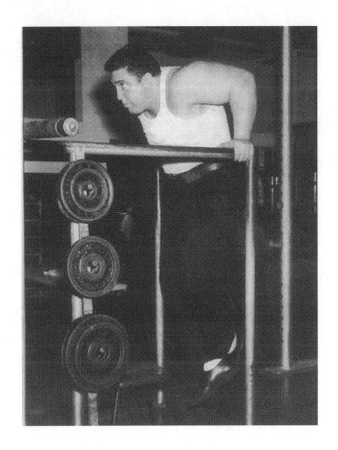

Of course, Pat was another icon of the original Westside era, though not a true "core member". Pat was also highlighted in "Forgotten Secrets of the Culver City Westside Barbell club revealed", and was seen in several of the older Weider publication articles written by Armand Tanny during those years.

Here is an early Muscle Builder (1954) piece on Bill;

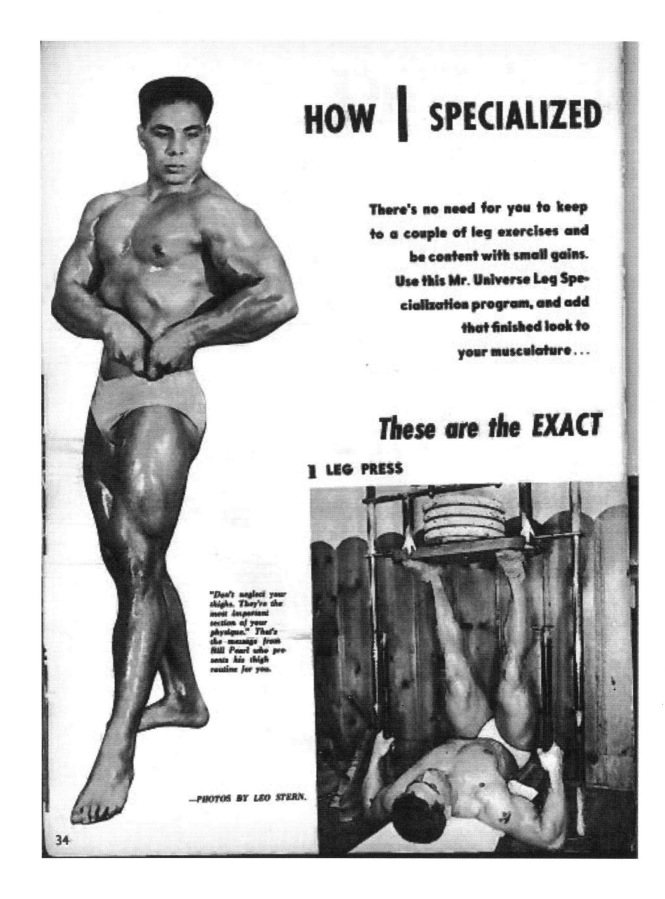

HOW I SPECIALIZED

There's no need for you to keep to a couple of leg exercises and be content with small gains. Use this Mr. Universe Leg Specialization program, and add that finished look to your musculature...

These are the EXACT

1 LEG PRESS

"Don't neglect your thighs. They're the most important section of your physique." That's the message from Bill Pearl who presents his thigh routine for you.

—PHOTOS BY LEO STERN.

"Don't neglect your thighs. They're the most important section of your physique." That's the message from Bill Pearl who presents his thigh routine for you.

TO ADD INCHES OF MUSCLE TO MY THIGHS

By
BILL PEARL
MR. UNIVERSE...MR. AMERICA 1953
as told to Leo Stern

IN NEARLY every gym, there's one or more bodybuilders working out, who have exceptionally well developed physiques, and are more or less, sources of inspiration to the other weight trainers. But there are also other who have the type of development that is open to criticism . . . and their training mates are always finding flaws . . . "Sure" they'll say . . . "So and so is terrific, has a nice build . . . BUT—" the ending of the sentence is sure indication that some body part lags behind the other muscle groups. With some bodybuilders it might be the biceps—or the triceps—but mainly it is the thighs.

For some obscure reason weight trainers will specialize month after month on their upper bodies, yet neglect the legs, which are just as important, if not more so, than large arms or deltoids. The thighs are usually clothed, not visible as the arms and chest are, but this is poor reason for a man to neglect them and work only on those muscle parts which are more noticeable. After *(Continued on page 55)*

EXERCISES I USED TO BUILD UP MY LEGS:

2 BENCH SQUATS   3 FRONT SQUATS

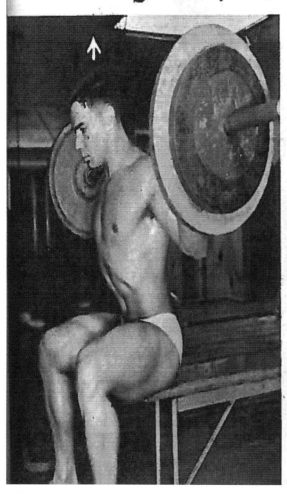
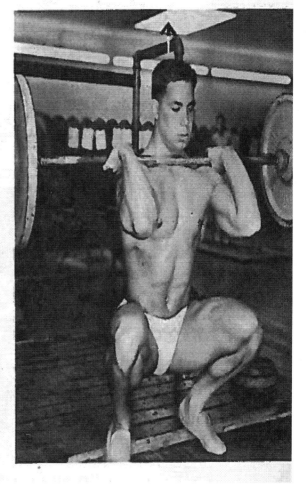

HOW I SPECIALIZED TO ADD INCHES

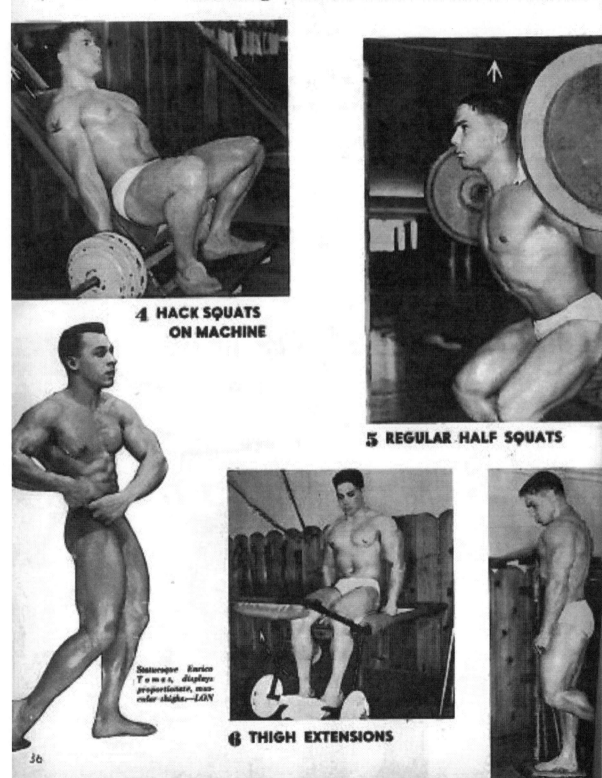

4 HACK SQUATS ON MACHINE

5 REGULAR HALF SQUATS

6 THIGH EXTENSIONS

Statuesque Enrico Tomas displays proportionate, muscular thighs. —LON

OF MUSCLE TO MY THIGHS

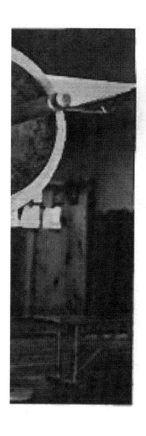

7 STANDING LEG CURLS

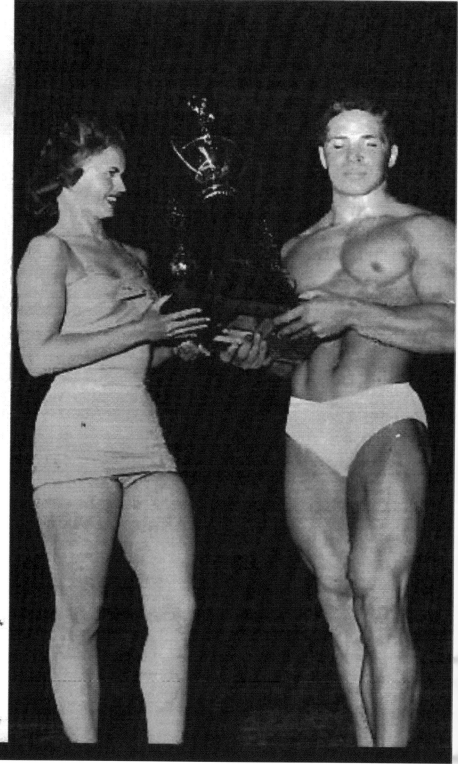

Pretty model hands Bill Pearl the Mr. America Trophy. Note the massive sweep of Bill's legs, the development peak above his knees.

How I Specialized To Add Muscles To My Thighs

(Continued from page 35)

all, we cannot see our internal organs, but we would never dream of neglecting them so that they failed to function efficiently, or keep them in the best possible condition.

You may have naturally large thighs, but that is no reason why they should not receive their fair share of exercise, because, as with other body parts, they can never reach their peak of shape and muscularity without a great deal of time and effort expended on their behalf. And with weight gaining being the goal of many bodybuilders, there is all the more reason for giving large muscle groups the major portion of the exercise in a workout. The thighs and hips comprise the largest muscles of the body . . . vivid proof of the important part they play in a weight gaining program.

While it is true that some weight trainers are interested only in building their upper bodies, they will find that leg work will also add inches to their chests because of the heavy breathing caused by the exertion of the thighs. Those whose legs are in poor condition, can be pretty certain that the rest of the physique is suffering because of this.

Every famous physique star, a man like Clarence Ross, Jack Delinger, Malcolm Brenner, to name a few, have large, massive chests and well developed thighs. They will tell you that developing them is a "tied-in" task, that the benefits of leg work are manifested in every part of the physique. Take Dave Sheppard, strictly an Olympic Lifter. His development is outstanding yet practically every exercise he does is for the thighs and the other large muscle groups.

Never forget that thigh exercise is one of the best ways to develop great body power. If you specialize on the legs for a good period of time, you will not only experience gains in leg power, but you will find you are able to handle more weight in your upper body movements . . . and . . . naturally add more size, shape and strength to the entire development.

If you are thinking of undertaking a period of intense leg specialization, it is always good to remember that they are just like the biceps or deltoids or any other muscle group, and must be trained for shape as well as bulk. If they get too heavy, or are without the requisite muscularity, they will lack proportion. It is common for physique contestants to forget this, and place lower than they would have done if they had spent as much time shaping the thighs, as they had on using bulk movements. Size is not enough. Few, if *any*, contests have been won with size alone. It is a combination of size, shape, muscularity, posing ability, skin texture and general appearance that takes the top award, and without any of these, your chances of winning are reduced.

The exercises I give in this article are strictly for the thighs and are designed to produce size and shape. They are the best I have ever found, and I have used all of them at one time or another. I suggest you insert some of these in a thigh specialization routine you are compiling. I know that you will obtain great benefit from them . . . as I have done.

EXERCISE 1. LEG PRESS. Here is one movement that will give your thighs a championship appearance and pack them with power. It is one movement in which you rapidly increase the poundage you use, and see good progress in a short time. My good friend, Pedro Calderon, of Mexico City, worked up to 1000 pounds ten repetitions in this exercise. While performing the leg press, it is best to place your feet fairly wide on the platform and make sure your legs are directly under the machine. Breathing in this exercise is the same as in any regular leg work. You take a deep breath while lowering the weight and exhale while returning to starting position. Three sets of ten reps are sufficient for this exercise.

EXERCISE 2. BENCH SQUATS. The bench squat is an excellent way to perform leg work if you are troubled with bad knees. It relieves a lot of pressure and discomfort from the area, and you can handle a much more heavy poundage than in the ordinary deep knee bend. Many bodybuilders are afraid to perform heavy squats, because they do not want to increase the size of their buttocks. The bench squat will eliminate this possibility. When performing this exercise, use a sturdy bench of sufficient height so that when you sit on it, your upper thighs are level with the ground. There's no sticking point as in ordinary squats and you'll experience rapid poundage increases. I recommend 3 sets of 10 squats after a few warm up sets with a light weight.

EXERCISE 3. FRONT SQUATS. This exercise is performed by many weight lifters and is similar to regular squats except that the weight is held across the upper chest, instead of the back. The elbows are kept high, to maintain the position of the bar. While the amount of weight you can handle is considerably reduced, the effectiveness of the exercise is not in any way adversely influenced. It is a terriffic exercise, brings fast results, and since it is "different" than most thigh movements, introduces the element of change and variety when you are tired of the standard type of leg work. Three sets of 10 repetitions should be performed.

EXERCISE 4. HACK SQUATS ON MACHINE. I've been performing this exercise for the past two years, and have found it the best for building the muscles around the knee and front of the thigh, (vastus internus and externus). It is a very good "remedial exercise," fine for strengthening a bad knee. I believe it was the main factor in building up my knee I had injured while playing football. It is good for shaping the thigh muscles as well as packing on added size. Breathe the same as you do when performing squats . . . in before going down, and out while returning to starting position. Three sets of ten repetitions is enough in this movement.

EXERCISE 5. REGULAR HALF SQUATS. Here's a terrific movement for building power and one you mustn't leave out of your routine if you are trying to improve your all round strength. Paul Anderson does set after set of this exercise and credits his enormous regular squat of 820 pounds, and much of his lifting power to this exercise. It is a really good movement for gaining weight and adding size to your thighs. Again use three sets of 10 repetitions.

EXERCISE 6. THIGH EXTENSIONS.

Here's another good thigh shaping exercise and should be done in conjunction with squats and other heavy leg work. It not only adds size but will make every muscle stand out in the thighs when they are flexed. This is practically the only type of leg work I performed before the 1953 Mr. America contest, to get my thighs into shape. The amount of weight you use is relatively unimportant, but the repetitions should be fairly high. Three to five sets of 15 to 20 repetitions should be performed in this exercise.

EXERCISE 7. STANDING LEG CURLS. This movement is excellent for building the muscle at the back of the thigh, the Biceps Femoris. Very few bodybuilders give any time or thought to improving this group. But if you do so, you will gain additional fullness to the thighs, and as they increase in size and muscularity, they will have the effect of making the buttocks appear less prominent. This muscle is just as important to leg development as the triceps is to the arms. While working the biceps of the thigh, you should keep the knee of the leg you are exercising, on the same level as the knee of the leg you are standing on. Three sets of ten to fifteen repetitions is sufficient, and the manner of breathing is of little importance in this movement.

Now that you have a variety of fine exercises for the thighs, there is no reason why you should stick to a few movements and be content with small gains. Use a wide variety of exercises and make really rapid progress. Add that finished look to your musculature by building the thighs of a physique champion. Make sure no one can criticize you for poor thigh proportion, so get working on those under developed lags today and obtain a flawless physique.

This next piece is taken from the September, 1967 Muscle Builder issue;

The Muscle Building Techniques that Made Bill Pearl Great

as told by Bill Pearl "Mr. Universe" to Richard Simons

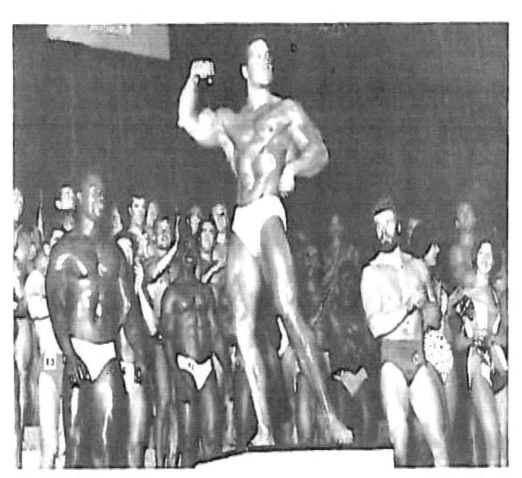

MR. UNIVERSE

Bill Pearl at his best, displaying the "BIG 4" combination: Massive Size, Sharp Definition, Symmetry, Muscularity that are essential for championship glory. Bill had them all the night he won the "Mr. Universe" title in London. The techniques he used to mold this perfection are clearly explained in this article, and you should listen to what this great has to say, if you want Herculean perfection.

Editor's note: Since 1948 every bodybuilding champion has used Weider training principles in his workouts. Sure, some will claim that this isn't so. They'll even go so far as to endorse other methods. Methods that are about as progressive as a snail in a pan of grease. They'll do this for many reasons. Some don't like to give credit to anyone but themselves, feeling that if they didn't invent it, it doesn't exist. Then there's always the guy who'll endorse anything for the almighty buck. Whatever the reason, the facts can't be changed. But don't believe us, you might think we have an axe to grind. Learn the truth from the archives of history. Read Weider publications of years past. See for yourself all the exciting training innovations that were developed through the Weider Research Clinic and given to the bodybuilding world first through Weider Publications. After you've done that, check on other physical culture magazines of that or any time. Those phrases, the ones you and the champs use so glibly today—"super sets," "Tri-bombing," "instinctive training" and "split routines," are just a few of the many that were developed by Weider yesterday. At the time, we were called "crackpots." After we had proved the value of Weider training the various principles would mysteriously materialize in different bodybuilder's routines. This is all in the past, but that past can be examined and analyzed. If you do this you will find that all worthwhile training principles were developed by Weider. This is a fact.

With the idea of keeping that record straight, the following is printed with the sincere hope that it will open the eyes of the younger bodybuilders and jar the memories of the older ones. Remember that the roots of the tree of bodybuilding were planted in Weider ground. That "tree" continues to grow and flourish and will bear the fruits of great future progress.

IT was a blistery cold day a few months ago. There I was, my teeth about to crack from the cold, standing at Kennedy International Airport waiting for a plane to arrive. It wasn't just *any* plane, for the one I was waiting for carried Bill Pearl. He was coming to New York to give one of his incomparable posing routines. Finally the announcement came over the speakers that Bill's flight was arriving. As the big bird with the golden tail moved up to the ramp, I began getting a little excited. I was anxious to see this muscular phenomenon. Well, it wasn't too hard to spot something like a Bill Pearl in a crowd. Just look for a set of massive shoulders. Sure enough there he was. It looked like he was trying to conceal his muscularity by piling clothes on it, but this, of course, only made him look bigger. After all, how are you gonna conceal 235 lbs. of muscle that sports a 20" cold arm, a 53" chest and 19¼" cold calves with striated definition that stands out like cables on the Brooklyn Bridge? Ah, if only you and I had such a camouflage problem.

We greeted each other and went into the coffee shop for a bite to eat. In talking with him, I was impressed not only by his obvious size but by the size of his personality as well. Too many bodybuilders today rely on physical size alone—not Bill Pearl. Here is a man whose mind can match his muscles. Now that's really saying something.

We touched almost all the bases as we discussed his many pastimes. Bill has a large library *(Continued on page 64)*

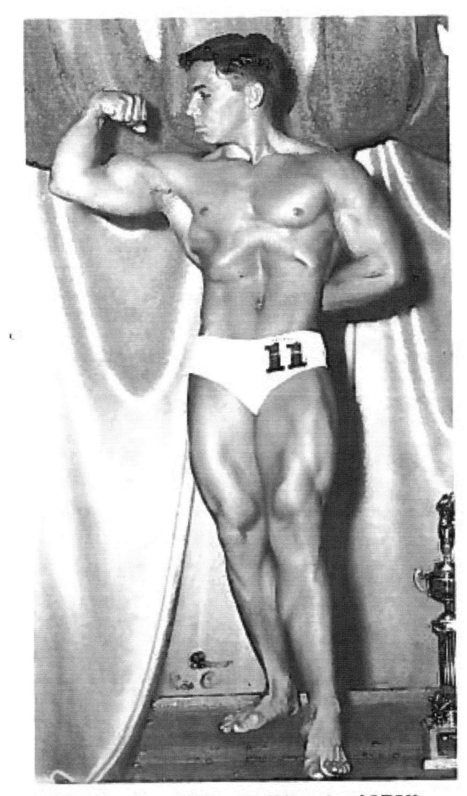

Bill Winning "Mr. California 1953".
In this early picture, he shows his potential for greatness. His arms were 18¼, chest 49, waist 32, 205 bodyweight. He always worked for symmetry and fine proportions.

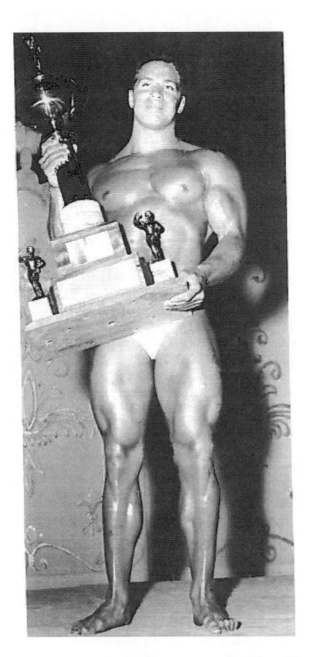

MR. USA

A smiling Bill Pearl displays the huge golden trophy he received for winning the 1956 Mr. U.S.A. contest. Although his physique was great then, he has managed to add massive bulk while retaining his fine symmetry and shape.

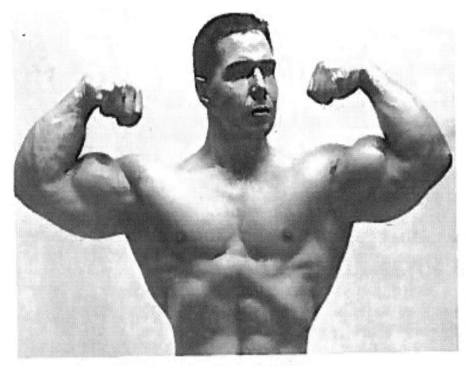

Bill As He Looks Today!

Titanic bulk, and excellent symmetry gives Bill the sensationally impressive body that he owns today. Scientific training and diet helped Bill keep the BIG 4. Although he is 37 years of age, he retains his massive bulk and perfect symmetry that have made him immortal.

BILL PEARL

(Continued from page 18)

covering many topics. One of its biggest departments being that on nutrition. He also collects coins and American antiques of all sorts. The antiques he loves best are the type that run on four wheels. Recently he was casting covetous eyes on a Stanley Steamer, but the price tag weighed more than the car did.

By this time we were well into our meal. I noticed that he was eating everything that was put before him without any particular regard to what it was. This made me wonder. "Bill," sez I, while munching on a piece of toast, "how have you been training for the show?" "Well, Rich," said Bill, "I'm a very busy guy and because of that, I've gotten in the habit of getting up at 5:15." He could see the look of surprise on my face. "I know it sound pretty rugged," he continued, "but once you get in the habit it isn't so bad. Of course, it's getting in the habit that's tough." (Weider Instinctive Training Principle—Ed.)

"I've been training for quite a few years now and I've found that hard work is the only answer for results. So I really hit it hard with four or five exercises per muscle group, doing about 30 sets for each of the groups. Since I don't have much time, I've found that I have to split my routine, doing my upper body one day and lower body the next. In this way I can concentrate on the parts I'm working on more completely. (The Weider Split Routine Principles—Ed.) "My workouts run 2½ to 3 hours and I vary the sets and reps from day to day. I was literally doing six different routines a week."

"With all those sets and reps you must really have to work like a demon. I'll bet you have to work pretty fast to get everything in before you open the gym." Bill nodded. "Personally I find that fast training is best for me. I don't even rest between sets." (The Weider Speed System —Pioneered by a member of the Weider Research Clinic, Leroy Colbert—ed.) "Well," I said, "the results are pretty obvious." "I want to emphasize, however," said Bill, "that you don't *have* to train fast to get a great physique. Champions like Jack Dellinger, Ray Shaefer and Marvin Eder took long slow workouts. I think each bodybuilder should experiment by trial and error until he finds the best combination of factors for himself. Make the routine fit your own personal needs."

The sun was beginning to break through the clouds making a shaft of light glare in my eyes. The warmth felt good though. I squinted across the table at Pearl. "How about cheating movements? Do you use any of them when you train?" Bill thought for a moment. "Cheating movements are good for some bodybuilders," he said, "especially those who need bulk and power. On the other hand, strict movements bring out shape and definition to a greater degree, which I feel is important to the finished physique. Now, I feel that I'm pretty well stocked in the size and power department so I concentrate on the strict moves with full extensions and contractions with every rep." (Weider Peak Contraction Principle—ed.) "When you cheat you're actually taking away the stress from the muscles you're trying to reach."

Bill finished off a large glass of milk. "You know, Bill," I said, "I've noticed that you have pretty 'normal' eating habits which makes me wonder about your diet. Do you use many supplements?" "No, I don't. Let me qualify that. I use supplements when I feel I need them. In other words if I need to bulk up before a contest, I've found I can put on as much as 25 lbs. in a month's time, by adding protein powder to my diet. Again let me stress that this is the way *I* respond. I know of many who can't do without a continual source of supply of all types of supplements. Again I must emphasize that we must take and do what is best for each one of us."

"Okay, now Bill, while I've got you here, tell me the 'secret' routine you must use to get all that muscle." "What?" said Bill in surprise. I laughed, "I'll bet you hear that a lot don't you?" "Yes, I do. And there *is* a secret." Now *I* was the one who was surprised. Suddenly I felt I might be getting in on something big as I leaned forward in anticipation. "What is it?" I asked eagerly. Bill smiled. "Ready? *Hard work!* That's the 'secret' of *any* success. I've worked out at least five times a week for the last 17 years. During that time I've never spared the horses with either weight, reps or sets. If there *is* any 'secret' I believe it's hard regular workouts."

The waitress brought us the checks and we left. As we walked through the terminal I asked Bil what he thought of the future of bodybuilding. He shook his head. "Rich," he said, "I think that within the next few years there will be thousands of Reg Parks, Larry Scotts, Harold Pooles and Bill Pearls. All over the country there are guys who could be the greatest if they would only train. Great physiques will be seen everywhere. Compared to the Mr. America of 1985, I'll look like a kid. The standard of excellence in bodybuilding is improving every day." "What do you consider the most important qualities in a physique?" I asked. Bill's answer was quick, "Cuts, shape and proportionate symmetry. I've been training for almost 20 years and I've specialized in almost every type of routine you could think of. Bulk, power, definition and shape routines, you name it and I've done it. Whatever the program, if the results you get bring you a symmetrical and proportionate physique with health and physical fitness then you've struck oil." "Yes, it is Rich, I plan to reach one hundred years of age in good condition. I believe that a strong heart and good circulation is more important than arm size, that's why I run two or three miles a day."

We were standing outside by now. Luckily we found a cab quickly and were on our way to Manhattan. On the way Bill told me of the activities of Pat Casey. Some of the things I found hard to believe. He told me that Pat does incline lateral flyes with a pair of *200*-lb. dumbbells for several reps. He's also done a full parallel bar dip with 400 lbs. At a bodyweight of over 300 lbs. it doesn't take a mathematician to figure that Pat was lifting over *700 lbs.* total. To top all this off, Pat has done a strict bench press with 620 lbs. in training. Before all these astounding facts could sink in we had reached Bill's destination. We said goodby and I went on to the Weider office in Union City.

I was feeling pretty good. I had a great time talking with Bill and now I was on my way to work at the Weider Barbell Company. I got to thinking of all the Weider principles that Bill has used and is using to build and maintain his great physique and I began to feel proud. I think I worked with a little more enthusiasm that day. And why *not?*—I was working for Joe Weider, the trainer of champions since 1936!

65

Chapter 7   Vince's Gym

Vince's Gym was in Studio City, California which he ran from 1948 to 1997. The exact address was; 11262 Ventura Boulevard, Studio City, CA. (Between Vineland and Tujunga Avenues.)

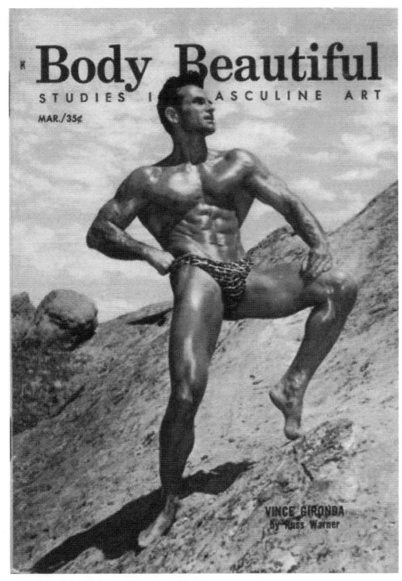

Vince in his heyday

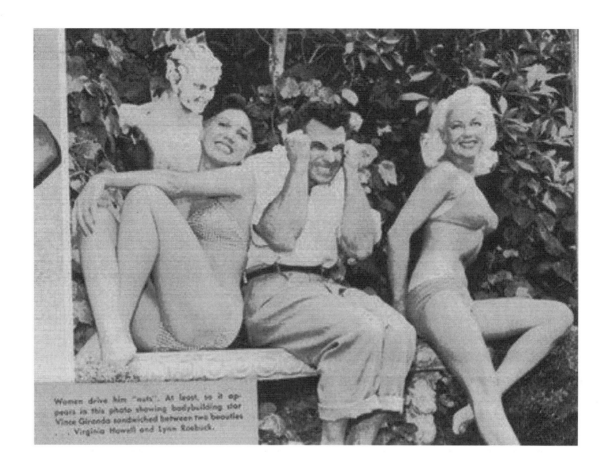

The caption says something about women driving Vince nuts.

This author wrote a book about Vince and his gym, and trained there in the '80s;

http://whowasvincegironda.com/vince-gironda-gym.html

For over 50 years in Hollywood and throughout the fitness universe there was only one place to be... "Vince's Gym". His small almost museum like health club was always packed with bodybuilding wanna be's and many big name TV and motion picture stars. I was trained by Vince Gironda in the early eighties and did my own workout there at 11 am each day, usually you were paired up with someone on training days, quite often it was a star but in Vince's eyes even the big names were nobody's in his gym, in this small little space he was king and made ALL the rules. It was common place for him to simply decide he didn't want to deal with your face that day and he would throw you out and tell you to come back tomorrow, I think all totaled in the 2 years I was there he threw me out over a dozen times, but there were others that got the boot more times than I did. After 50 years in the business Vince definitely had his own ideas on how things should be run, he never allowed cable for the cross- overs he only allowed rope, I asked him once why, big mistake....he got right up in my face and said machines made cable "Man" makes rope and then I was told to leave for asking a stupid question. If you were lucky enough to make it through your workout before he tossed you out it was common place for him to be visited by great old time bodybuilders, politicians and movie stars. Vince had a fondness for beautiful starlets and I recall a time there were 3 men in the gym including me and 5 well known TV and movie female faces in the room, out of the blue in the middle of a bench press he told all the guys to leave "today is women only day", so much for your workout but there was no place else in the world you could learn more than Vince's Gym so you always came back for more. I owe a lot to Vince for all he taught me, I have been a Personal Trainer for 30 years now and many of my concepts are a trickle down from the Great One, I have been a Masters Bodybuilder since 1989 and still hear his voice in the back of my head every rep telling me never forget..."Everything works, but Nothing works for ever". His concepts are still the ultimate for contest prep at any age and are used daily with my clients. I am proud to say I knew this man and will never forget my days at Vince Gironda's Gym.

Ken P Babich
Personal Trainer 30 years
Business web site http://www.quadfather.com
57 years old, 55 and over Grand Masters Pro WNSO/Fame

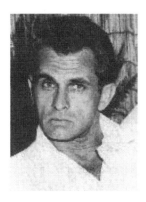

Born November 9th, 1917
Died October 18th, 1997

Vince Gironda's bodybuilding contest history includes:

1951 Pro Mr. America 2nd
1956 Mr. USA Did Not Place
1957 Mr. USA 3rd
1962 NABBA Pro Mr. Universe Short, 2nd

Vince's Gym was a small, old school gym. The motto was - No fancy machines, no music, just basic free-weights and hard training. All the top bodybuilders and many movie stars trained there.

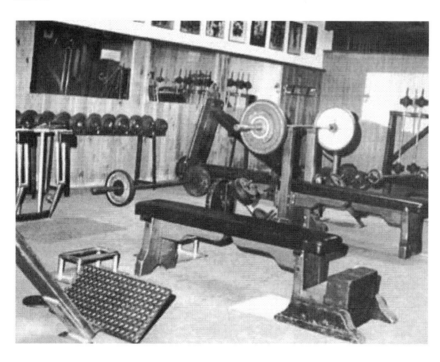

Vince's Gym in the early days

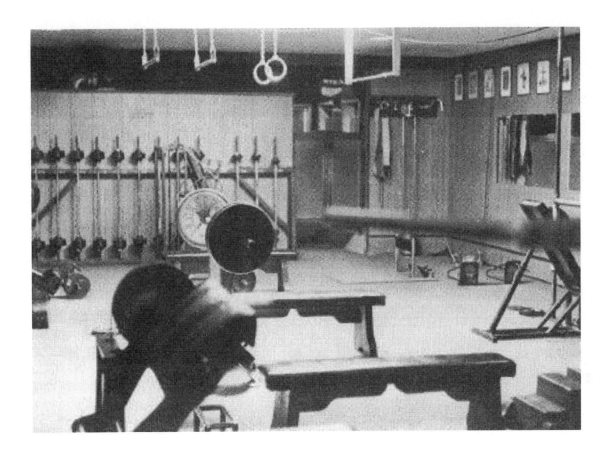

Here's another shot of Vince's gym.

How much did Vince charge to join his gym? It cost $300 to start to as a member.

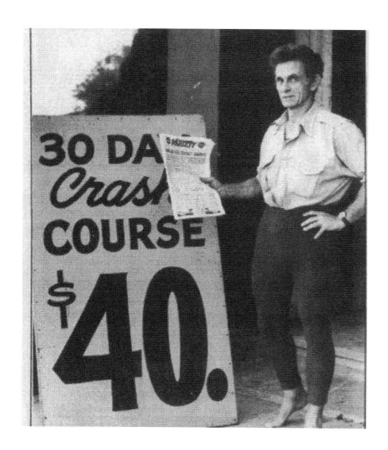

Special deal!

Many top bodybuilders and movie stars trained under Vince Gironda at his famous gym.

The **Bodybuilders** included:

Arnold Schwarzenegger, Don Howorth, Don Peters, Frank Zane, Freddy Ortiz, Jake Steinman, Larry Scott, Lou Ferrigno, Mohamed Makkaway, and many more!

The **Movie Stars** Included:

Burt Reynolds, Cher, Clint Eastwood, Carl Weathers, Denzel Washington, James Garner, John Schneider, Kurt Russell, Shawn Penn, Tommy Chong, Erik Estrada, and many more!

Another website dedicated to Vince is this one;

http://ironguru.com/vinces-gym/

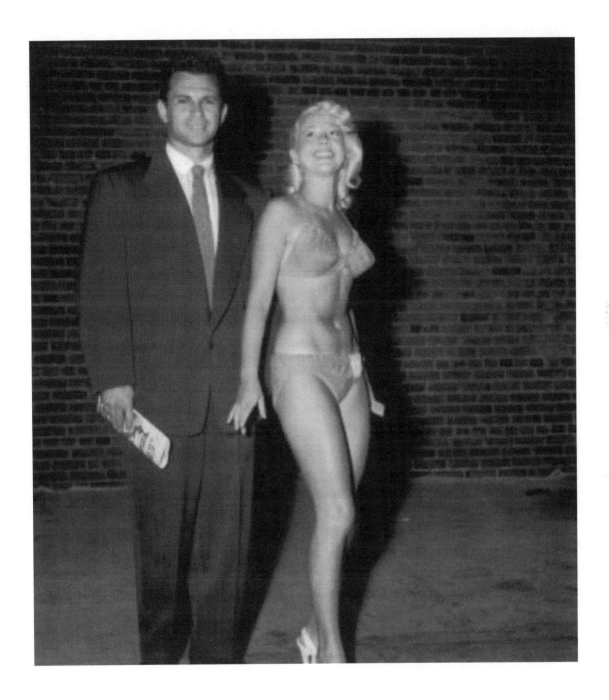

Vince in 1950 with one of his lovely pupils; Lynn Roebuck.

You may recall Lynn's name mentioned as one of the winners in a muscle beach pageant

In my "**Forgotten Secrets of the Culver City Westside Barbell club revealed**", I retold a couple of stories about Vince & his gym that were told to me by Joe DiMarco. Joe confirmed the fact that Vince would routinely toss out anyone he pleased to for whatever reason he deemed reasonable. Here is an excerpt from my book, from the Joe DiMarco chapter; Joe and I talked about Vince Gironda, who had a column in the **Muscle Builder** magazine during the same era as the Bill West and Joe DiMarco articles. Joe never met Vince, but said he did actually meet his son, Guy, and actually trained with him a bit. Joe thought it ironic that he actually got Guy to do squats, which was a pet peeve of his dad's, who advised very strongly against them. Guy was pretty strong on the squat, in fact, starting with around 400 pounds in the lift. Joe also said that Vince was against neck training for the bodybuilder, saying that an overly developed neck makes the shoulders appear less wide, but Joe was amused by the fact that Guy had a pretty well developed neck himself. Joe said Vince was very particular about the way people at his gym trained, and that he actually would run guys out of his gym with a baseball bat if they used what Vince regarded as unsound methods, or otherwise got out of line in any way. Squatting was one of the taboos, and in fact there were no squat stands at Vince's Gym. One of the men that was a victim of such treatment was actually **Robert Blake**, the bird loving detective we all remember well, told Joe. Word has it that **Clint East**wood got a similar treatment from Vince.

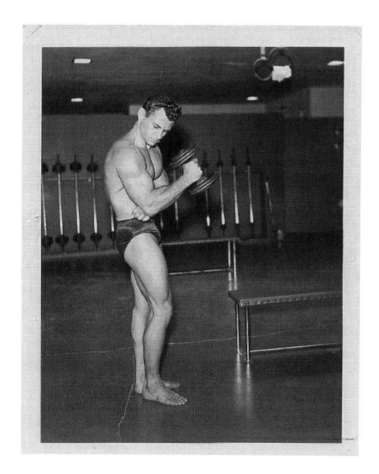

Vince using one of his own special arm training techniques

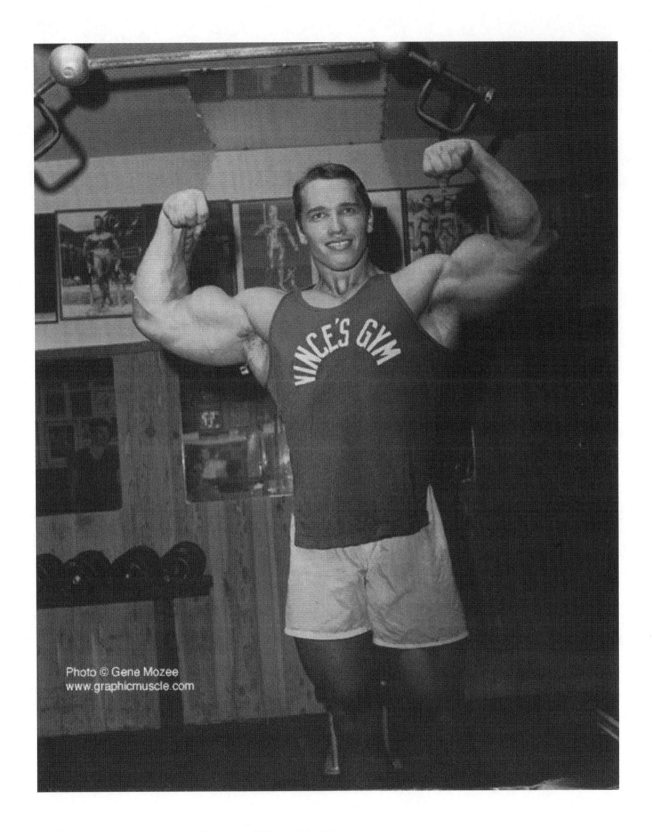

This guy spent some time at Vince's Gym

Arnold reportedly was introduced to the preacher curl, AKA the "Scott Curl" at Vince's, and he took to it like a fish to water

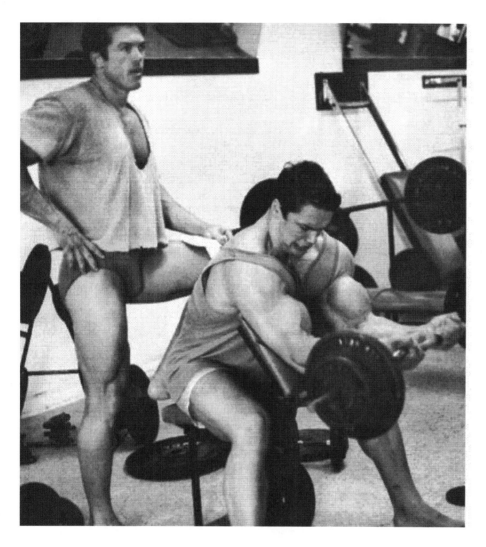

The guy behind Arny was pretty popular in the '60s, too.

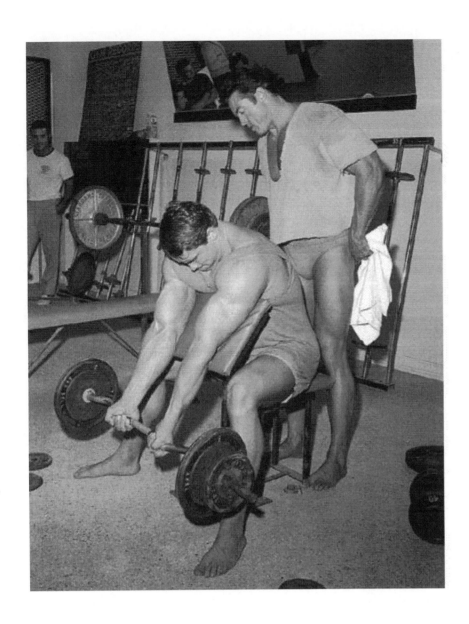

Here is another shot of Arny at Vince's, with Don Peters looking over his form.

Here is an early article on Vince when he was just "coming into his own"

Muscle Power, Vol 11 No 6, Page 16, May 1951

Meet Vince Gironda

By Barton R Horvath

From sunny California, the cradle of hundreds of physique stars, the fame of Vince Gironda has engulfed the globe. Here are intimate details of the man, his career and his opinions. Exclusively YOURS in this inspiring story.

AT the borderline of San Fernando Valley, California, there is a spot where the weak are made strong. Known as "Vince's" gym, the sparkling enthusiasm of its owner, Vince Gironda, combined with his technical "Know-how" of modern physical training, makes possible an enviable record of SUCCESS cases among his many clients. His personal victory over previous physical inferiority and puny weakness makes him a sympathetic teacher whom his pupils worship. The knowledge they have that he too started from SCRATCH...and used the very same methods of weight training to rebuild his own body that he teaches them, immediately secures a common bond between instructor and pupil, and one look at his present flawless physique is more than enough inspiration for anyone. A bodybuilder for more than 10 years, his first taste of fame came in 1941, when at 22 years of age he won the Mr. California title. Vince admits that he could hardly believe it as being true, when he was presented the trophy that great night 10 years ago. As a beginner he had been so much weaker and thinner than the average, that his victory left him breathless, unbelieving that the magic of weights had actually performed another of its miracles... and that this championship body was really his.
[MUSCLEMEMORY NOTE: I have Vince Gironda born in 1917, which would make him 24 in 1941. I also have Harold Zinkin winning the 1941 AAU Mr California.] As reality took hold and Vince found that he had actually rebuilt his body to outstanding perfection, he felt a deep sense of gratitude for the methods of weight training which had made this possible. It was right then that the seed of desire to help others was sown. He KNEW that a kind fate had pointed out his future career to him.. a career of helping others to be strong and healthy. From that point on he dedicated himself to the future realization of this goal... which presently has reached a ripe maturity. While Vince was adding the finishing touches to his splendid physique, his fame spread to Hollywood where his fine appearance and fearlessness placed him in strong demand as a double and stunt man in the movies He still accepts an occasional part, his latest appearances being in the movies JET PILOT as well as in a gymnasium scene in a new Larry Parks picture. Frequently he works together with his good friend Armand Tanny in the movies and their rough and tumble action keeps the public on edge whenever they appear.

Despite all his success he has remained sincere and humble always. It is this undivided attention he pays to every pupil, feeling each of their problems as strongly as though they were his own which places such a demand on his time that frequently he misses work-outs, just so that he can give his full attention to assuring the success of others. This unselfish attitude gives you some idea of his entire personality. Soft spoken, mild mannered, intelligent and a perfect gentleman, he represents the BEST in physical educators. Possessor of a magnetic, charm, his happy marriage to his beautiful wife Peggy, who also is a keen health enthusiast, represents the ideal union and sets a perfect matrimonial example for others to follow. This majestic Adonis, now 32 years of age, is always in perfect condition. He can be seen actively taking part in dozens of contests and exhibitions yearly and has justly built up a following of fans who insist that he represents PERFECTION. Standing 5'9" tall, weight 175 pounds, neck, arms and calves each approximately 16 1/2" in size, his artistic form and clean-cut muscularity is greatly admired. His slim 30" waist, spreading out to a massive 49" expanded chest, supported by powerful 24" thighs, lends an impressively strong quality to his body, and others unconsciously sense his immense strength. His unusual ability in the bench press, with a personal record of 325 pounds, largely explains the massive formation of his thick pectorals and balloon-like deltoids. Always fast to accept modem training methods, Vince has every type of apparatus in his gym. He feels that the time required to build physical perfection today has been cut in a third . . compared with the less modem methods and equipment of years ago. In particular he approves of specialization as a means of rapid progress. A change of pace in the program is highly recommended by him. In this manner the muscles develop more all around utility and serve one better for all physical activities. While he changes the actual exercises he performs from time to time, his manner of performing sets and repetitions is interesting. For three weeks out of each month, he performs all exercises 6 repetitions and in sets of three. The fourth week, he performs all exercises 30 repetitions in sets of five. This varied repetition program builds power, bulk, and endurance, and keeps the physique well defined and not too bulky in appearance, according to Vince. Certainly it has worked ideally in his case. A believer of moderation in all things, Vince is annoyed at those bodybuilders who force themselves to eat and drink to extreme in their desire to pack on body weight fast. Such a program will end up in disaster if continued indiscriminately. A more sensible diet will bring sure and safe gains, so his advice is to never stuff. Personally, Vince is rather indifferent to his prize-winning muscles. Of course he is proud and thrilled to possess an outstanding and world famous physique, but his greatest pride rests in the success of those he trains. Conscientious, ambitious, and progressive, the career of Vince Gironda to date may well be summed up with this incident. One day, not too long ago, a young advertising salesman paid Vince a call. He asked Vince if he was interested in placing an ad in his publication . . . adding, "I'll of course be glad to write the ad for you." Vince smiled and said . . . "My best ads aren't written. My pupils wear them wherever they go." Vince of course was referring to the muscles, good health and happy attractiveness his pupils always carry with them Custom made health and physique . . . created by a great craftsman. . . Vince Gironda . . . the Adonis of San Fernando Valley . . !

This **Muscle Builder** article is a pretty good example of Vince's writing and his training philosophy;

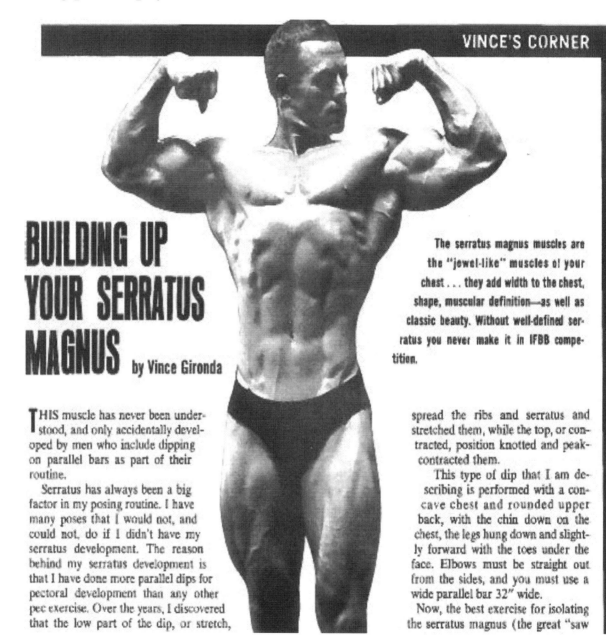

BUILDING UP YOUR SERRATUS MAGNUS
by Vince Gironda

The serratus magnus muscles are the "jewel-like" muscles of your chest... they add width to the chest, shape, muscular definition—as well as classic beauty. Without well-defined serratus you never make it in IFBB competition.

THIS muscle has never been understood, and only accidentally developed by men who include dipping on parallel bars as part of their routine.

Serratus has always been a big factor in my posing routine. I have many poses that I would not, and could not, do if I didn't have my serratus development. The reason behind my serratus development is that I have done more parallel dips for pectoral development than any other pec exercise. Over the years, I discovered that the low part of the dip, or stretch, spread the ribs and serratus and stretched them, while the top, or contracted, position knotted and peak-contracted them.

This type of dip that I am describing is performed with a concave chest and rounded upper back, with the chin down on the chest, the legs hung down and slightly forward with the toes under the face. Elbows must be straight out from the sides, and you must use a wide parallel bar 32" wide.

Now, the best exercise for isolating the serratus magnus (the great "saw

SPECIAL DIPPING TECHNIQUES FOR SERRATUS DEVELOPMENT

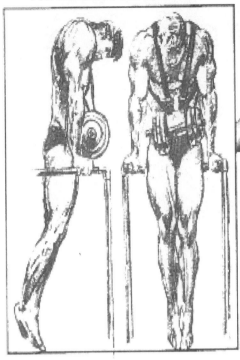

tooth" muscle) is to hang a heavy dumbbell around the waist and perform the top or round back contracted position of the dip. This is a peak contraction movement, and the weight employed should be one that is actually too heavy to dip with. So, in order to get into proper position to perform this exercise, you must step up on a high box or a ladder to get up high enough to perform this top part of the dip only. I also suggest that this exercise be performed after your pectoral work, preferably paral- *(Continued on page 54)*

The serratus, a small muscle group compared with other body parts, is nonetheless impressive; its "saw tooth" appearance lends a finishing touch to the chest. Ken Waller, who performs the kind of dips explained in this article, possesses excellent serratus development.

To be completely effective in developing the serratus, dips must be performed with a concave chest and rounded upper back, chin down on chest, legs hung down and slightly forward. Use a 32" wide grip.

VINCE'S CORNER

(Continued from page 35)

lel dips done in the form I have described in the earlier part of this article.

The function of the serratus magnus muscle is to spread and contract the ribs and to hold the rib cage in place. So you can readily see that any stretching of the chest and contracting movement of the chest will bring the serratus into play.

Here is another one;

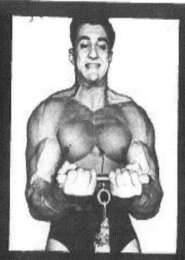

VINCE'S CORNER

BUILDING MUSCLE THROUGH CONCENTRATION

by Vince Gironda

Former "Mr. America" Tom Sansone shows the intense concentration the champs apply in their workouts—total mental and physical concentration—that really builds muscle.

THE bodybuilder of the future will exercise much less than we do today. Every top bodybuilder I have ever observed used concentration to the extent that he is oblivious to the activity around him. Needless to say, such bodybuilders work-out alone because they are aware of individual capacity and need no pushing or encouragement. I, personally, have worked out a program employing 6 sets of 6 reps, getting the same benefit I used to get from 8 sets of 8 reps—and now I use only 70% of my poundage capabilities.

To get maximum benefits from your workouts you must first know the workings of every muscle . . . how and where the muscle is attached to bone, and what exercises involve the various parts of each muscle. Every muscle has a low, middle and high area. The slow-growing areas call for maximum concentration, while the faster-growing areas call for considerably less. This is one reason for choosing the naturally-attributed areas to work on; do not destroy confidence by selecting areas that do not have a natural tendency to build.

Concentration is confidence. The more confidence you build, the greater concentration you are capable of.

All the champions I have observed have one shared quality—an unshakable belief that they will succeed. Should you ask a champion bodybuilder how he gets into shape, he (9 chances out of 10) will reply, "I think about it." He uses a form of self-hypnosis to develop maximum muscle size. Thus, positive thinking opens channels in his mind and allows positive building; his muscles respond.

You can see such men grow day by day—and you can do the same by first knowing your muscles and then tackling them with undaunted determination—*CONCENTRATE!*

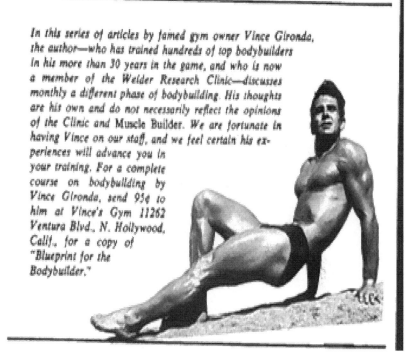

In this series of articles by famed gym owner Vince Gironda, the author—who has trained hundreds of top bodybuilders in his more than 30 years in the game, and who is now a member of the Weider Research Clinic—discusses monthly a different phase of bodybuilding. His thoughts are his own and do not necessarily reflect the opinions of the Clinic and Muscle Builder. We are fortunate in having Vince on our staff, and we feel certain his experiences will advance you in your training. For a complete course on bodybuilding by Vince Gironda, send 95¢ to him at Vince's Gym 11262 Ventura Blvd., N. Hollywood, Calif., for a copy of "Blueprint for the Bodybuilder."

Vince on Training philosophy

Philosophy Of Champions

by Vince Gironda

CLANCY ROSS used to say, "Don't talk to me during my workouts—talk to me after I am finished, and then I'll help you." Clancy would also advise people to never talk to him about training after he left the gym.

Dwelling on the subject of training all day long causes *endocrine tension* which can upset the chemical balance of your nervous system. This form of tension can be absolutely destructive to the muscle-building process and hinder formation of new tissue. For the growth process to function to its optimum level, all of your glandular processes must operate with maximum efficiency. Worry and anxiety over constantly dwelling on your workouts can prevent the free flow of endocrine secretions which is necessary for the rebuilding of *nervous energy force*. Remember—nerve force is essential for rebuilding tissue.

When you are in the gym, you are there to concentrate on training and work; but the minute you step out of

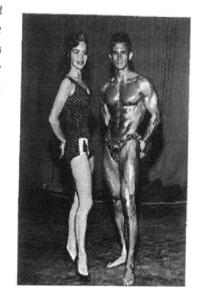

Editor's note: *MUSCLE BUILDER is proud to present this monthly series of articles in which one of the all-time great bodybuilding experts has been invited to freely present his own unique ideas, which are the product of more than three decades of experience in weight training, as a participant and instructor. Although many of his early contemporaries have retired from the field, Vince Gironda continues to both practice and preach. That he practices what he preaches is attested to by the fact that he has a physique that would not be out of place in top-flight modern competition with men half his age. That he preaches well is attested to by the many superb physical specimens who have trained under his direction. Have you purchased his course, "Blueprint for the Bodybuilder" yet? If not, rush 98¢ to Vince at 11262 Ventura Blvd, N. Hollywood, Calif.*

there to concentrate on training and work; but the minute you step out of the door when the training session is over, fret not, "turn it off." Give your subconscious mind a chance to perform its mystical job. Over-enthusiasm is the bodybuilder's worst enemy. You must always remember that *tranquillity* is the first rule of good health—I have never observed a champion who did not subscribe to this fact.

It is my honest opinion, based on thirty years of bodybuilding experience, that you cannot fail to make gains if you see yourself as you wish to be. Changing your workouts around constantly is not the answer, but a proper mental attitude is. Never doubt or lose sight of the fact that you will reach your goal. I personally agree

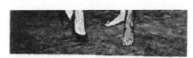

Vince's career spans 35 years of muscle-building. He has won numerous titles—has trained with the world's best—designed unique training equipment and is here seen with pretty Nicki Gibson, taking 3rd in the MR. USA CONTEST . . . losing to bigger and heavier men—at least 40 pounds heavier . . . champs like Ross and Pearl. He's truly an all-time great!

with Reg Park who contends that there are only one or two good exercises for each given muscle. The rest of the exercises are only variations.

Most of my training is done with workout partners and the training program is changed often to keep them interested and enthusiastic. I normally change the exercises each month only because my training partners are not capable of real concentration. Whenever I have a show or photo session coming up, however, I always revert back to my own specialized training program which works best for me. I also work out alone with as few people as possible in the gym and take the phone off the hook. Training without interruption allows maximum concentration and full attention to be focused on my workout. Any interruption can ruin a workout by dissipating nervous energy. Concentration such as this is not a conscious thing except for the surface awareness of the proper amount of sets, repetitions and weight to use in such exercise. All great champions have this ability of complete concentration which allows them to use their nerve energy force to its maximum.

A Bodybuilding Team For Vince?

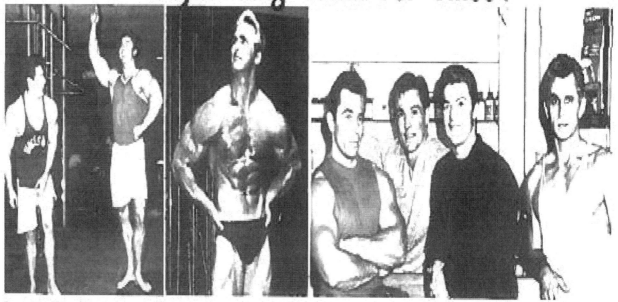

Gym owner Vince Gironda (extreme right) boasts so many star members that he's divided them into "teams." When one such team competes, the others cheer. His "first string" comprises Don Howorth, Larry Scott (you see them clowning in photo at left), Bill McArdle (middle photo), and John Tristram (left end, right photo). In the group photo you see Bill Smith, muscleman television star, between Tristram and Scott

FROM DICK TYLER . . . "Vince Gironda has so many great physique stars training at his world-famous gym, that he's gotten to refer to it as his 'football team.' He even has a 'first' and 'second string.' First string consists of Larry Scott, Don Howorth, Bill McArdle and John Tristram. These are well-established stars. The newcomers who are rising swiftly in the ranks of bodybuilding are the second string. They are such men as Gable Boudreaux, Mike Coleman, Fred Sills and Don Peters. When a local contest is on the whole 'team' goes. The first string sits in the audience and roots the second string, posing. This sounded like a great idea so I asked if I might join the team. 'Sure,' Vince replied, 'we need another man.' Without saying another word, he went into the back room. A minute later he came out with a bucket in his hand and tossed it to me. 'Good luck,' he said."

Here is something from Vince but retold by another author;

By Tom Venuto for Ironman Magazine

When Joe Weider brought Arnold Schwarzenegger to America, the first thing Weider did was to send him to Vince's Gironda's Gym in North Hollywood to whip the over-bulked Austrian into top shape. Legend has it that when Arnold walked in the door, he introduced himself to Vince by saying, "I am Arnold Schwarzenegger, Mr. Universe." The inimitable Vince replied, "You look like a fat f*** to me." Yes, Vince had a way with words. He was also known for a mercurial temper and complete intolerance for anyone who refused to follow his rules. The list of reasons for expulsion from his gym included offenses such as laziness, squatting, bench pressing, taking steroids, mentioning the word jogging and asking for advice and not following it. Personal foibles aside, Vince Gironda may have been the greatest bodybuilding trainer who ever lived. Vince was brilliant - decades ahead of his time. Some of his ideas about training and nutrition were controversial, if not downright bizarre. But no matter how peculiar his methods seemed, the results spoke for themselves. During his heyday, Vince was credited with turning out more Mr. America and Mr. Universe champions than any trainer in history. Two of Vince's most famous pupils were Larry Scott, the first Mr. Olympia, and Mohammed Makkawy, twice runner-up in the Olympia (behind Samir Bannout in 1983 and Lee Haney in 1984).

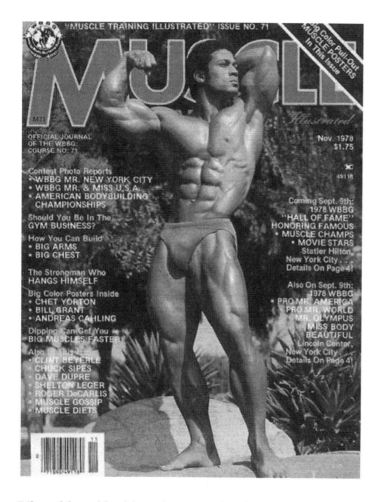

Makkawy

Vince himself achieved an amazing level of muscularity and definition long before being shredded was in vogue. It's speculated that the reason Vince never won a major physique title was because he was too ripped for his day and age!

Trainer of the stars

Before it's doors closed after nearly 50 years in business, Vince's Gym was the number one destination for Hollywood stars that had to get in shape in a hurry. Movie execs would often send their flabby leading men and women to Vince so he could work his magic on them. Although it was located conveniently on Ventura Boulevard in Studio City, Armand Tanny once said, "If Vince had his place on a Tibet mountain top instead of near the major motion picture studios, his followers would make the pilgrimage." Vince had the ability to get the movie stars in shape so fast it was almost uncanny - not in months - but in weeks or even days! Cher, Erik Estrada, Clint Eastwood, Denzel Washington, Michael Landon, Kurt Russell, Burt Reynolds, Carl Weathers and Tommy Chong were just a few of the names on his star-studded client roster. Vince was one of my very first mentors. When I was a teenager just starting in bodybuilding, I cut out and saved every one of Vince's articles from Ironman and the other muscle mags. I purchased all of Vince's mail order courses and studied every word as if my life depended on it. I experimented extensively with his techniques and came to the conclusion that Vince possessed esoteric knowledge about the art of bodybuilding that few others ever had or ever will have.

Vince's most powerful training system: The 8 X 8 "honest workout"

Vince was known for his unusual training methods. Some of his unique exercises included the bench press to the neck, the sternum chin up (touching the chest to the bar), "drag" curls and sissy squats with what he called a "Burlesque Bump." His training systems included 15 sets of 4, 3 sets of 12, 6 sets of 6, 10 sets of 10 and 4 exercises in a giant set - one for each "side" of the muscle. Of all Vince's techniques, the 8 sets of 8 program was his favorite for the advanced bodybuilder. "I have a definite preference for the 8 X 8 system of sets and reps," wrote Vince. "I come back to this high intensity "honest workout" more often than any other for maximizing muscle fiber growth in the quickest possible time for the advanced bodybuilder."

8 sets of 8 might be the most effective set and rep combination ever developed for rapidly building muscle fiber size while simultaneously shedding body fat. Vince called it the "honest workout " because of the pure muscle fiber size that can be achieved on it. "Keep to 8 X 8 and your muscle fiber will plump out, giving you a solid mass of muscle density as a result," promised Vince. 8 sets of 8 is so effective that as a 20 year old novice competitive bodybuilder, I was able to gain 17 pounds of muscle drug-free (contest weight from one show to the next) in under nine months using this system. To this day, I still use the 8 sets of 8 system whenever I need a "shock program" to bring up a lagging body part. Vince warned that this set and rep combination is not for beginners: "You have to build up to the stage where you can benefit from this extremely advanced form of training. I doubt if anyone with less than two years of training experience could benefit from this method."

How it works

8 sets of 8 is a high volume, fast tempo, size building workout. It is not designed for strength development - it's purely for bodybuilding or "cosmetic" improvements. 8 sets of 8 will also help you get leaner. The short rest intervals stress the cardiovascular system to the point where calories are burned, the metabolism is stimulated, hormones are stirred up and fat is melted away. Here's how it works: You will select three or four exercises per muscle group and perform 8 sets of 8 on each exercise. Yes - that's 24 to 32 sets per body part! You will work two or three muscle groups per session and rest only 15 to 30 seconds between sets. Each workout will be completed in approximately 45 minutes and never more than 60 minutes. Although this apparently excessive volume might seem reminiscent of the Steve Michalik and John Defendis "Intensity or Insanity" style of training - it's NOT the same thing. These are not two or three hour marathon workouts. You are completing this routine in under an hour. The reason this doesn't constitute overtraining is because you're not exceeding the workout duration that begins having a negative effect on recovery and anabolic hormones. You are simply overloading the muscles by condensing more training into less time.

Why it works: More work in less time = higher intensity and bigger muscles

Many people are under the impression that the only way to make a muscle larger is to increase the amount of weight you use. This is not true. Overload is an absolute requirement to build muscle, but the overload can come in more ways than one. Progressively adding weight may be one of the best ways to provide an overload, but it's not the only way. Vince was all in favor of adding weight to the bar, (provided good form was maintained), but he believed that performing more work in less time was a better method of overload. The Iron Guru's advice: "To acquire larger muscles you must increase the intensity of work done within a given time. This means minimum rest between sets. Push yourself. I feel workouts should be timed and you should constantly strive to shorten the time it takes to get through your routine. This is another form of progressive resistance, and is more important than raising your weights. This principle of overload explains why sprinters have bigger muscles than distance runners. Although it's more work to run a mile than it is to run 100 yards, the sprinter is doing more work per second. Consequently, his muscles will become larger."

Why use 8 sets of 8 instead of "conventional" training ?

The most popular method of training for advanced bodybuilders is to choose between two and four exercises per muscle group and perform three or four sets of 6-12 reps on each exercise. The rest intervals range from 60 seconds to four minutes, depending on the goal. So why bother with such an "outrageous" program as 8 sets of 8?

The answer is because this type of "honest," high volume, fast tempo training will be a complete shock to your body, especially in the beginning when you are unaccustomed to it. An advanced bodybuilder will adapt to any training program within a matter of months and often within just weeks. Once adaptation occurs, you must seek out new types of stress to coax your muscles into continued growth.

Although Vince did not advocate over-training in any way, shape or form, he did advocate using "muscle confusion" for stimulating gains, even if this meant, "temporarily overtraining." 8 sets of 8 is simply an unusual and effective method of overload and muscle confusion. Obviously, this program is not intended for constant use. It's a "shock routine" you can use for brief periods to kick-start a new growth spurt when you need it most. After completing a cycle of 8 sets of 8, you can go back to more conventional methods. How long should you use 8 sets of 8? As long as it keeps working. Another advantage of 8 sets of 8 is that it can be used to work around an injury. Heavy training with 5-6 rep maxes is impossible when you're babying a strain, pull or soft tissue injury. But you can do 8 sets of 8 because you get such an "honest" workout with a fraction of your usual weight. 8 sets of 8 is a fantastic method for pre-contest definition training because 50-60 sets in under an hour is decidedly aerobic. You can easily count each weight training session as a cardio workout. Fast-metabolism types may not even need any other aerobic work while using 8 sets of 8.

How much rest between sets?

Vince advocated "a very businesslike approach towards tempo." He said that using the 8 sets of 8 format is not enough to ensure muscle gains.

What's more important is the speed with which you get through the program. "Minimum rest between sets is a must," said the master. When Vince was training Mohammed Makkawy for the Olympia, he had Mohammed conditioned to the point of doing 8 sets in as little as 5 minutes or less. Your goal is to reduce your rest intervals to 30 seconds or less, ultimately cutting them down to just 15-20 seconds between each set. Once your conditioning has adjusted to the demands, you'll need just five to ten deep breaths between each set, and then it's on to the next set. If your tempo on each exercise is 2-0-2-0 (2 second eccentric, no pauses and two second concentric), then each rep will take you four seconds. Eight reps per set means that each set will take you 32 seconds. With a 15-20 second rest interval, 24 sets will take only 18 to 21 minutes to complete and 32 sets will take 25 to 28 minutes to complete.

Tempo tips

The proper tempo combined with the correct resistance is the key to the success of this program. Vince defined optimal tempo as "the evenly spaced sets (time-wise) without any distractions and complete concentration on when to pick up the next weight and do the next set."
This means no magazine reading, no walking around the gym, no gossiping, no changing the CD in your Walkman, and no - not even going to the bathroom. This program requires 100% total concentration. If you get interrupted or distracted, you might as well pack up your gym bag and go home. Do not put the dumbbells down between sets. Rest them on your knees, but don't put them down or re-rack them. Also, don't release the bar between sets; rack it, but keep your hands on it. If you're using straps, don't unwrap them. Stay on the bench or machine until all 8 sets of 8 are completed. Take no rest between body parts. When you finish the last exercise for the first muscle group, move directly into the first exercise for the next muscle group. By the way, to follow these tempo guidelines means you'll have to ditch your training partner. This program must be done alone.

How much weight ?

Using 15-20 second rest intervals will limit the amount of weight you can use, but that's ok. Initially, there will be a large drop in your normal training poundage. Most people will need to reduce their normal 8 rep max by about 40% to successfully complete 8 sets with such brief rest intervals. For example, if you normally perform dumbbell flyes with 55 pounds for 8 reps with a 60 - 90 second rest interval, you're going to have to reduce your weight to about 35 pounds to successfully complete 8 sets of 8 with 15-30 second rest intervals. you become more conditioned, it will amaze you how much weight you will be able to build back up to while maintaining the short rest interval. Amazingly, you may even get close to your original poundage. At this point, some serious growth will begin to occur. Proper weight selection is critical. The first workout should be made intentionally easy. If you attempt too much weight too quickly, you won't be able to complete 8 reps on the last several sets nor will you be allowing room for progression over a period of weeks. Vince cautioned that the same weight for all eight sets is imperative. If you fail on the sixth or seventh rep on the last set or two, that's fine, but if your reps drop below 8 by your 4th or 5th set, the weight you selected is too heavy.

For the whole body or for body part specializing?

8 sets of 8 is excellent for body part specialization. You don't have to use 8 sets of 8 for the entire body. You can use it for ONE body part a time. For example, if your chest is lagging, you could do the 8 sets of 8 routine to specialize on chest and do conventional training for the rest of your body. If you decide to use 8 sets of 8 for large muscle groups such as legs and back, be warned: it's brutal beyond belief. 8 sets of 8 for compound, large muscle group exercises is extremely difficult because cardiovascular failure may limit your performance. Prepare to be huffing and puffing. You may have to start with longer rest intervals (about 30 seconds) and work down to the 15-20 seconds. Alternately, you'll could start with very light weights and build up gradually.

Which exercises?

Your exercises should be selected carefully to hit the aspects of each muscle you want to target the most. For example, if it's side deltoid and shoulder width you're after, you would select side deltoid movements such as side lateral raises and wide grip upright rows instead of front raises and military presses. Machines and single joint movements will be easier, but don't shy away from the big compound movements just because they're more difficult. As with any training program, the basic exercises will always produce the best results. For example, if you want a massive back, think rows and chin ups, not one arm cable pulls and machines. 8 sets of 8 works as well for calves and abdominals as it does for any other body part. However, Vince was always partial to 20 reps for calves. He would often suggest staying with 8 sets, but keeping the repetitions at 20.

Intensity: "training over your head"

Most of your sets will not be taken to failure, and none of them will be taken beyond failure. On your last set or two of each exercise, it's normal to fail at the 6th or 7th rep. When you can easily complete a full 8 sets of 8 reps, and then increase the weight on the next workout. Although you won't be reaching failure on most of your sets, make no mistake - this is some of the most difficult training you will ever undertake. Training large muscle groups and doing multi-joint free weight exercises are especially difficult. You will face the burn of local muscle fatigue, the challenge of oxygen debt and the difficulty of maintaining mental concentration. 8 sets of 8 is a test of strength, endurance and mental toughness. Gironda called this "training over your head." At times, you won't be sure if you can go on, but once you start, you cannot stop.

How many sets & exercises?

As a general rule, Vince suggested limiting your total sets to no more than 12-15 per body part. He said that if you can't get a workout in 12 sets, you're not concentrating properly. However, he also said there are certain occasions where this rule could be broken. The 8 sets of 8 program for the advanced bodybuilder is one of them.

As far as how many exercises, Vince recommend anywhere from one to four exercises per muscle group, depending on the circumstances. For this particular variation of the program, you will perform 8 sets of 8 reps on two to four exercises per body part. Generally, you will aim for three or four exercises for large muscle groups and two or three exercises for small muscle groups. This is the way Vince had Makkawy do it when he was training for the Olympia. Vince was quick to point out that Mohammed was a "genetic superior," and that not everyone can handle this kind volume. The optimal number of exercises and total sets per muscle group will depend on your level of training experience, your tolerance to stress, and your recuperative abilities. The number of exercises per body part will also depend on what type of split routine you choose. The most important factor is to do only as many exercises as you can fit into the 45 minute time limit.

What type of split routine?

Vince advocated different types of split routines for various purposes. Sometimes he had his pupils train as often as six days in a row with each muscle group being worked three times per week! More often, Vince was partial to routines split two or three ways so that each muscle group was trained twice per week. He advised advanced bodybuilders to use a three-day split with 72 hours of recuperation between maximum-intensity workouts. These days it's more popular to split a routine four or even five ways. With a four or five day split, each muscle group is worked once every five to seven days. If Vince were around today, he would surely give me a verbal beating for saying this, but I've discovered that 8 sets of 8 works with nearly any split routine whether you work each muscle group once a week or twice a week. The important thing is to adjust your volume so you can observe the tempo and time limit rules. If you have a split routine that works well for you, by all means stay with it. For example, if you're on the popular four-day split where you train two days on, one day off, you'll get great results on 8 sets of 8. With this type of split, you can perform seven or eight exercises for 8 sets of 8 reps and fit it all inside of forty-five minutes. If you are on a two or three day split as Vince often recommended, you may have time for only one or two exercises per muscle group, each performed for 8 sets of 8. The sample routine I've outlined is based on a four day split.

The Routine:

DAY 1
Chest
Decline low cable crossover (touch hands at waistline) 8 X 8
Bench press to neck 8 X 8
Incline Dumbbell Press (palms facing each other) 8 X 8
Wide Grip V-Bar Dips 8 X 8

Biceps
Drag Curl 8 X 8
Preacher curl (top of bench at low pec line) 8 X 8
Incline Dumbbell Curl 8 X 8

Forearms
Zottman Curl 8 X 8
Barbell Wrist Curl 8 X 8

DAY 2
Shoulders
Dumbbell Side Lateral raise seated 8 X 8
Wide Grip upright row 8 X 8
Front to back barbell shoulder press 8 X 8
Dumbbell bent over rear deltoid lateral 8 X 8

Triceps
Kneeling rope extension 8 X 8
Lying Triceps Extension 8 X 8
2 Dumbbell Triceps Kickback 8 X 8

DAY 3
Back
Sternum Chin up 8 X 8
High bench two dumbbell rowing 8 X 8
Low cable row with 18" high pulley 8 X 8
Medium Grip Lat Pull-down to Chest 8 X 8

Abs
Double Crunch (pull in knees and elbows together at same time) 8 X 8
Weighted Crunch 8 X 8
Lying Bent Knee Leg Raises 8 X 8

DAY 4
Quads
Front Squat 8 X 8
Hack machine squat 8 X 8
Sissy Squat 8 X 8
Leg Extension 8 X 8

Hamstrings
Supine Leg Curl 8 X 8
Seated leg Curl machine 8 X 8

Calves Standing Calf raise 8 X 20
Seated Calf raise 8 X 20

Conclusion

8 sets of 8 is a little known and very misunderstood program. This is partly because Vince never explained it clearly in great detail- not even in his famous mail order courses. Even when fully understood, most people will never even attempt this type of training because it seems like too much volume and the weights seem too light to get anything out of it. Too bad for them! The real reason most people never finish a full cycle of 8 sets of 8 is because it's too damn hard! 8 sets of 8 reps performed in five minutes for a large muscle group can test the grit of the toughest bodybuilder. You don't have to agree with all of Vince's teachings to use this program. It's natural to resist concepts that are so radical. Vince was quite used to it. Nearly all of Vince's ideas met with a certain degree of skepticism initially, yet eventually - sometimes two or three decades later - many of his methods became accepted as standard bodybuilding truths. When questioned, Vince advised, "If in doubt, try these concepts and try others. Results count. Examine. Test. Then make up your own mind. The secret to success is to believe that the course I give will work and it will. If you have doubts, you will find it won't work." Regardless of whether you think Vince was the greatest trainer of all time or just a crusty old curmudgeon, I urge you to give this "honest workout" an "honest" try.

http://bodybuilding.com/fun/kosloff3.htm

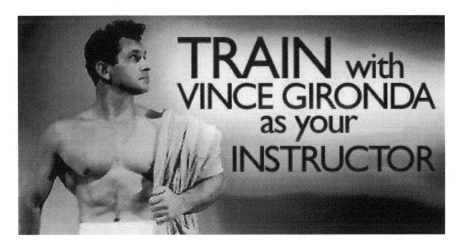

Vince Gironda's Body Drag Curl

If you've ever read any of Vince Gironda's courses you may remember his "barbell body drag curl" movement. I never gave this much thought until I tried it one day out of boredom. To my surprise, and Vince's credit, it is truly an outstanding movement for the biceps. It also takes the pressure off the deltoids entirely. Last and certainly not least, you'll get a killer pump from the puppies!

The Technique

You'll be using a light barbell. Don't worry your muscles have no idea how much weight is on the bar. Men, start with the 45lb bar (or lighter if you haven't been training long). Ladies, find a 25lb straight bar. Begin the movement in a normal curl stance: bar at your thighs with your grip about shoulder-width. During this exercise you'll bend slightly at the waist, unlike normal barbell curls. Now, here's where it gets tricky. Instead of curling the weight up in an arch away from the body, as in a normal curl, DRAG the barbell up, keeping your elbows back at all times. Keep the bar in contact with your body throughout the curl. You'll drag the bar up to about mid-chest level (or a little higher if you can) and control it back down to your thighs. Concentrate on flexing your biceps the entire time. After about 4-5 reps you'll really feel this in the belly of your bicep and you won't feel it in your delts. Just feel your way around the movement and you'll find the groove that suits you best. Standard barbell curls didn't do much for my biceps, but my front delts grew like crazy! Now my biceps are growing. Give this movement a shot.

A Variation

Vince actually performed this with a reverse grip. To me this works the brachialis more than the belly of the bicep. (The brachialis is the muscle that runs between the bicep and triceps on the outside of the arm). However, increasing the size of the brachialis will definitely make your arm larger, so give this movement a place in your routine. The only difference in form is that you grip the bar with your hands facing toward you rather than away from you when the bar is in the starting position. This movement works great performed body-drag fashion or traditionally, arching the bar away from the body. Concentrate by focusing on the side of the arm rather than the forearms to contract and lift the bar.

Vince Gironda 8x8 Routine

Try this exercise and work up to 8 sets of 8 reps with the same weight resting only 30 to 45 seconds between sets.

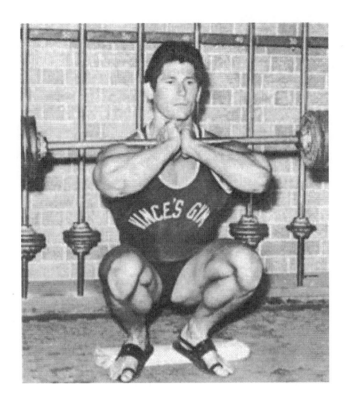

This next article from the January 1968 Muscle builder issue shows Don Peters training at Vince's;

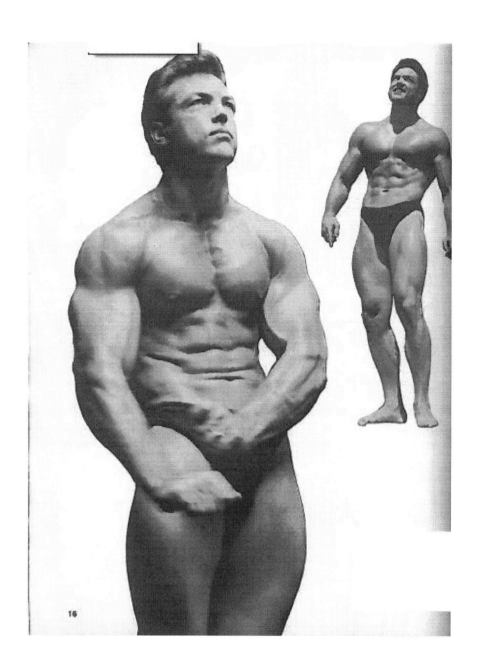

Here is a blown up version of the text box:

The kind of iron-willed determination that makes a champion can be read in every line of Don's face, as he takes this tremendously impressive most muscular pose. Note the finger-like striations in his inner pec region and the very full biceps contour, like Scott's.

TRAINING AT VINCE'S GYM IS A NEW MUSCLE STAR THAT WILL CARVE MUSCLE GREATNESS ON THE WALLS OF MUSCLEDOM

A Future Mr. America DON PETERS

By DICK TYLER
West Coast Editor

YOU know, looking at the title and lead I just wrote, I might have laid things on a bit thick. After all, who can be that great? Answer—Don Peters. I make the fearless prediction that Don Peters will be one of the greatest in a few years... *IF*, and that's a pretty big word, he continues to train with the same desire and purpose he has now. All too many bodybuilders with great potential peter out whenever things don't come their way with the speed they want. Suddenly they stop training, chuck in all they've worked for, and drop off the earth as if gravity vanished on the spot where they were standing. What a pity and what a lousy waste.

Don Peters is not this type of person. He's one of those whose purpose is fixed and whose potential won't be denied.

I first remember seeing Don around a year ago at one of the local contests. At the time I was impressed with his size and shape, but not enough to remember his name. It wasn't until last month that I first heard the *name* of Don Peters.

MON.-THURS.-SAT. BICEPS ROUTINE

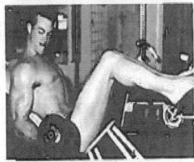

INCLINE DUMBBELL CURLS
Don works his lower biceps with 5 sets of 10 reps of this Reeves favorite.

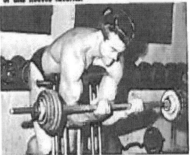

PREACHER BENCH CURL
You can see intense concentration in Don, as he does 4 sets of 10 reps of this Scott all-time biceps favorite.

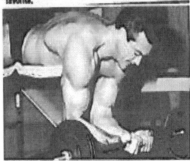

GIRONDA BICEPS BLITZING BENCH CURL
This special biceps blitzer is used for 4 sets of 10 reps by Don.

Reg Lewis and I were sitting in his gym discussing the new crop of bodybuilders that seem to spring up like rows of corn every year.

"You know, Dick," said Reg, "you should do a story on Don Peters."

"Who's that?' I inquired.

He looked at me in surprise.

"Aw, come on, Reg, I can't remember every new bodybuilder that comes along."

"I suppose not, but you should remember the good ones," he said reproachfully.

I figured I'd change the subject by talking about one of Reg's favorite topics.

"Reg," I said, "you've made such great improvement that I think you'd be hard to beat in any contest."

more ▶

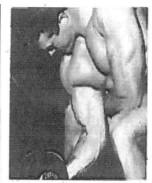

ONE ARM CONCENTRATION CURL
Carves out a very high peak and deep definition. Don does 4 sets of 10 perfectly executed reps.

17

TRICEPS ROUTINE

MON.-THURS.-SAT.

LATS ROUTINE

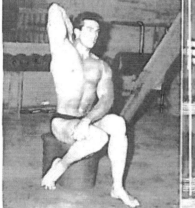

ONE ARM SEATED TRICEPS PRESS
Really works the lower triceps region. Don does 6 sets of 10 strict reps, elbow close to head.

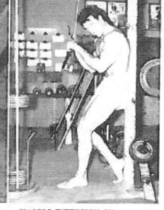

TRICEPS EXTENSION ON THE LONG PULL
Another very strict definition movement, done for 5 sets of 10 very strict reps.

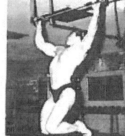

WIDE GRIP CHIN
Don's basic back exercise for width. He does 5 sets of 6-8 strict reps.

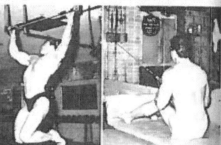

LONG PULLEY LAT EXERCISE
Don gets that streamlined look with 5 sets of 10 reps.

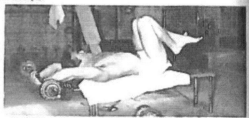

STRAIGHT-ARM PULLOVER
This works just about every muscle in the rib cage, also the lats. Don really hits them hard with 5 sets of 10 reps, done strictly.

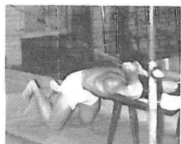

LAT BAR TRICEPS EXTENSION
Strictly isolates the triceps and carves out deep cuts. Five sets of 10 reps is Don's quota for this.

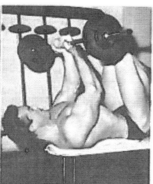

SUPINE REVERSE GRIP TRICEPS PRESSES
A really great bulk builder for the triceps. Don bombs on this one for 5 sets of 10.

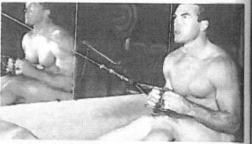

LAT PULLEY PULLINS
This Scott favorite for tapered lats gives Don's torso that 'long line' look, and he carves it out with 5 sets of 10 complete reps.

DON PETERS continued

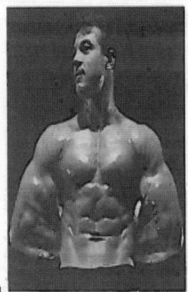

There was silence

"I can't believe you've never heard of Don Peters," said Reg as if I had said nothing. Then I tried another subject.

"That beauty contest you just had sure had some beauties in it."

"You think so," said Reg as his eyes lit up. "How about that girl who came in third. Of course, the winner wasn't bad either . . . ."

I had found Reg's favorite subject. It happens to be mine as well. So who was Don Peters from then on!

Last week I stopped by Vince's for my weekly "lesson" on bodybuilding from the "spaghetti king" himself. After listening to a few of the gems of wisdom he periodically imparts, I came up with a brilliant "What's new?"

"Why don't you do a story on Don Peters?" was Vince's answer.

There was that name again.

"Look, Vince, what or who is a Don Peters?" *(Continued on page 57)*

TUESDAYS FRIDAYS

SHOULDER ROUTINE

SEATED DUMBBELL PRESS
Delts are Don's best bodypart and he begins bombing them with 6 sets of 10 reps.

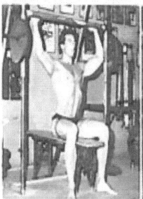

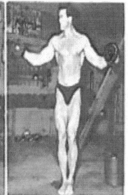

SEATED BEHIND THE NECK PRESS
Don really blasts the lateral delts with 5 sets of 6-10 reps.

STANDING SIDE LATERAL RAISE
This builds massive roundness into the delts. Five sets, 10 reps.

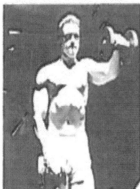

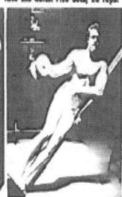

ALTERNATE FRONT LATERAL RAISE
This isolates and works the delt-pec tie-in. Five sets, 10 reps.

ONE ARM RAISE ON THE INCLINE BENCH
Another Scott delt exercise. Do 4 sets of 10 reps.

CHEST ROUTINE

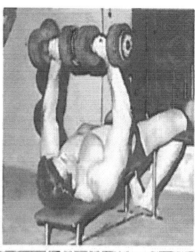

DECLINE DUMBBELL PRESSES
Don carves out shape and cuts with 5 sets of 10 reps of this one.

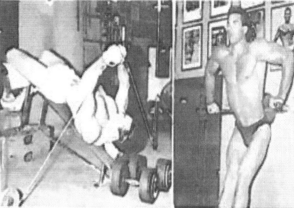

DECLINE PULLEY FLYES
Don Super-Sets this exercise with previous one, set for set.

REVERSE GRIP DIPS
Works the delts, pecs, triceps, the entire upper body. Don does 5 sets of 8-10 reps.

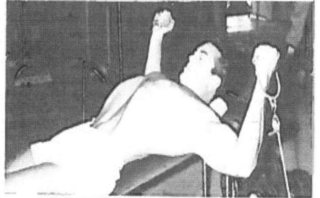

INCLINE PULLEY FLY
Carves out shape and cuts all around the pecs. Do 5 sets of 8-10 strict reps.

EVERY OTHER DAY, ABDOMINALS AND LEGS

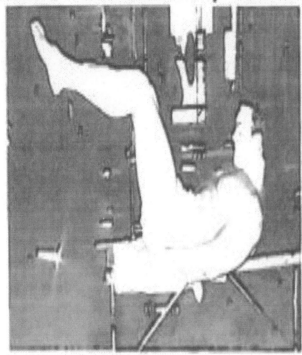

GIRONDA ABDOMINAL SQUEEZES
Carve out abdominal shape and form. Don does a complete movement, doesn't follow sets and reps pattern, just does many sets, many reps.

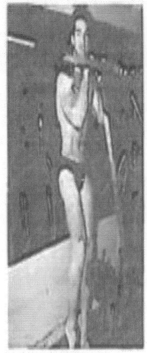

TOE RAISES ON THE CALF MACHINE
Don does 50 reps the first set then 4 more sets of 25-50.

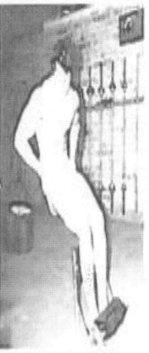

ROMAN CHAIR SQUATS
Don prefers slim hips, so he does 5 sets of 20-30 reps in Roman Chair Squat.

Chapter 8   Ed Yarick's Gym

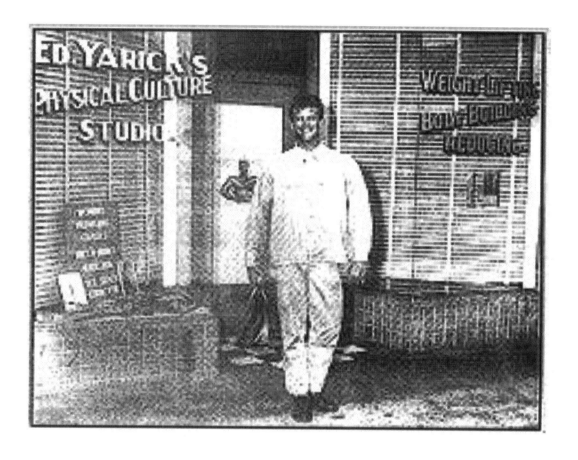

This little gem was found at this guy's site;

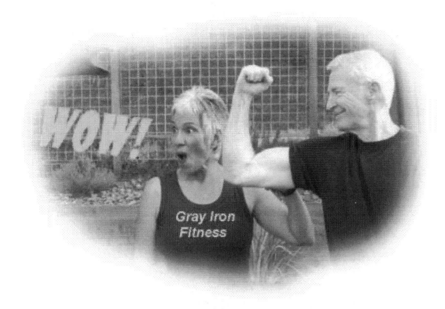

http://www.senior-exercise-central.com/index.html

In the early 1950s, I lived in what was then rural Danville, California, over the hills east of Oakland. At 16, I got a driver's license and once a month would drive to Oakland to DeLauer's newsstand for the latest issues of *Strength & Health* and *Iron Man* (Peary Rader's *Iron Man*, not the magazine of today with the same name). I owned a York barbell set. In those days most people thought lifting weights was pretty strange behavior. Coaches even warned athletes that weights would make them "muscle bound." Today's athletes would laugh, of course. But that's the way it was. Steroids had yet to offer up their ugliness and muddy clear waters. So I was going against conventional wisdom. The muscle magazines promised that weight training would make me big and strong and I believed them. They also introduced me to bodybuilding's superstars, and I began to wonder if there was somewhere nearby where they trained. I found out that a place called Yarick's Gym in Oakland was a gathering spot on the West Coast. Several Mr. Americas and Olympic weightlifting team members had worked out there. It was the legendary Steve Reeves' first gym and Ed Yarick had been his trainer. I scraped together enough money for a month's worth of workouts and drove to Oakland. Now to imagine the Ed Yarick Gym you have to block out any image you might have based on today's modern health clubs. For better or worse, times have changed. As well known as it was in the subculture of bodybuilding and weightlifting, Yarick's was a tiny space, the blinds pulled down over the windows, and sandwiched between other small storefronts on a busy block of Oakland's Foothill Blvd. Inside and immediately to your right were a small wooden desk that was Ed Yarick's office. That's where you paid your dues and he marked you down as a member.

When the financial transaction was out of the way, he would measure and record the size of your arms, chest, waist and legs, and then walk you through the beginner's routine. If you read the muscle magazines you reasoned that you were being given the very same treatment he gave to Steve Reeves only a few years earlier. Man, you were ready to fly. Like other gyms of the day, Yarick's had few exercise "machines." There was a lat pull-down, a cable row, a leg extension device, a vertical leg press, and a couple of basic wall pulley arrangements. That was it. Along one wall the fixed weight barbells were racked vertically. Against the other wall was a long rack of dumbbells that went from fives to well over 100s. Above the weights were mirrors and framed photographs of famous bodybuilders and weight lifters. There were a couple of flat benches and inclines. Basic stuff. More or less in the center of the room was a slightly elevated wooden platform. On it were two Olympic sets, lots of plates, a squat rack, and a heavy-duty flat bench. There was a rubberized kind of mat to protect the platform when weights were dropped during unsuccessful overhead lifts. There was a small box on the floor with chalk in it. The lifters would reach in and chalk their hands before gripping the Olympic bar. Beyond the platform and farther back in the room was a slant board for sit-ups and the leg extension apparatus. The room was a narrow rectangle and couldn't have been more than 40 or 50 feet deep. At the far end you entered the dressing room. Inside, there were two small, metal stall showers with plastic curtains, a tiny bathroom, and several old lockers. There was a bench to sit on. If you didn't have a locker, you hung your clothes on a hook. A door next to the stall showers opened to a small back yard. Outside, there were a few more dumbbells, barbells and benches. The attraction to Yarick's was not its ambiance. It was the man himself, Ed Yarick. He knew his stuff and people liked him. He treated everybody the same, Mr. America winners and nobody teenagers like I was. I remember that he liked soy nuts and always offered them to the kids. "Have you tried these?" he would ask. "They're good and good for you." He was a big guy, at least 6'4" and probably 250 lbs. If he wanted to be intimidating he could have been. But instead he was kind, good natured and friendly. He liked jokes. For a while he not only trained Steve Reeves but was also his training partner. By the time I arrived, Reeves had won Mr. America (1947), Mr. World (1948), and Mr. Universe (1950), and had moved on to Los Angeles for opportunities in television and movies. Another Mr. America (1949), Jack Delinger, was still a regular. Delinger was only 5'6" but weighed 195 and was powerful. He was also a super-intense trainer and the word around Yarick's was that he didn't go for any horseplay. One afternoon some young guys got too noisy and Delinger shouted out just two words: "Shut up!" And the gym went silent. It was the only time I ever heard him speak. John Davis and Tommy Kono were members of the U.S. National Team and stopped to train while traveling through. I watched them one night practicing the Clean and Jerk with huge weights, weights approaching world records, while I, not 10 feet away, curled a ponderous 40-lb. barbell. A Little Leaguer tossing a ball around while a few feet away Ted Williams and Joe DiMaggio took batting practice. The evening that topped them all involved the great Canadian heavyweight, Doug Hepburn. Hepburn was born with a clubfoot that left him with one slightly deformed lower leg. It seemed a minor flaw but I guess he was self-conscious about it because he always pulled one sock halfway up the calf. People said he was the strongest man in the world. While visiting, he and a few local strongmen got into a friendly competition of oddball feats of strength. One of the events was trying to explode a hot water bottle by blowing into it. Hepburn did it and no one else could. Another event required balancing on your chin a tall ladder while walking around Yarick's backyard. Hepburn handled it with ease and grace, but one of the others was also successful. The tie had to be broken.

So someone got a 12-inch ruler from Ed Yarick's desk. Hepburn won the contest by successfully balancing the ruler on his chin while walking around the gym as everyone cheered.

So it went in the first gym I ever belonged to. And I was hooked.

Something from Ed himself:

Strength & Health, Page 28, January 1952

The 1,001 Exercise System

By Ed Yarick

THE axiom, "One man's meat is another man's poison", is the basis of this article. There has been much controversy over the so-called "set system" and the 1001 exercise systems. After 15 years of experience in physical culture work, in competition and the judging of strength events, I have assembled a series of observations on the form and other qualifications that mark the strongman and the "Mr. America" of front rank caliber. Today most of the fellows, beginners and advanced barbell men, are using the set system, where you do from one to twenty sets of one exercise. I have yet to see a man use that system and become a "Mr. America" or a contest winner. I have trained three "Mr. Americas" and many fellows that have won city and state contests and not one of them had used the Set systems. I do not believe you can build a perfect, all-'round body combined with speed, coordination, strength, lifting ability, suppleness and symmetry unless you use the "1001 exercise system". You have to build every muscle on your body from every angle possible. Instead of doing eight to ten sets of one exercise, I teach my gym members to use three or four variations, with three or more sets of each exercise. There are a hundred different ways to vary each and every basic exercise. By basic exercises, I mean the deep-knee-bend, military press, rowing motion, supine press, regular curls, calf raises, and the abdominal sit-up exercise. Prior to "Mr. America 1947" contest, that Steve Reeves won, "Mr. America 1949", won by Jack Delinger, and "Mr. America , 1951", won by Roy Hilligenn, I have planned courses that included many different exercises to work the muscles from all angles for the greatest benefit. A muscle developed in this manner can attain maximum size and strength, combined with suppleness. A muscle built in this manner has a supple texture and more power than the "hard as iron" muscle. Both John Grimek and Roy Hilligenn have this extra fine quality of muscle. And both these men are the best all around men I have ever seen. I have witnessed their performance of splits, back bends, standing somersaults, running, swimming, dancing, and colossal feats of strength with lightness and grace. Grimek's bent press of almost 300 pounds, over 500 pounds squats, over 300 pounds continental presses, amazing crucifix lifts; Hilligenn's 490 pounds squats, 270 pound military presses, dumbbells clean, of 142 pounds in each hand, and 350 pounds clean and jerk. Steve Reeves has amazing power in using dumbbells, and very few can beat him in exercise lifts. So has Jack Delinger. He has military pressed 250 pounds, squatted well over 400 pounds and can curl tremendous poundage.

I have George Brignola working on just such a program. George was considered the strongest 15-year old in the country. He became one of the first to lift 300 pounds overhead. He has squatted with close to 500 pounds; supine pressed 350 pounds, has totaled 750 pounds in competition, and has won physique contests. Men like these just don't happen. They come only as a result of following a correct system of training. I firmly believe that, for maximum strength and development, you have to use a 1001 exercise system in your program. For the squats there are, to mention a few variations, the flatfoot squat, squat on low bench, half squats, partial squats, one legged squats, step on box, hack squats, lunge squats, wide and narrow squats, etc. For every exercise, many variations can be found. Roy Hilligenn is a fine product of this system. He has exceptional lifting ability, all around strength, and a great physique. It has been said that you cannot train for body building and lifting at the same time. Hilligenn and Grimek both have disproved this fallacy, so have Dan Uhalde and George Brignola who train at both. John Davis included many body building exercises in his program, and so do Stan Stanczyk and Dave Sheppard. The "high set system" is a one-sided affair. It builds in one direction only. It definitely does not build maximum strength and development, particularly symmetry. It is monotonous, and the program gets stale too fast. I will, however, agree on this system for specialization purposes only. Without well balanced shapeliness, the greatest strength loses its beauty of form in execution, which distinguishes the finest athletic performance. Therefore I would recommend Bob Hoffman's York Courses No. 3 and No. 4 as the finest courses written to combine strength and perfection in physical development. Only the all around strongman would be able to refute the erroneous, but nevertheless widely accepted theory that big muscles are slow, by a few feats that require speed, agility and strength. There are probably thousands of body builders who believe differently, but as I said, I still have to see a "Mr. America" that successfully used such a program. It is especially bad for a beginner. Many of my members and members of other gyms have adopted the combination of lifting and body building; since Roy Hilligenn won the "Mr. America" title, the combination has become even more popular. Another fallacy, in my estimation, is the cheating way of training. If you cheat, you're not cheating anyone but yourself. It is essential to keep the muscles alive by using training that offers progressive resistance and exercises the muscles from extreme contraction to extreme extension. A Muscle that is being built by cheating exercises cannot obtain its normal elasticity. To do a half curl, a half deep-knee bend, half supine press, half a military press; these will never build a body. It is the combination of many exercises performed correctly that builds the finished athlete of strength and beauty. After all, anything worth doing is worth doing well. Proper training will make you a finished athlete and a disciple of the weight training game. You will then be able to do your bit to improve humanity, to show the way to all that is desirable in a physical way. In that way you can obtain much that is worthwhile from life, and will be an inspiration to others. The body that becomes immortal and serves as inspiration to advanced barbell men is the physique that has been created through proper and intensive training over a considerable period of time.

Steve Reeves

The Ultimate Classic Bodybuilder!

To many Steve Reeves is considered the pinnacle of the male physique. Without the aid of anabolic steroids Steve relied on determination and hard work. He forged a solid 215 pounds of muscle on a 6'1" frame. Winning every major title of his era he retired from competitive bodybuilding at the age of just 24. Steve went on to become a famous movie star and ambassador of bodybuilding. His life was as amazing as his physique. Steve Reeves is truly an Iron Age legend!

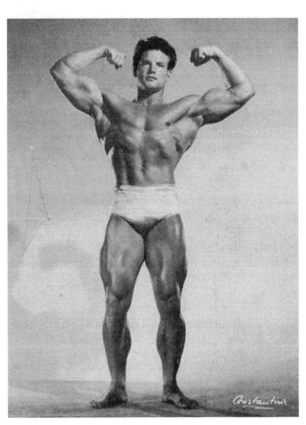

The Early Years

Stephen Lester Reeves was born January 21st, 1926 in Glasgow, Montana. His father died from a farming accident while Steve was just a baby. Steve's early years were spent moving from place to place as his mother tried to find work. He and his mother eventually settled in Oakland, California when he was ten. This move would place Steve at the right place at the right time.

At one point Steve was shocked after being beaten at arm wrestling by a smaller kid from school. He later found out the kid's secret....weight lifting! He found the boy, Joe Gambino, working out in a homemade gym in his garage. Steve also saw his first bodybuilding magazine, Strength and Health with John Grimek on the cover. He'd never seen a bodybuilder before but sure wanted to look like Grimek did. John Grimek sported muscular legs, broad shoulders, bulging biceps, and a thick chest. It was at that point that Steve Reeves knew he wanted to become a bodybuilder. Steve worked out with the other boy for a short time and then began putting together his own gym. He filled his Stepfather's one car garage with weights and make-shift equipment and began his quest for muscles. He responded quickly to weight training. Soon the little garage wasn't enough for an up and coming bodybuilder. It was time for Steve Reeves to join a real gym!

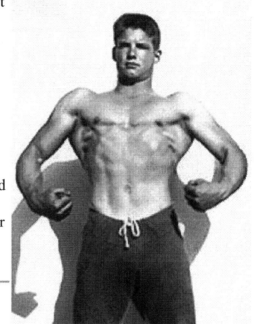

The Gym Scene

His move to Oakland was a lucky thing for Steve since it happened to be the Mecca of bodybuilding in those days. He joined Ed Yarick's gym on the east side of Oakland. It was a real bodybuilding gym with all the equipment a Mr. America would ever need. Yarick was a bodybuilder himself and took Steve under his wing. Ed became the father figure Reeves never had and a life long friend. He put Steve on whole body routines three days per week. Steve entered Yarick's gym at 6' 163lbs. After four months of the full body workouts he was 193lbs! His genetics for bodybuilding were incredible. Most men would be happy to gain that kind of size in four years if they could at all.

The Steve Reeves Workout!
Click here to see the routine Steve used to pack on muscle fast.

His mother helped fuel Steve's workouts with her good knowledge of nutrition. He believed that healthy eating contributed to his success in bodybuilding. Reeves ate lots of fruits and vegetables along with lean meats. Nothing complex; just a good balance of healthy foods. After another year of bodybuilding Steve reached 203lbs and was beginning to make an impression on the local bodybuilding community.

Duty Calls

In 1944 after graduating from High School he decided to enter the U.S. military. In the middle of World War 2 at the time, Steve went through basic training and headed off to the front against Japanese forces. He did manage to acquire a 100lb York barbell set and continued training as much as he could. Reeves caught malaria and remained ill for some time. Losing 25lbs and the incentive to train, his body suffered till wars' end. During the occupation of Japan he was able to acquire more weights and began building himself up again. He gained twenty pounds of muscle relatively quickly. He left the Army at nearly the same weight in which he entered.

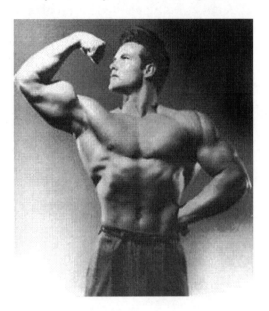

Reeves the Competitor

Once back home in California Steve returned to Ed Yarick's gym and hit the weights hard. He brought his body weight up to 215lbs for the first time and set his sights on the 1946 Mr. Pacific Coast contest. Steve and a friend traveled to Oregon by train to compete in the contest. In his first bodybuilding competition Steve easily won the show. It wasn't even close. Now a title winner Steve Reeves started to become known outside of Oakland. He now thought about the big one, the Mr. America contest. In the mean time he entered and won the 1947 Mr. Pacific Coast contest defending his title. Steve not only took first place, but also won trophies for Best Chest, Best Arms, and Best Legs!

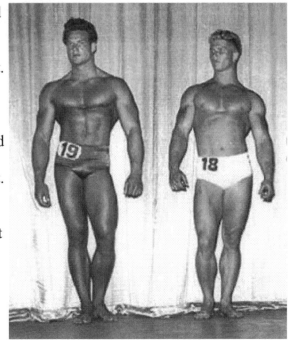

One look at any of Steve Reeves photos of the event will tell you he had deserved every single award.

The 1947 Mr. America Contest

For the 1947 Mr. America Steve flew to Chicago, IL and competed against the best bodybuilders of the day. The America was the biggest title in bodybuilding. He came out on top after initially tying with Eric Pedersen whom he had beaten earlier in the Mr. Pacific Coast contest. With each of them tied at 72 points a pose off decided 1st place. Pedersen came out first and wowed the crowd. Then Steve took the stage and it was clear that it wasn't Pedersen's day. Bronzed to perfection, at the peak of development, and with a graceful posing routine Steve took top honors.

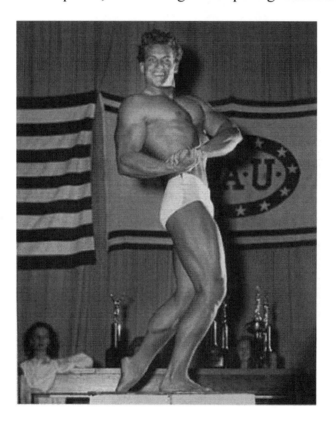

Steve Reeves' measurements on that day were:

Height: 6'1"

Weight: 215lbs

Biceps: 18.5"

Chest: 52"

Neck: 18.5"

Calves: 18.5"

Waist: 29"

Now What?

Steve Reeves had risen to the top of the bodybuilding world having won the 1947 Mr. America title. Not sure of his future Reeves began acting classes in New York. He also worked out at Sig Klein's gym and made guest posing appearances as the newly crowned Mr. America. In 1948 Reeves made a last minute decision to enter the Mr. USA contest. Steve had been lured by the $1000.00 top prize but did not allow time to prepare properly. Rushing a tan, he burned himself badly which affected his appearance and posing ability. A polished and prepared former Mr. America Clancy Ross won the contest.

Reeves had been delivered his first defeat and knew he deserved it. Ross was the better man that day.

The USA, the World, and the Universe

The 1948 Mr. USA was the first in a series of ups and downs for Steve. For the man with probably the best genetics in bodybuilding history he didn't have an easy time of it. He entered the new NABBA Mr. Universe contest in London but took second to legendary John Grimek. Although huge and muscular, John didn't have the aesthetic looking body Steve possessed. The judging seemed influenced by Grimek's gymnastic ability rather than only his physique. After the loss, but still in top shape, Reeves flew to France to compete in the Mr. World contest. Here is footage of Steve Reeves pumping and posing in Cannes, France and winning the 1948 Mr. World title: It's hard to imagine someone beating Steve sporting this physique! However, in 1949 Steve once again was defeated by John Grimek. Steve not only lost to John but actually took third behind Clancy Ross. Grimek was booed and many thought he had received a gift winning first place. Bob Hoffman, Grimek's good friend, was a big figure behind the scenes and that might have influenced the win. This may have been the most controversial bodybuilding event until the much heated 1980 Mr. Olympia 3 decades later. Reeves took time off from competition after the USA and focused on his career outside of bodybuilding.

One More Competition

In 1950 Steve Reeves decided to make another run at the NABBA Mr. Universe title. It had now overshadowed the Mr. America as the biggest title in bodybuilding and Steve wanted it bad. After his recent losses he felt he owed it to himself to once again be on top.

He trained for this competition at the famous York Barbell Club in York, PA with his good friend George Eiferman. Reeves had lost a great deal of his previous muscle and few thought he could get into shape by contest time.

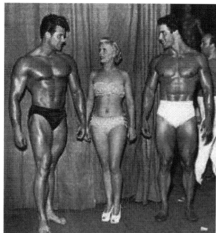

In a few weeks, however, Reeves genetics and muscle memory combined to add slabs of muscle to his frame. Reeves was also motivated by the fact that the new British sensation Reg Park would be competing in the contest. (Park would later follow Reeves starring as Hercules in his own series of films.) Reeves flew once again to London confident in victory. The British crowd had their favorite in massive Reg Park. It was a tremendous battle for sure. Once again, as with the 1947 Mr. America, the contest was a tie for first place. It came down to just Steve and Reg Park. The two were called out for final pose downs. Both men were in top shape and it could have gone either way without much complaint. At the end of the day Steve once again captured the top prize in bodybuilding. Announced the 1950 Mr. Universe, Steve Reeves was presented a very special trophy. A bronze statue of Eugene Sandow. After the contest Steve announced he was retiring from bodybuilding competition to pursue other interests. With no real money in the sport those days he had to think of his future. Acting seemed to be his focus now. No one could have imagined how Steve's physique would impact the movie business. At 24 years old Steve Reeves future was bright indeed. Forever immortalized as an Iron Age bodybuilding champion he would soon become famous the world around as the mythical Hercules!

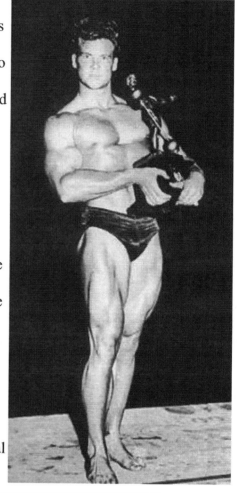

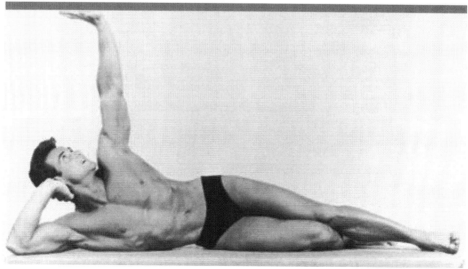

Iron Age Home

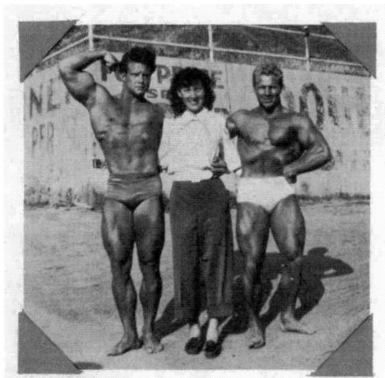

Jack Delinger and I clown around with Ed Yarick's wife. He owned the gym where we trained.

Here's something about Steve penned by Yarick himself;

Ironman, Vol 7, No 5, Page 7, est. fall 1947

Steve Reeves - "Mr. America" 1947

By Peary Rader

We are happy to present this interesting story of Steve Beeves the new "Mr. America". The information contained in this article was obtained from the man who has trained Steve through almost all his exercising career, Ed Yarick, so the information can be considered quite authentic.

On the night of June 29, 1947 at the Auditorium of the Lane High School in Chicago about 3,000 people witnessed the crowning of a new and sensational "'Mr. America". Most of the audience left the Auditorium amazed that such a muscularly perfect specimen existed. It was unbelievable that anyone could have such huge muscular size and yet retain the perfect balance in proportions, the excellent separation that Steve Reeves displayed. Here was a man who combined the massive muscular development that appeals so much to barbell men with the broad shoulders and slender hips that the average man prefers. Here was a man who not only had a magnificent physique, but also combined it with a very handsome face crowned with beautiful jet black, curly hair. a magnetic personality and a flashing smile that showed his ivory white teeth. We have never seen a man who looked finer in his street or dress clothes than Steve Reeves. Everywhere he goes people, turn to stare at this handsome young giant with the very broad shoulders and the erect carriage and lithe step. Steve Reeves was born January 21, 1926 of Irish Scotch and English descent. He grew up as any normal, healthy boy would with an interest in general sports and play. However, he acquired a desire to be larger and more powerful at an early age and missed no opportunity to increase his knowledge on any subject concerning bodybuilding. Steve was not introduced to barbell exercise until the age of 16 when he visited the home of a friend, Joe Gamina. Some of the boys at Joe's house were having a wrist wrestling contest and Steve, knowing that he was much larger and heavier than Joe, decided to try himself. Much to his surprise he was turned down. Upon inquiry concerning this turn of events, Joe told him of his weight training and showed Steve his outdoor gym and weights in his back yard. Steve at once realized that here was what he had been looking for and immediately began training with Joe. The progress he made from the first was very inspiring. and, having a fine framework for a well developed physique, Steve secretly started training for the top reward -- the "Mr. America" title. Barbells became to him what baseball, football, etc. are to other young fellows. Steve literally lived for his training. He began buying all the magazines he could find, both new and back issues, with information on bodybuilding and today has a superb collection. Steve realized his need for the best information available if he was to make the greatest gains toward a perfect physique. To this end he sought out Ed Yarick who has one of the oldest and most successful barbell gyms in California. Steve placed himself under Ed's expert supervision for several months, then was away for a time only to return again to the gym to resume training. After two years training here, he enlisted in the army. During this period he had gained from 166 pounds to 190 pounds of super physique at 6 feet in height. After six months training, Reeves was shipped to the Philippines. While there he contracted Malaria. He lost 20 pounds bodyweight from his first attack. Thereafter he had 7 more attacks. This placed him in very bad physical condition. It was shortly after this that he was sent to Japan. It was here that he was able to obtain a barbell set from the Japanese. For the first time in many months he was able to train again.

He knew that his training would help him develop resistance to disease and return his lost bodyweight. It was just 2 years and 2 days after he entered the service until he was discharged. When he returned home he went at once to Yarick's gym and trained with Ed again. Here he remained training hard until one month before he went to Chicago for the big "Mr. America" Contest. Little had been heard of Steve until he won the "Mr. Pacific Coast'" contest staged in Portland of last December. Steve has always been very regular in his workouts and any misses were noticed by Ed and the other pupils. One Sat. of December '46, Steve failed to show up for his workout. Ed thought this very irregular but thought he would wait until the next workout period before inquiring into the matter. On the next workout period for Steve, Tuesday night in he walked with two fine trophies for having won the "Mr. Pacific Coast" contest in Portland No one but Steve's Mother and a friend, Bob Weilick, who went with him, knew where he had gone. This is quite characteristic of Steve. He would much rather make his plans quietly and leave the shouting until after his victory. Not knowing that he was eligible for the '"Mr. California" contest until too late, Steve did not enter. However he did enter the "Mr. Pacific Coast" contest held in Los Angeles. This was for the 1947 title. This he won also. Eric Pedersen, who won the "Mr. California" contest placed second to Steve in this as he also did in the ""Mr. America" contest, the two of them tying in the latter contest and Steve winning by vote of the judges. Steve was quite confident of winning the '"Mr. America" contest and knew that he had trained the best he and his teacher knew how to win it. Steve's mother has cooperated in every possible way to help her boy realize his ambition by giving him all possible encouragement, helping him keep his training and cooking the things he wanted the way he liked them. How fortunate other boys would be if their mothers took as much interest in their training efforts. She is very happy about Steve's triumphs and thankful for the kindness shown to her son wherever he has been. Steve is not fussy to cook for and likes plenty of salads, meat vegetables and milk. Previous to the training period for the contest, Steve drank one quart of milk per day, but while training for his big event, he greatly increased the quantity of milk consumed, realizing its value. He does not eat white bread, white flour products, candy or white sugar. He likes a lot of fresh fruit, and uses honey for sweets. He always gets lots of sleep each night for he needs plenty of rest when working out so heavily. His mother tells us that he has never had to have a doctor for he has always been in perfect health. His teeth are very beautiful and have not a single cavity. Other than his training with barbells, which is his passion, he likes horse-back riding and likes to visit his aunt and uncle who have a ranch in Montana. He also likes swimming and sunbathing and has a very beautiful tan and a fine textured skin denoting vital health. Steve has no favorite barbell exercises. He just likes lots of all kinds of exercise and hard work because he knows that only by hard work can one succeed. He has followed many programs during his 5 years of exercising but just before he left for the '"Mr. America" contest he was performing the following very strenuous program:

 3 sets prone presses with wide grip.

 3 sets of incline presses (a favorite invention of Ed Yarick)

 2 sets of side presses.

 2 sets of front raises.

 2 sets of curl and press 3 sets of chins behind neck.

3 sets of Latissimus rowing on 45 degree pulleys. .

2 sets of triceps curls on the dorsi bench. .

2 sets of bent arm curl behind neck 2 sets of triceps bench curl.

6 sets of incline bench curls.

4 sets of squats.

4 sets of leg curls for leg biceps.

4 sets of calf raises on leg press machine.

2 sets of good-morning exercise on roman chair.

Steve has never gone in for Olympic lifting in any form being interested only in bodybuilding. In his exercises he has worked up to 20 reps in half squats with 400 pounds. He did 6 repetitions with 70 pound dumbbells on the incline curls. 20 reps in the calf raises with 450 pounds.

His before and after measurements are as follows:

	Before	After
Weight	166 lbs	213 lbs
Height	6 feet	6 feet
Neck	13½	17½
Chest normal	37	49½
Chest expanded	39½	51
Waist	30	29
Thighs	22½	25½
Calf	16	17¾
Arm	12¾	18

Although Steve has been a barbell man 5 years, yet only 3 years of this have been spent in hard training under Yarick. He is sure to improve a great deal more as the years pass. With his broad shoulders and narrow hips, he has acquired the nick name of "Lil Abner". We wish him the best of everything in a life that is just beginning for him.

Jack Delinger

A Mr. America Built Like a Tank!

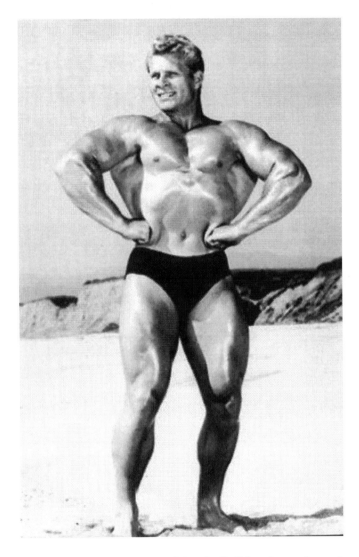

Jack Delinger was born on June 22, 1926 in Oakland, California, a place that would later become *the* place for bodybuilding. The combination of location, weather, and genetic specimens was ideal. At 16 he began training at the YMCA to become a powerful athlete. He was inspired no doubt by the great John Grimek. Grimek, an Olympic team weightlifter combined athletic skill and speed with an outstanding physique. Jack also wanted to improve his gymnastic prowess since he was a member of his high school's team.

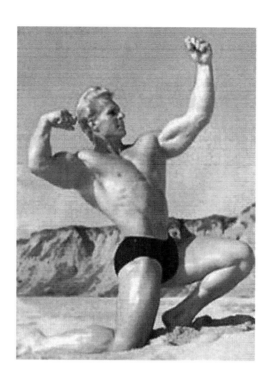

Soon after this he joined Ed Yarick's gym. Yarick was a 6'3" 230lb giant of a man who was a great role model for the young lifters entering the bodybuilding scene. The Great Steve Reeves also trained at Yarick's and was mentored by Ed. Jack was in good hands and achieved his goal of becoming a powerful athlete and more. By winning his first contest, Mr. Northern California in 1946, he was further encouraged to develop a top level physique. He would eventually display a very thick and muscular build, outstanding for his era. It is interesting to note a young Steve Reeve's first impression of Delinger, who was a high school gymnast at the time. Steve was watching Jack's gymnastic routine and noticed that although he had tremendous arms and shoulders, his legs were underdeveloped. Reeves thought, *"If I had his upper body and my legs, or if he had my lower body with his incredible upper body, then we'd both be well built."* **Steve Reeves - Worlds to Conquer**

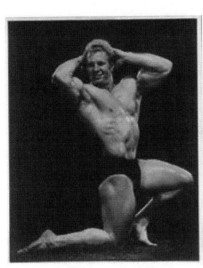
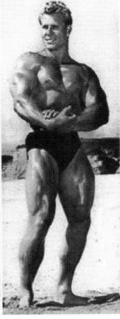
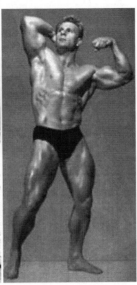

This imbalance, noted by Reeves, did not continue. Delinger devoted himself to producing a balanced muscular build. His legs came up to par and he was eventually known for his great underpinnings. Looking over his finished physique it is tough to spot a weak point. He was massive from all angles with calves and thighs to match. Jack went on to win the AAU Mr. America in 1949 earning his place in bodybuilding history. At 23 years old he was at the top of the bodybuilding game rubbing shoulders with other greats such as Reeves, Ross, and Grimek. Later that year he married Loretta Soper on December 18th. Five months later his only child, John was born on May 28th. He named his son after the great John Grimek. Jack continued to train hard. He refined and molded his body into a masterpiece of muscle and symmetry. At 30 years old he won the top title of the day, the NABBA Pro Mr. Universe in 1956. While winning that contest he defeated the great Bill Pearl in the process.

Training

Ed Yarick typically advised his young students of bodybuilding to train 3 days per week. Whole body routines were utilized which gave them a solid foundation. They would later refine their workouts to suite their specific needs as they progressed up the competitive ranks.

A fan of basic compound movements, here is a typical workout Jack later advised for gaining muscular bulk:

Jack Delinger Workout for Muscular Bulk

Exercise	Sets	Reps
Bench Press	3	9-15
Barbell Cheat Curls	3	9-15
Bent Over Rows	3	9-15
Squats	3	9-15
Upright Rows	3	9-12

Cheating was advised for rows and curls. Once 15 reps are reached on all 3 sets, increase the weight to bring you down to 9 again.

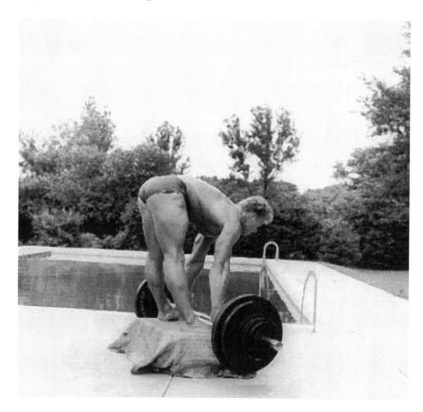

With his bodybuilding stature secured, Jack and Loretta opened their own gym in Oakland, California and continued a healthy natural bodybuilding lifestyle for many years. Unfortunately, tragedy struck the Delinger family in later life. His son John died at age 42 (November 23, 1992) from a cerebral brain hemorrhage. Jack, heart-broken, died a month later of a heart attack on December 28, 1992. Loretta is now nearing 80 years of age but is an active dog trainer and dog show judge in Orinda, California. Jack Delinger, with his classic brawn, will always be considered an Iron Age champion.

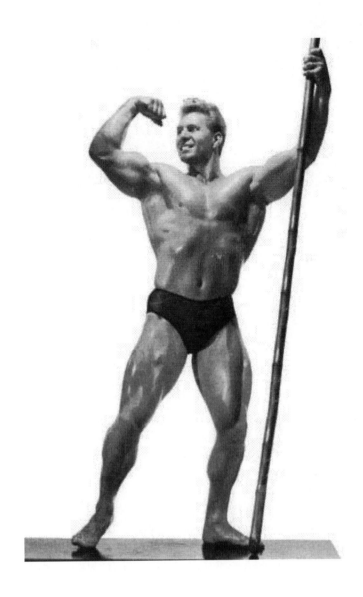

This Strength & Health excerpt, from John Grimek is a nice piece on Delinger;

Strength & Health, Page 12, August 1949

Jack Delinger - "Mr. America" - Achieves Ambition

by John Grimek

ONCE again another conscientious, hard working fellow achieved his goal; the winning of an official Mr. America title. The evening of May 21st at the Masonic Auditorium in Cleveland was warm when most of the contenders for the Mr. America title vied for sub-divisions. It was obvious that more contestants took part in this contest than in recent years. A count indicated that 40 contestants were entered. Many of them were impressive from the point of muscularity and symmetry; therefore Delinger's victory proved to be a big feather in his cap. Jack Delinger, our new 1949 Mr. America, had his heart set on winning the title in Los Angeles last year after successfully winning the "Mr. Western America" contest and nosing out some notable physique champions. Although Eiferman beat Jack by a small margin in the 1948 contest, the fault could be placed on Jack himself for accepting some false advise urging him to approach the pedestal more effectively. This, he lamented later, proved his downfall and cheated him out of the victory he felt so sure of getting. His exaggerated stride invoked a few hoot calls and whistles and he could feel the title, he worked so hard to gain, was slipping from him. This defeat didn't discourage Jack, however, but made him more determined than ever to train harder and longer to win the following year. A brief rest from all barbell work would prove helpful, he thought. So, accordingly, he devoted the next several months of his leisure time to hand balancing, sunbathing and other forms of recreation. About a year ago Ed Yarick was formulating plans to sponsor a huge physical culture show in Oakland and subsequently invited me as special guest to this affair. He also asked Delinger to be one of the feature attractions feeling quite certain that Jack would win a Mr. America title soon. Jack consented and immediately he and Ed began training in earnest, Ed training along to help and encourage Jack. In order to train without any interference, Jack and Ed rose early and started their workouts around 7:00 A. M., consequently would be finished by the time the gym was opened to his regular pupils. During this time I corresponded regularly with Jack and Ed and they wrote much about their early morning training. It was difficult to believe that anyone could survive such workouts, let alone make gains. Everyone who saw their program expressed skepticism and I admit I seemed a bit dubious. I had the pleasure later of watching them go through their routine and I can truthfully vouch for their integrity. Came the evening of the "Big Show" last October and Jack opened the program with his posing. Everyone at the show remarked "how improved" he looked. This was the first time I saw him under favorable lights and I felt quite certain that here was our next Mr. America. During my brief sojourn in Oakland Ed and I discussed Jack's possibility in the coming Mr. America. I had to admit that in my opinion I knew of no one to top him. Jack and Ed were pleased by my remarks and, I know, they started their early morning training with even greater enthusiasm. When Jack first appeared in the Mr. America sub-divisions in Cleveland the audience gave him a vociferous reception. He looked wonderful even though no special lighting was arranged for this occasion; the judges wanted to study each man "as he was" without the flattering effects of prearranged lights. However any man with a good physique doesn't need lights to offset his development. Even under the adverse conditions Jack's development was hard to conceal.

His chest, back, arms, shoulders, thighs and calves were all massively developed in symmetrical proportions. His muscularity was evident as he assumed each pose in a nonchalant but effective manner. It was fairly apparent whom the audience favored and this was the man they wanted to see win...they got their wish. The following night we arranged a more suitable posing light to give the setting a more "professional" look. Although Jack looked wonderful the previous night, he certainly looked "in his glory" this night, the finals of the Mr. America contest. One could almost detect a trace of grim determination as you saw him change from one pose to another. You could almost read his thoughts as he struck each attitude. There was only one thing in his mind this night-TO WIN! Once before he let the title escape him through some misguided advice, but now nothing must interfere with his chances...Nothing did. Before leaving Oakland Ed and I did everything to encourage Jack to continue his training. He was with us constantly, before and after the Big Show. I found him to be very quiet and pleasant company. We had a lot of laughs, but I became quite irritated when it took us over three hours to go from Oakland to San Francisco via the Bay Bridge...how I fumed! How they laughed at my impatience. 'Frisco and its Saturday night parades! I don't suppose the incident of losing the 1948 title ever left Jack's mind because during the days when he felt sluggish and training was a bore he would simply allow his mind to wander to the coming Mr. America contest and suddenly would be charged with renewed ambition. Added pep would envelop him. He would train like a Trojan, finishing his training with abundant energy. Though he is quiet he is very attentive and absorbs everything. During my stay in Oakland I suggested that he come to York several weeks before the Mr. America contest to become thoroughly acclimated, since this would be his first trip east. He took this advice and arrived in York on an unscheduled plane flight. The following morning, after a good night's rest, he walked into my office...a very pleasant surprise...I was happy to see him. I introduced him to some of the fellows he didn't meet. He looked over the layout of the gym and made plans to begin training the following day. A week later Pepper Gomez from Tanny's Gym also came to York to complete his training and prepare for this contest, so Jack had a fine training partner. They roomed at the same house, ate meals at the same places and trained together. They had only one thing in mind; to make as much added improvement as possible-if this was possible. These fellows really trained hard. Where they got all that endless endurance was difficult to understand. Most of us got tired just watching these fellows train, but they had a task to accomplish and they weren't missing any opportunities. They realized in another week or so they would meet some of the best men of the nation in a physique competition. They continued to train like demons. Jack's sweat clothes were wringing wet after every workout so that perspiration dripped from his sweat suit. He didn't wear sweat clothes to lose weight, but as an added protective measures against drafts and chills. We saw how Pepper forced himself to follow Jack through his training even though at times he altered poundage and repetitions in some of the exercises. Pepper is a fins fellow and possesses a fine symmetrical physique. In spite of this huge expenditure of energy neither of them was ever tired, suffered any setbacks or muscular aches. One could almost see their muscles grow; taking on fuller and better contour. Often after a workout they would strip and practice a few poses just to be sure they knew which to feature. In such poses their herculean muscles would stand out sharply and their muscular appearance would be arresting. Everyone agreed, especially after seeing Jack, that here was the next Mr. America. This unanimous prediction turned out to be a fact! It was our luck for Jack to arrive before the Middle Atlantic Championships and we were eager to present him to the crowd. We felt this would be a good chance to see how he clicked before an audience who heard much about him but never saw him perform.

Bob Hoffman who acted as M. C. for the lifting gave Jack a splendid introduction, adding, he felt pretty certain that Delinger will take top honors in the coming Mr. America contest. Just as we expected the crowd gave him a thunderous ovation and everyone felt they were getting a preview of the new Mr. America. How right they were. Jack won the competition by a large lead. Jack was born in Oakland, California on June 22nd, 1926. He is of Swedish extraction and his general appearance-light hair and blue eyes betrays this fact. He is inclined to be tranquil and doesn't like to have his training interrupted. While training at the gym one time he became quite upset when someone deluged him with questions. He prefers to concentrate on his exercises without interruption. Born of sturdy stock he had the misfortune of losing his father before he was born. His father met death when the scaffold on which he was working broke, which plunged him to his death. Jack is the "baby" of the group. He has two older sisters and one brother. None of them has the bulky symmetrical physique he has, be each possesses a fine natural development and good health. None of the others followed any special training. Jack is the only exercise enthusiast in his family. Ever since he can remember he wanted to be a powerfully built athlete and chose gymnastics as a means to achieve his dreams. He seemed to possess a natural ability for gymnastics and was strong enough to perform a "crucifix" on the rings the first time he tried it. He made the high school gym team with flying colors. Jack started his weight training in a rather odd way. It was while attending Technical High school in Oakland that he was indirectly introduced to weight training. While practicing on the gym apparatus two of his team mates suggested he come and try the weights at the local "Y" where they trained. He expressed reluctance and felt assured gymnastics would achieve the type of physique he was striving to develop. Nevertheless he accepted the invitation one day and met the others at the appointed hour. He was mildly impressed by the barbell movements the fellows demonstrated, but later was tempted to lift a barbell. Standing off-center in the gym was a 150 pound loaded barbell which he cleaned and pressed overhead with comparative ease. This amazed his team mates who felt they had discovered a potential lifting champion. It wasn't till months later; however, that Jack finally signed up and began using the weights as a medium for furthering his development. His ambition to become huskier and better built was beginning to materialize. Through coincidence he met Ellwood Holbrook on the beach who was then active in lifting, still is for that matter, who took an interest in him. Holbrook in turn introduced him to his friend, Ed Yarick, who operated one of the best gyms in that locality. Instantly a friendship sprung up between these "two Swedes" and Ed invited Jack over for a workout sometime. Previously Jack had heard much about Ed's knowledge to prescribe exercises for certain fellows which brought them results in record time, and because his own program was "growing stale" he was anxious to train under Ed's guidance. Immediately they formed a working-out partnership. For a year and a half they trained with the regularity of a clock, rarely ever missing a training session. During this time Jack's weight increased from 163 to 195 and his development was phenomenal, Ed was proud of this fine progress Jack was making and told Jack that some day he will reap fame for his physique. A massive but symmetrical development was his goal. He always trained hard and specialized on parts of his body which he felt were not in proportion. His arms and chest grew larger and rounder; his legs attained prodigious proportions. He was now ready to make his "debut" by entering and winning the "Mr. Northern California" contest. Earlier, however, to gain some "stage experience" he entered the 1945 Mr. America contest and, while he did present a fine appearance, he didn't finish in the first five. His posing ability was poor, his carriage was awkward which hurt his chances, but he entered mainly for experience and profited by it.

Prior to March 1948 he prepared himself for the coming "Mr. Western America" contest held in Los Angeles as the amateur portion of the great Mr. U.S.A. show. Several well known bodybuilders were entered and Jack realized he must appear at his best if he was to win. When the final scores were tallied, lo and behold, Jack Delinger's name headed the list. He won the fight and he well deserved the victory. Now he pointed to the Mr. America contest just a few months away. A setback resulted, however, when three months later Eiferman nosed out Delinger in the '48 Mr. America contest but this defeat, tough as it seemed to Jack, made him more determined to come through the following year. In Cleveland he did come through and thus achieved the goal he had long ago set out to accomplish; winning a Mr. America title. Upon his return after the contest Stanko asked: "How do you feel, Jack, now that you're Mr. America?" "You know," he slowly went on, "I don't feel any different than I did before I won the contest. I thought winning would be different!" During the few weeks he spent in York with us we had a lot of fun with him. Every time you saw Jack or Pepper you would see a quart of milk in their hands. They drank a lot of milk daily. When they went on the roof to sunbathe they would always take along a quart of milk under each arm to quench their thirst. Even when they went to a movie they would sport a quart of white fluid under their arms. The ticket seller noting this unusual procedure exclaimed: "Now I've seen everything!" But Jack likes milk. He doesn't drink it only because of the food value it contains, but he enjoys every swallow. Tea, coffee and other drinks are taboo with him. Milk is his main beverage. Now that he has achieved his goal, the winning of a Mr. America title, he has other things in mind. Already he has had some stage offers and being a very excellent hand balancer he is considering entering this field. Without a doubt he should do excellently on the stage in a herculean balancing act. His physique is extraordinary and he has showmanship on the stage. His partner Sam Buss and he do some wonderful balancing tricks, assuring their chances of success if they pursue this vocation. Before flying back to the west coast we discussed his chances in a Mr. Universe contest, but he indicated that he might not rate. Personally we all feel that he would stand an excellent chance and many others feel this way too. Anyway if he should enter such a competition the judges will decide that - they always do. One thing certain, Jack is more muscular and better built than lots of other men who make such claims, and having known him personally for the past few years, I know he has "plenty on the ball" whether he wins another contest or not. People watching him in training or doing his balancing routine on a stage invariably remark, "That fellow is really built!" When Eiferman surrendered his crown on May 22nd in Cleveland he gave it to another worthy fellow, Jack Delinger, to reign as the current Mr. America. We know Jack will be a very worthy title holder and uphold the honor it represents. We feel, as everyone else does, he deserves the success he has finally achieved and wish him loads of luck during his reign. Good luck, Mr. America 1949!

Before leaving York Jack stopped by the York Precision Co. to bid Bob and some of the others goodbye. Bob explained some of the intricate uses of the precision machinery in this place which interested Jack very much. Bob wished him safe journey and every success in life before he departed from "Muscletown", which ended a very happy stay for him.

JACK DELINGER, who likes to "take it easy", watches DICK BACHTELL, former national featherweight weightlifting champ many times, preparing shipments for parcel post. Jack found it easier to watch than to do the job. He expressed amazement at the quantity of shipments made daily.

Coincidentally, Jack and Stan walked into Terpak's office to pick up his trophy when Jules Bacon, who is out in California making final arrangements for our west coast branch called. Jules extended congratulations to Jack via long distance. The huge trophy rests on Terpak's desk.

MuscleMemory

Another Denizen of Yarick's was this great one;

Ironman, Vol 11, No 3, Page 8, September 1951

Roy Hilligenn "Mr. America" 1951

By M Kirchner

ROY HILLIGENN started his winning ways in physique competition at the tender age of six months when he won a trophy for being a beautiful baby. Since then he has continued with his winning ways by winning the "Mr. South Africa" title for three years from 1943 to 1945 inclusive as well as the "Most Muscular" man title in the 1946 competition. Roy was born in South Africa November 15, 1922. When he was 4 years old his father died leaving the rearing of the five children to his mother. The going was difficult and after two years it was necessary to send the children to an Orphanage. Roy lived here until the age of 15 during which time he attended a trade school, learning to be an electrician. After this he left the school to earn his living at this trade. Until the age of 17 Roy had but little interest in sports. However, while working on a roof of a four story building fitting a neon sign and bending a piece of pipe, Roy slipped. He woke up twelve hours later in a hospital with a fractured wrist, broken fingers and ribs and serious internal injuries. Roy lost weight down to 83 pounds. He was too weak to work when he recovered. It was while walking by a news stand at this time that he saw an American physical culture magazine. Roy had just enough money to purchase it. Reading the magazine that night Roy was fired with zeal to develop his pitiful physique and the next morning started out on his quest for exercising equipment by searching all the junk heaps for weights. He round some trolley wheels, pieces of iron of various weights and a punching bag which he hung In the back yard and started his outdoor training (incidentally, this was the chicken yard). Roy trained hard and soon weighed 101 lbs. with the great measurements of 12½ neck, 28 chest, 26 waist and 17 thigh and a terrific 8 1/8 inch arm. A short time later Roy showed a photo of a set of weights to a foundry man who immediately cast up a 145 lb. set and Roy trained with such zest with the new set that he was so sore he could hardly walk for awhile! Another four months brought his weight to 135 lbs. and he began wrestling, soon winning the 1943 wrestling championship.

Roy was now training four nights per week and devoting more attention to his legs which he had been neglecting before. His bodyweight rose to 149 lbs. and he won the lightweight lifting title of South Africa even though he had never done much training on the three Olympics. It was this year that he first won the "Mr. South Africa" title. His photo began to appear in magazines all over the world and he became quite famous for his wonderful development and amazing definition. During the war years, Roy worked 1800 feet underground in a gold mine. A chance meeting with Ivor Kirston, a South African film director lead to several parts in the movies. Previous to this Roy had been using three sets of 10 reps in all his exercises but now realizing that he needed more bulk he changed to five sets of five reps with much heavier weights. By September 1945 he was weighing 165 with a 17 neck, 46 chest, 16 arm, 29 waist, 23 thighs and 15¼ calves at a height of approximately 5' 6". He now decided to concentrate on lifting which he did for a year finally making a 240 press and snatch and a fine 320 clean and jerk. This latter poundage was made at a bodyweight of 160 lbs. making Roy the first man in South Africa to clean and jerk double bodyweight and placing him with that exclusive few in the world who have performed this great feat. Roy later made a 250 snatch, 400 squat, 175 curl, 510 dead lift, 170 one hand snatch, 205 side press and 305 press on back. All these were done at a bodyweight of 160 to 165. Roy used a method of lifting training similar to the Americans with several sets in each lift with increasing poundage starting with 5 reps on the first lift and reducing one rep with each increase in poundage until he makes one rep with maximum poundage then dropping to the starting weight for high reps again. During this time, Roy followed a careful diet of healthful foods. He believes in eating when hungry rather than at stated times, sometimes eating five times per day and other times only two meals per day. About this time, Roy decided he would like to see some of the world so he began traveling going to many countries for a visit and making quite a stay in England, then coming to Canada where he lived with and trained with John Bavington. Roy says he owes much to John for teaching the American training methods and much about America itself. Roy first appeared on the John Terlazzo show where he was a sensation. This was in January 1948. He then appeared in John Fritshe's show, the George Yacos' show in Detroit and the Norb Grueber show in Chicago. In January, 1949 he arrived in Los Angeles and began training at the Tanny gym with Gomez, Eiferman, Reeves and other famous stars. A short time later he obtained work in Trona in the Mojave Desert where he again trained in a homemade gym with Bill Meyers as a training partner. He worked here two years and during this period he won the "Mr. Pacific Coast" and the "Mr. Northern California" contest. The first of April, 1951 he quit his job to train for the 1951 "Mr. America" contest and decided on the Yarick gym in Oakland as being most suitable as they taught both bodybuilding and lifting. The majority of the other gyms have no lifting whatever. He and Ed Yarick carefully laid out a training program with Cal Craddock as upper body training partner and Sam Ulversoy as his leg training partner. Uhalde, Brigonola and Terry were his lifting partners. Three weeks later he won the "Mr. San Francisco" contest and the Pacific Coast 198 pound lifting title although he weighed but 177 and had to eat bananas and milk to bring his bodyweight up to 183 for this class. He made a 235 press and snatch and a 335 clean and jerk. Roy trained three days per week on bodybuilding and 3 days on lifting, always under the careful guidance of Ed Yarick who has developed three previous "Mr. America's." He was living at the Yarick home during this two months and enjoying the fine meals prepared by Alice. Knowing that readers like to know how these men train we herewith present the training programs used by Roy. Monday, Wednesday, and Friday mornings he did upper body work.

Starting at 10 o'clock he did 3 sets of 10 reps of dumbbell rowing motions with 105 to 155 lbs. 3 sets of 12 reps front pulley weight exercises for lats. with 180 lbs. 3 more sets to back of neck with 170 lbs. 3 more sets of straight arm pull downs while kneeling with 100 lbs. 12 reps. Two dumbbell press together 3 sets of 10 reps with 70 to 90 lb. dumbbells, 6 sets of alternate dumbbell presses with 75 to 95 lb. dumbbells, sitting down lateral raises, front and sidewise, alternate and together, 6 sets with 30 lb. dumbbells. Incline press with leg press machine for 3 sets with 170 lbs. of 10 reps. Pulley weights for deltoids, 3 sets of 15 reps. Dislocates with pulleys for shoulders, 2 sets 60 reps. Dislocates on narrow bench with 30 lb. dumbbells, 3 sets of 25 reps. Incline bench press 3 sets 10 reps with 75 to 95 lb. dumbbells, 3 sets of barbell bench presses with 225 to 250. Flat bench lateral flying exercise 3 sets of 15 reps 45 to 50 lbs. 6 sets of pectoral exercises with pulleys, similar to flying exercise on bench but standing up. This was 25 reps with 60 lbs., sitting down curls with two dumbbells 2 sets of 12 reps with 60 lbs then 2 alternate curls of same type and weights. Incline bench curl 12 reps with 50 lbs. Then concentrated curl with one arm with 45 lb. dumbbell 4 sets of 10 reps. Curling from overhead pulleys while lying on bench on back, 3 sets of 15 reps. Triceps press with dumbbell from behind neck 115 to 135 lbs. 15 reps and 3 sets, both arms at once. One arm triceps curl with 25 lb. dumbbells for 20 reps and 3 sets. Triceps curl on overhead pulley 3 sets of 12 reps. Dipping between parallel bars with 50 lbs. Sit ups and leg raises for abdominals with 60 lb. dumbbell 3 sets of 20 reps. The above finishes his upper body workout and takes 5 hours. Roy then went home for lunch and to sleep an hour then back to the gym for his leg workout. This started at about 5:30 P.M. After a little warm up he does the flat footed squat with 350 to 420 lbs. for 4 sets of 10 reps each (he has made a single rep squat with 490 lbs.). He then squats on a low box; 3 sets of 10 reps with 300 to 360 lbs. Then the Hack squat, 3 sets of 12 reps with 300 to 360 lbs. Squats with weight on chest 5 sets of 3 reps with 320 to 400 lbs. Partial squats for strength 4 sets of 15 to 20 reps with 500 to 700 lbs. One set of wide knee squats with 320 lbs. Leg curls on incline bench 4 sets of 15 reps with 130 lb. bar. 5 sets of single leg Iron Boot curls with 25 lbs. 5 sets of calf raises on calf machine, 4 sets of leg extensors with Iron Boots. The above leg workout lasted 3 hours after which he had a hot dinner and was in bed by 11 o'clock. He slept 10 hours and was ready the next day for his lifting workout. This began with military press working up from 135 to 240 and starting with 3 reps and finishing with 1 then working down in singles to 200 again. Then the snatch with same weights and reps. In the cleans he did the same schedule of reps starting with 225 and working up to 330. In the jerk he took weight from racks and worked up from 225 to 350. He then did heavy pulls with snatch grip of 300 to 400 lbs. then pulls with clean grip up to 500 lbs. always pulling as high and as fast as possible. He would try his limit in the lifts on Saturday. His best lifetime lifts were a 255 press, 250 snatch and 350 clean and jerk, with a 360 clean. The above programs, both lifting and bodybuilding are of course not for the beginner. They are only used even by super men like Roy for a very short period to put them in top condition with maximum definition and shape. It is certain that Roy would have been much stronger had he concentrated on lifting alone, because his intensive bodybuilding program with high reps is not conducive to greatest strength development. Roy put in 155 training hours each of the two months he was specializing at Yarick's gym. Now that he has won the "Mr. America" title it is his ambition to win the lifting title of America and the world and I for one am sure that he will do it. He is capable of 270, 270, 360, 900 total with about two months specialized training on the lifts only. This would put him near the top of the light heavyweights. Roy tells us that he is a very light eater. For breakfast he has a glass of orange juice, cereal with honey and 1 banana, two eggs and one apple.

For lunch 3 scrambled eggs, cold ham or hamburger meat, 4 slices of whole wheat, glass of milk and a glass of yogurt. For dinner he might have a steak with vegetables, salad, fruit and milk. "Mr. America" gives all credit for winning the 1951 title to his trainer, **Ed Yarick**, who he says is the best liked trainer he has ever met. Roy's measurements at the time he won the contest were, neck 17½, chest 48½, waist 31, calf 16¼, arm 17¾, (18 warmed up slightly), forearm 14½, wrist 7½, thigh 24½, ankle 8. His height is but 5' 6" making him the shortest man to ever win the "Mr. America" title which still further emphasizes the perfection of his physique for a tall man usually has quite an advantage. His bodyweight was 178. Roy has a personality second to none. He is bubbling over with enthusiasm and has a bright smile for everyone. He is a real credit to our game. Roy is again employed as an electrician in Oakland where he can train regularly at the Yarick gym.

The following excerpt from Charles Poliquin's site was more or less his eulogy to Jack, and it notes Jack's own gym, which was one of those early California gyms, but was not really exceptionally notable as a gym; LaLanne would make his mark elsewhere. The excerpt does mention Jack hanging out at Yarick's, however.

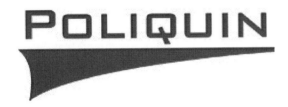

Training Articles

Strong to the Finish: Jack LaLanne

A tribute to a true fitness pioneer

By Charles Poliquin's
1/25/2011 10:40:22 AM

If there is one person who exemplifies physical fitness and vibrant health, it's Jack LaLanne. A lifelong bodybuilder and fitness celebrity, Jack practiced what he preached, every day of his life, and performed amazing feats of strength and muscular endurance throughout his entire life that few can equal. Jack passed away on January 23, and this is his story. François Henri LaLanne was born in San Francisco on September 26, 1914, the son of Jennie and Jean LaLanne, who had emigrated from France. His mother was a maid, and his father was a dance instructor and a worker for a phone company. His brother Norman, who lived 97 years, nicknamed him "Jack." The media called him the "Godfather of Fitness." Jack was not always a health and fitness fanatic, and he characterized his early teen years as being a "sugarholic" and a "junk food junkie" – he joked that he was sought out by little girls who wanted to beat him up. That unhealthy lifestyle changed at age 15 when he heard a lecture by nutritionist Paul Bragg, at which point Jack became determined to become strong and healthy through proper diet and exercise. He became a voracious reader and graduated from Chiropractic College. In 1936, at just 21 years of age, Jack rented an office building for $45 a month in Oakland, California, and converted it into a gym he called LaLanne's Physical Culture Studio. At that time many health care professionals regarded Jack as a crackpot, and he claimed that doctors were telling their patients that training with weights would give them heart attacks and make them impotent, and would make women look like men. Even sport coaches were against him, telling their athletes that training with Jack would make them muscle-bound – but the athletes came anyway, and Jack would accommodate their secret training by giving them keys to the gym so they could train after the gym closed. Along the way Jack claimed to have invented several popular pulley machines using cables and weight selector apparatus – and even the leg-extension machine – but never bothered to patent his inventions. Although he was known more for general fitness, Jack exerted a big influence in the bodybuilding community. Recalls fitness writer Laura Dayton, the sister of former competitive bodybuilder and strongman Mike Dayton, "One of the good things about being born and raised in Oakland was that Jack LaLanne was a part of my life from an early age. Of course I'd run to get my mom so we could exercise with him in the mornings [on TV]. He influenced my brother Mike to pursue a career of bodybuilding and feats of strength, and he was there when Mike performed many of his shows. **He'd hang out at [Ed] Yarick's gym with 1950 bodybuilding greats like Clancy Ross and Jack Delinger. As a matter of fact, Oakland would have been the Mecca of Bodybuilding had a young Joe Weider not moved to Southern California.**"

Birth of a Fitness Celebrity

In 1951 The Jack LaLanne Show debuted on television, and Jack's natural charisma and sincere desire to help people made him a welcome visitor in people's homes. One of his early fans was Richard Simmons. Writing for CNN, Simmons recalls watching his mother, Shirley, exercising along with Jack on the show; she encouraged her 200-plus-pound son to join in. Simmons says at first he was jealous of Jack, but eventually he regarded him as a role model and followed Jack's career path. "He told people the truth about eating and exercising long before anyone else. And he was matter-of-fact. You see, Jack walked the walk and talked the talk.

And when he spoke, people really listened to him." A master at self-promotion, Jack would make his TV show entertaining with his excellent singing voice and inspirational lectures. He would bring his German shepherd "Happy" on the show to attract the kids, and then would encourage those kids to get their parents and grandparents in front of the TV to exercise with him. Along the way he would come up with mottos, which he called "LaLanneisms," that promoted his beliefs. Here are a few:

- "Your waistline is your lifeline."
- "Exercise is King, nutrition is Queen; put them together and you've got a kingdom."
- "Don't exceed the feed limit."
- "Ten seconds on the lips and a lifetime on the hips."
- "Better to wear out than rust out."
- "People don't die of old age; they die of inactivity."
- "First we inspire them, and then we perspire them."
- "You eat every day, you sleep every day, and your body was made to exercise every day."
- "I can't die; it would ruin my image."
- "If man makes it, don't eat it."
- "If it tastes good, spit it out."
- "It's not what you do some of the time that counts; it's what you do all of the time that counts."

And then there were the stunts. To promote his show and ever-expanding health club business (which eventually grew to more than 200 clubs before he sold them to Bally's), Jack would perform feats of strength and muscular endurance throughout his life. Here are a few:

1956 (age 42): Appeared on the television show *You Asked for It* and broke a world record by performing 1,033 push-ups in 23 minutes.

1959 (age 45): Completed 1,000 jumping jacks and 1,000 chin-ups in one hour and 22 minutes.

1974 (age 60): Handcuffed and shackled, he swam from Alcatraz Island to Fisherman's Wharf while towing a 1,000-pound boat.

1984 (age 70): Handcuffed and shackled, he swam one mile while towing 70 rowboats, one with several passengers.

Jack LaLanne's show went into syndication and remained so until 1985, and he also appeared on many other television shows, including Batman, The Addams Family, Peter Gunn and The Simpsons. His on-screen success led to him receiving a star on the Hollywood Walk of Fame in 2002, and his continual promotion of healthy living and physical fitness earned him lifetime achievement awards from many prestigious organizations, such as the State of California's Governor's Council on Physical Fitness and the Arnold Classic Lifetime Achievement Award. And speaking of the former "Governator," Arnold said that he met Jack in 1960 in Muscle Beach in Venice, California. Jack challenged the bodybuilders to match him in chin-ups and push-ups, but, as Arnold said to a news reporter, "No one even wanted to try." For 53 years LaLanne was married to Elaine LaLanne and they had three children. For Jack's 90th birthday party, Laura Dayton presented Jack with a plaque from then-governor Arnold Schwarzenegger. Says Dayton,

"Always dressed in tailored suits to show off his still enviable physique, Jack made it a point that day to go to every table and talk with every guest.
\With his crazy sunglasses, he also treated us all to a beautiful acapella version of Louis Armstrong's 'What a Wonderful World.' Not a dry face in the crowd." Many of Jack's television shows can be found on the Internet. If you haven't seen them, I encourage you to watch a few segments to see Jack doing what he did best: exercising and encouraging the world to eat well and live healthy. I also encourage you to watch at least one show to the very end, where he would sign off by singing the following jingle:

"It's time to leave you.
Let's say goodbye.
These precious moments just seem to fly.
Now here's my wish for you.
May the good Lord bless
and keep you too."

And goodbye to you, Jack. We'll miss you.

Here is another article from Ed Yarick;

Training for Bulk
by Ed Yarick (Coach, 1952 National Jr. Weightlifting Team)

How do you gain bulk? This is probably one of the most discussed questions in physical culture circles, and there have been hundreds of books and articles written on the subject. Now I have been around this business a long time, and in my time I have seen many a man gain weight – some too much and in the wrong places! And I've seen others breaking their backs without results. So I ask myself, "Why is it people crave this bulk in the first place?" There are too many fellows who spoil the looks of their physiques by gaining way too much weight indiscriminately. I can't help agreeing with my friend John Grimek who said, the last time he visited us in Oakland, "You know, Ed, a well-developed 15 inch arm looks much more impressive than a hammy 19 inch one." I have noticed that the fellows who win most physique contests are the ones with the most muscularity.

Naturally, you have to have size to have a shapely, defined physique, but how do you know when to stop gaining bulk? At what bodyweight do you look the best for what you aim to do? The same applies to the weightlifter. It would be folly for the man who plans to lift in a certain bodyweight class to deliberately "bulk up" to the point where it would weaken him to reduce to his most efficient lifting weight. The heavyweights, of course, can afford to carry as much bulk as they need for power, but must keep from getting too heavy and losing agility and speed required in the quick lifts. Now some guys, like George Eiferman and John Grimek, seem to be more muscular as they put on weight. They are exceptions, however, for most men who strive for bulk become "round" and lose every bit of definition. Sure, it's wonderful to brag about a 19" arm, a 50" chest and a 28" thigh, but it doesn't mean anything if they're accompanied by a 45" waist and mainly composed of soft, adipose tissue, Take, for example, the case of Roy Hilligenn, Mr. America, 1952. Roy started training in 1942 weighing a mere 83 pounds, after two years of serious illness. He weighed 160 when he won the Mr. South Africa title for three consecutive years. And last year at the winning of Mr. America he weighed only 178 pounds. He also became the only man to win both the Mr. America and Most Muscular titles in the same contest. In these contests there were fellows weighing 200 and more, and many had bigger measurements. So you see, the tape measure doesn't mean as much as you may have been led to believe. Only a beginner should record his gains by inches, and that just to give him early motivation until he knows better. Symmetry of physique and strength in lifting are the main factors. Bulk must be combined with proportion and structure; bodyweight gain should yield strength and power. To achieve the combination of bulk and muscularity does not mean that you should overstuff yourself, or that you should spend six hours a day in the gym sweating it out. There is great truth in the axiom, "One man's meat is another's poison." It takes careful planning to work out a bulk gaining routine. The best way is to experiment with yourself on every author's opinion of such a course and finally work out your own program that will suit your individual needs. I know for a fact that Roy Hilligenn can gain 30 extra pounds in two months if he trains on a course consisting of a few main exercises done in 4 sets of 15 to 20 reps. On the other hand, Jack Delinger, Mr. America, 1949, gains by using similar exercises but much heavier weights and lower repetitions. Each man determined on his own what kind of routine or combination of routines worked for *his* particular needs.

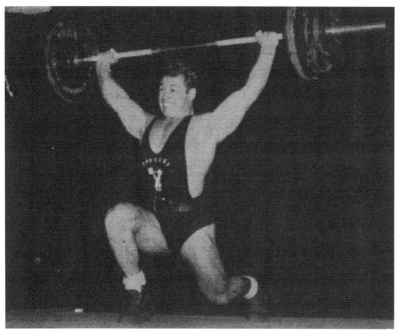
Roy Hilligan

A lot of men believe the best way to gain muscular bulk is to stick to heavy weight and do no more than 5 repetitions on each set – and this arrangement can work for some. It doesn't always work for everyone, so if the lower rep sets don't produce much at this time for you, try lighter weights and higher-rep sets. A combination of both schemes may be what you need for now. Never write off an idea – store it for later and utilize it when the proper time arises. Get plenty of rest and relaxation, and remember, eating is important for success in bulk gaining. Eat three to four sound meals a day, Get plenty of rest and add a few snacks if necessary. For heaven's sake, don't go gulping quart after quart of milk. Now I am a big man myself, standing 6-4 and weighing 250. I drink two or three quarts of milk a day and when I order half-dozen eggs for breakfast, people stare at me. Maybe that is too much, but I feel that my body can handle it. The average weight man seeking to gain, the man perhaps 100 pounds less than I, needs only a couple of eggs and a quart of milk a day. Once he has increased his muscle mass, and only then, should he add to the quantity of his daily food intake. Don't think for a minute that your body will simply turn excess food into muscle in a short time. It is a complicated process, one that takes time. You should have plenty of substantial, wholesome food, especially dairy products such as cheese, milk and yogurt. Balance your meal for best results, but remember not to go overboard when seeking added muscular weight. Eat fish at least once a week, as well as liver, beef, ham and steaks. Include green and yellow vegetables in your diet, as well as fruit, nuts, cereals, beans, etc. Eggs, peanut butter, yogurt, etc. mixed with milk and protein powder will help you add nutrition to your diet, no matter how busy your schedule. But don't think for one minute that eating and training cannot be overdone. You can overdo both. If you overdo training, you will tear your body down and if you overdo eating, you will find you have become soft, flabby and sloppy. Three training days per week may be best for you, two days for some, and four or five for still others. It is up to each individual, over time, to find what combination of training and eating works to fulfill his aims and desires.

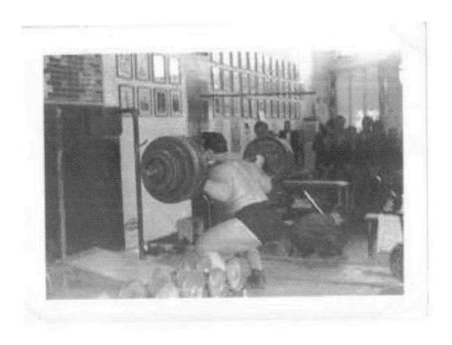

Doug Hepburn Training at Yarick's gym

Here is a little Iron Game history excerpt about Alyce Yarick;

Three years ago, Alyce Yarick's husband, Ed, died, and on December 4, 1991, Alyce passed away. Born Alyce Stagg on April 18, 1921, she wrote for **Muscle Power, Your Physique,** and **Strength & Health.** Ed had owned a gym in Oakland, California since 1939, and after he married Alyce, they remained together in the gym business, though they changed locations, until 1978. Alyce, as Alyce Yarick, began writing a women's column for the **Reg Park Journal** in January 1954, and a women's column for **Iron Man** that same month; the former column ran until September 1955, the latter until March 1958. In 1946 Alyce was reported to have squatted 100 reps with 100 pounds, a report which caused much skepticism, but seven years later, on April 11, 1953 (about a month before her son Bart was conceived), at one of the famous Yarick strength shows, she surprised the audience and silenced the critics by placing her heels on a two-by-four, placing a barbell of 105 pounds on her upper back and, as husband Ed counted, knocking out 105 repetitions! **Iron Man,** in a September, 1954 story, showed Alyce demonstrating the exercises she used during her pregnancy; the story includes seven photos of her using some hefty weights. Alyce (and Pudgy Stockton) had been warned that lifting weights could thwart pregnancy, but Pudgy and Alyce paid no heed; each had healthy offspring. (Alyce's son Bart was born on February 1, 1954.) According to Bart, Alyce ceased lifting weights in the mid-1960s, but she would walk for exercise, in later years accompanied by her pet dogs, along the canal banks of Modesto, California. She was suspicious of some of the performances of more recent barbelles, and she did not believe that the current crop of female bodybuilders could have attained the degree of muscularity often seen on the dais these days without the help of chemicals. This made her sad. When Alyce Yarick died, we lost a great "natural" strength athlete and pioneer.

Chapter 9   Zuver's Gym

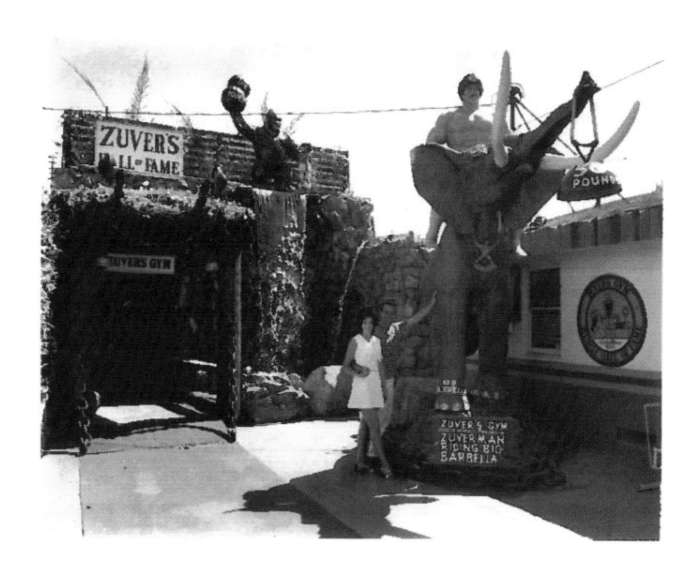

Is this the entrance to the greatest hard-core lifters gym that ever existed?

This chapter definitely fits into the category of "last but not least". In fact, it is my humble opinion that I have saved the best for last here. You may or may not agree with me on this point, but I think you'd be crazy to not at least list it with all the other great gyms of the "Golden Age" that we have already covered.

If there was ever such a thing as an adult, hard-core lifter's version of training "Disney Land", there is no doubt in many minds that this place was it. Unfortunately, this writer/lifter/ iron historian wannabe was a mere lad and born on the wrong coast of our great country to have ever seen this hallowed place up close & personal-like. This does not deter me from making the above claim, as I have seen the original pictures, and read the stories from those who were there, including someone who was not just there as a casual observer or had perhaps taken a few workouts there, but was part of the family that built the place, none other than **Jean Zuver**. I came across the Zuver story on Dave & Laree Draper's "Irononline" forum, of which I am a member in good standing (at least I hope so). Jean Zuver & Laree Draper are good friends, it turns out. There were only so many gyms that catered to the crème dela crème of power & physique training in Southern California in the "Golden Era", and Zuver's was right up there with the best of them. Zuver's, the original Gold's, Vic Tanny's (a.k.a, "the pit", or "the dungeon"), Vince's (Vince Gironda's place), Peanuts West's garage gym, and a few others were in this class. While some guys would stick to just one or the other of these placers in their quests for iron glory, others would jump around from one place to another, or at least had a couple of favorites they would alternate between. One such man was **Leonard Ingro**, who was featured in my book, "**Forgotten Secrets of the Culver City Westside Barbell club revealed**" (yeah, I know, that title is long & maybe a bit awkward). Ingro Trained at Zuver's and was also one of the core group that trained with Bill West & the gang known as the original Westside crew. Leonard was one of the lighter guys that trained with the bigger guys like West, Frenn, DiMarco, Merjanian, Casey, Coleman, etc.. He was a 165 pound class guy, but could hang with the big guys pretty well, as illustrated in the following picture:

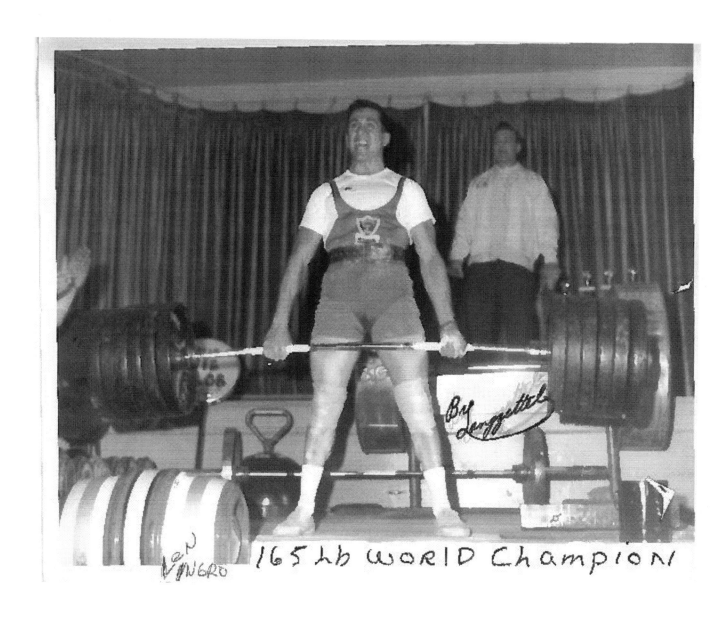

This looks to be a touch over 600 lbs here, so well over triple bodyweight. This lift took place at Zuver's, as you can see Bob in the background here.

Here is a shot of Lenny shaking hands with Bob;

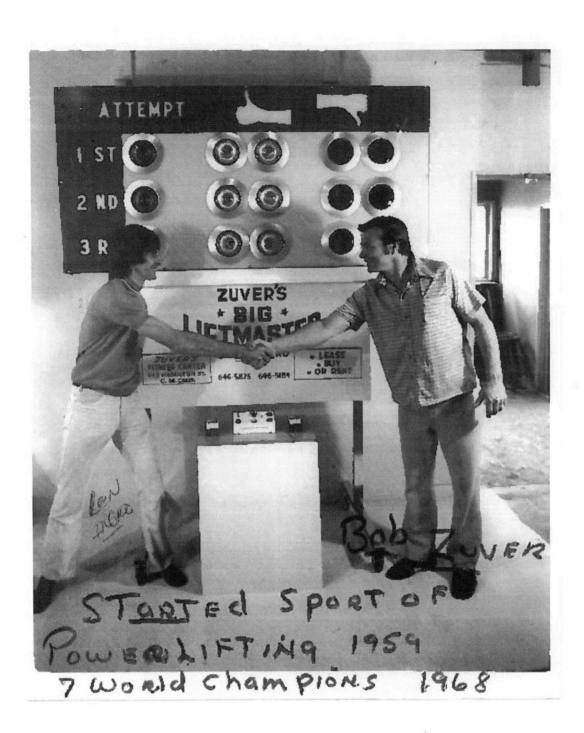

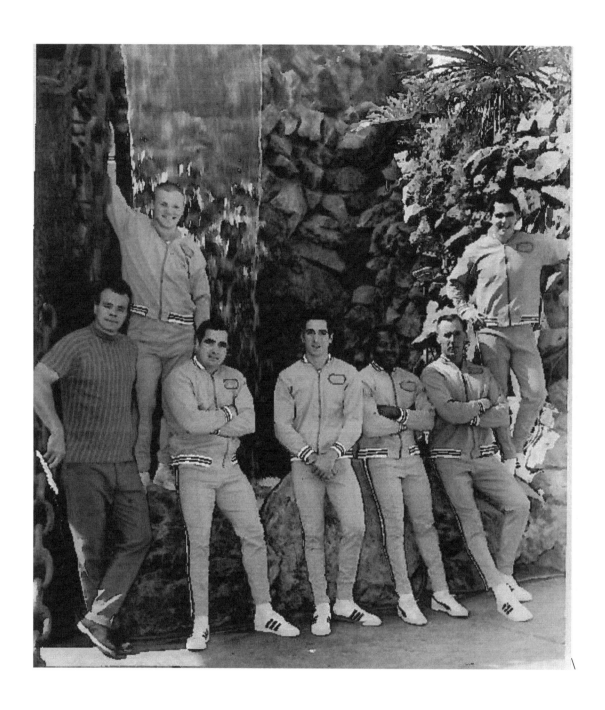

Zuver's Powerlifting Team

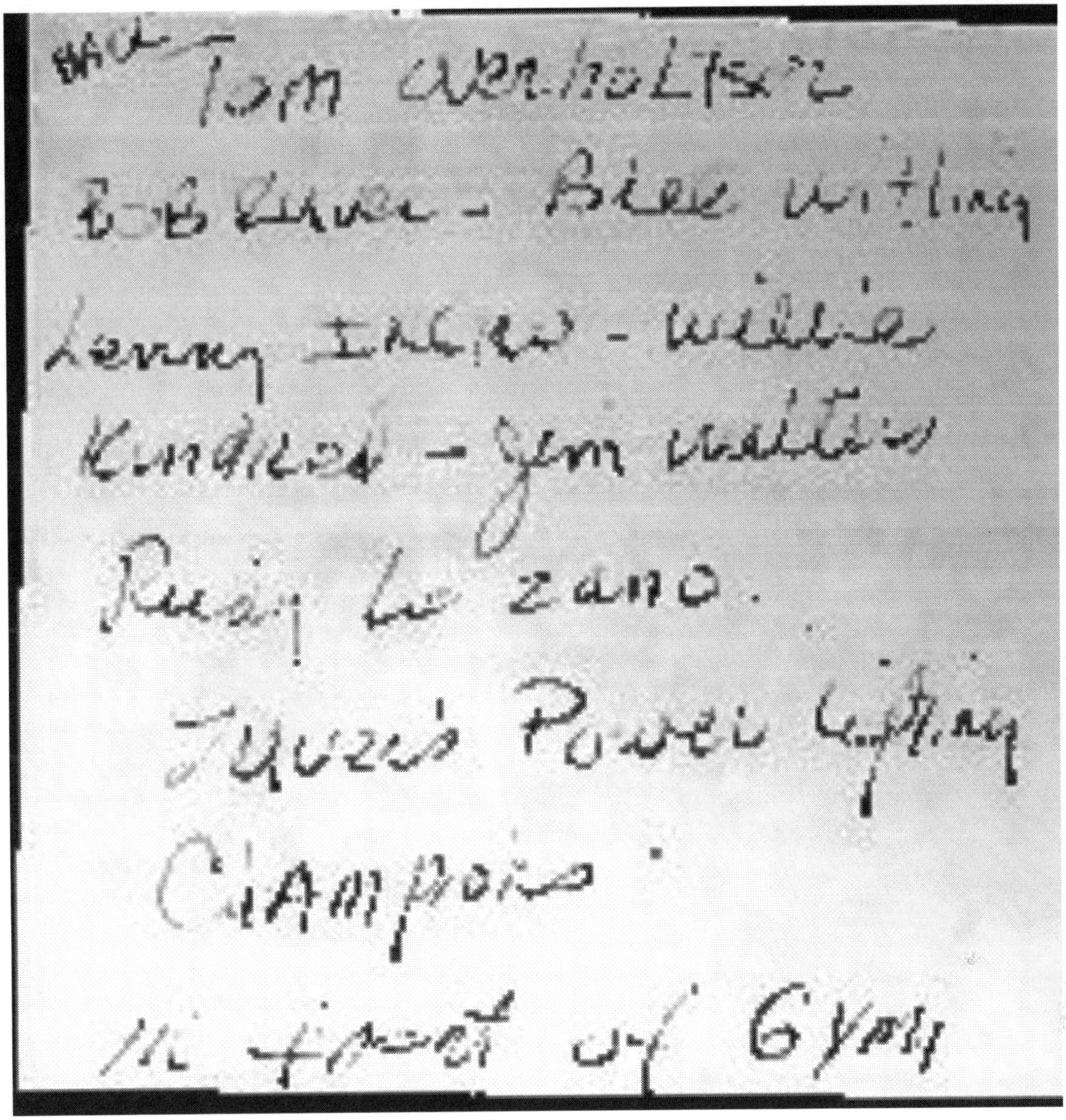

> BACK —
> Tom Wenholtz
> Bob Zuver — Bill Witling
> Lenny Ingro — Willie
> Kindred — Jim Walters
> Ricky Lezano.
> Zuver's Power Lifting
> Champions.
> The finest of Gyms

Lenny Ingro, dead center, was an integral part of the Zuver team, as well as the Westside crew.

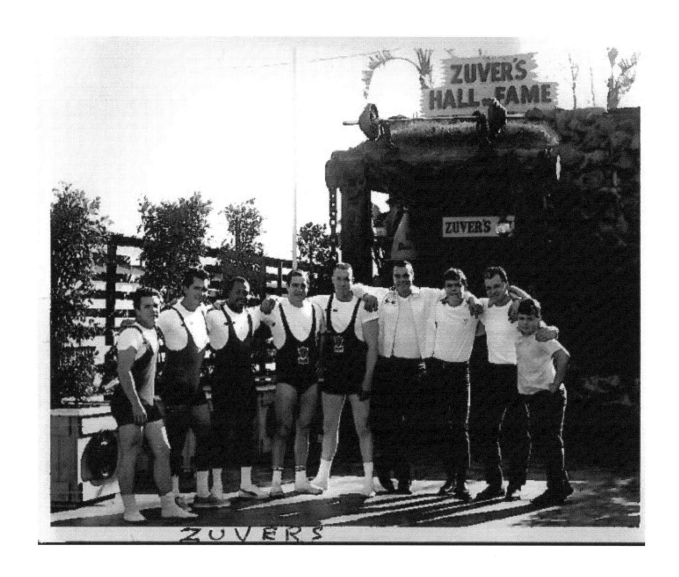

Here is another shot of the team, with the Zuver boys in tow.

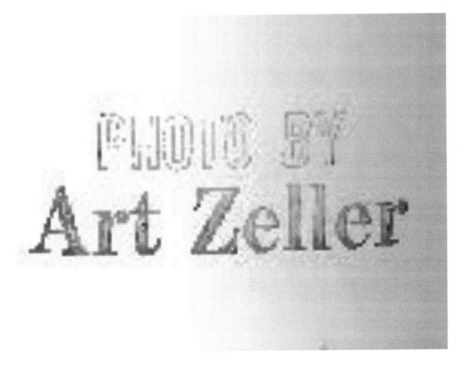

Bob, Bob Jr. & Ricky (our sons) with lifting team. I can't remember all their names.
- Bob Antlers
- Bill Witting
- Willie Kindred

PHOTO BY Art Zeller

Bill Witting made the California Lifting Hall of Fame;

From Orange County register news site:

Resident Bill Witting is inducted into the Powerlifting Hall of Fame.

Here is a shot of Bill in the big rack;

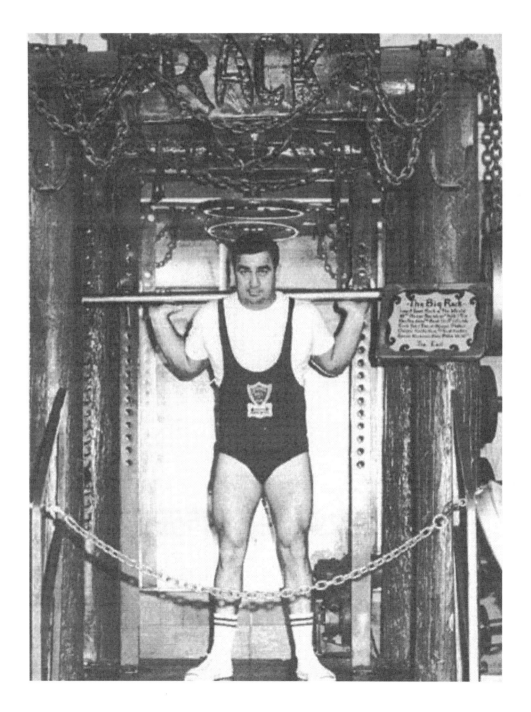

Here is Bill in the other big rack, with spotters;

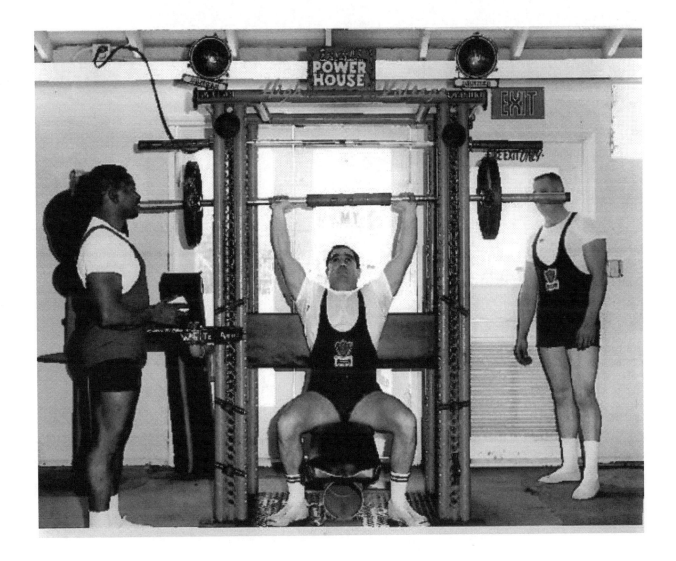

Tommy Overholtzer, another guy that was mentioned in "Forgotten Secrets of the Culver City Westside Barbell club revealed", was also a prominent member of the Zuver's team

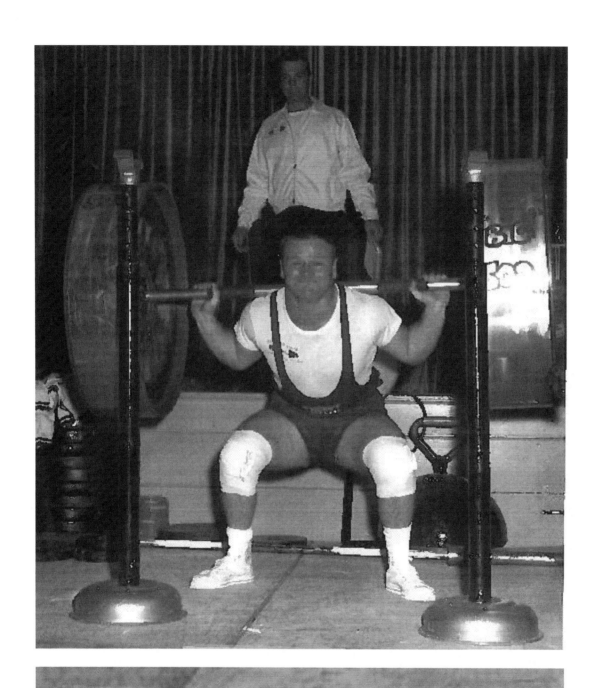

TOM OVERHOLTER - 181 POUNDS Nat. Record Holder in Hall Of Fame DOING FIVE REPETIONS WITH 500 LBS.

Yet another "Zuver man", Willie Kindred

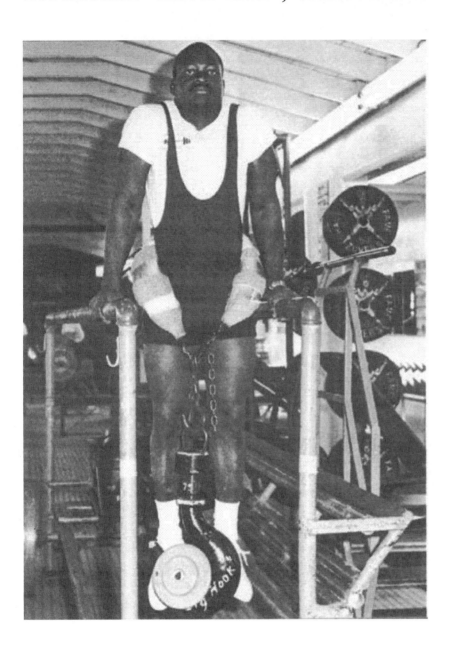

And another;

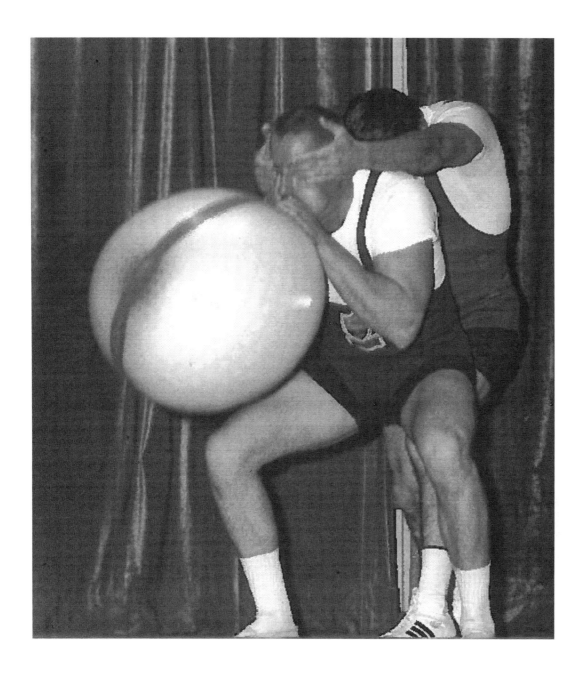

Jim Waters

In addition to the regular team members, there were many other men of renown that trained at Zuver's from time to time, or on a regular basis. The next picture shows one of the famous guys of the era that trained there and sent the Zuver's this Christmas card, which just exudes the warmth of the season;

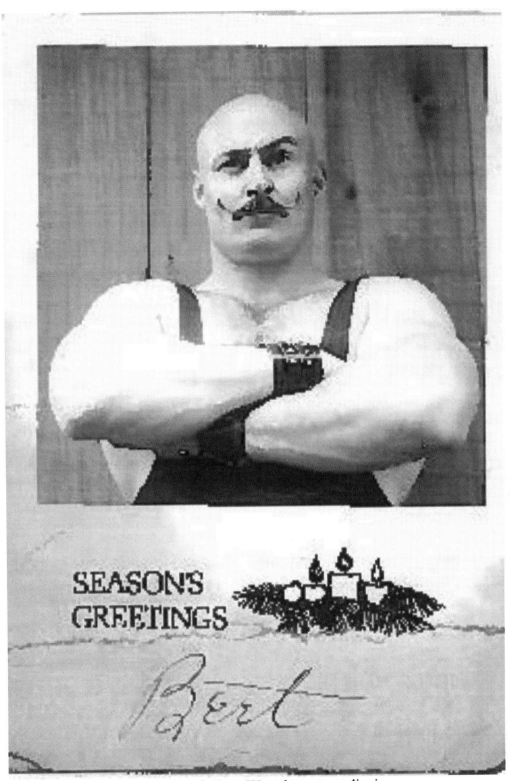

Bert Elliot, that is, Strongman & Arm Wrestler extraordinaire.

If you browse through various forums & internet blogs on the subjects of powerlifting, bodybuilding and weightlifting, you will now & then come across a mention of Zuver's gym, with one big exception being Dave & Laree Draper's Irononline forum, of which I am one of many members myself. They have a very nice picture spread & several related articles including an excerpt of Dick Tyler's book "West Coast Bodybuilding Scene, the Golden Era", which Dave wrote the picture captions for and gets quite a bit of ink from Mr. Tyler in. Another notable exception is Ken Leister's website; "History of Powerlifting, Weightlifting and Strength Training". Now, Ken's stuff is on Draper's forum, and the Irononline stuff is linked on Leistner's page, as one might expect. Another Old timer's forum, Ironage Forum, has quite a bit on the subject as well. The following forum post is interesting in that it keys on the methods primarily practiced at Zuver's, as opposed to its unique equipment, building and owners.

09-11-09 09:15 PM - Post#577601

Dan Martin posted the following on Cyberpump several years ago. Good and basic. Hopefully he doesn't mind me posting it.

Here is a most basic, and very good, result producing routine. It will work if you do. 3-6 months would be a good length of time to try it out. Think of this as the Garage Gym Anti-Westside Routine.

Monday
Squat
Bench Press
Pull-up

Wednesday
Bench Press
Dead Lift
Pull-up

Friday
Squat
Bench Press
Dead Lift

On Mondays, hit the squat hard, break a sweat on the bench and do pull-ups until you can't.

On Wednesdays, hit the bench hard, break a sweat on the DL, and you know the drill on the pull-ups.

On Fridays, break a sweat on the squat and bench, and let it rip on the dead lift.

What would be a good set and rep schedule? That's up to you. I wouldn't go for limit singles. But I would go for heavy 3's and 5's. A back-off set of 20 squats on Monday, and a back-off set of close-grip bench presses on Wednesday would be cool.

You think that three days of bench pressing would be too much? Do standing dumbbell presses on Monday instead.

Dr. Ken posted the following routines, I believe in the same thread as the above from Dan. Good and basic also.

Very Basic PL Routine

If you need to ask who these individuals are, there's no sense in trying to understand the point of the post:
Mike Bridges routine with almost no modification for his entire competitive career:

Mon-squat, bench press, deadlift
Wed-squat not as heavy as Monday, bench press moderately
Friday-heavy as heck on all three lifts

Hugh Cassidy

Mon-squat, bench press, deadlift, stiff legged deadlift
Wed-light squat, bench press moderate, upright row
Fri-squat, bench press, deadlift, shrug/heave
Lat pull downs and dumbbell curls on occasion

Standard NY City PL program 1960-1980s:

Mon-squat (heavy) and bench press (light)
Wed-Squat (moderate to light) and deadlift-heavy
Fri-bench press (heavy) and deadlift-light stressing speed

Lat pull down, curls, dips, dumbbell incline press each once per week. Ab work all three days. This program used by about a thousand guys, all of whom did very well in competition.

Here's the pertinent section;

Zuver's Hall Of Fame Gym, Costa Mesa, CALIF circa 1966-1971 routine that produced Tom Overholtzer, Bill Witting, Rudy Lazano, Willie Kindred (all record holders and/or Cal state champions, national level competitors)
Mon-squat (heavy), bench press (heavy)
Wed-squat (moderate to light), incline press (heavy), bent over row
Fri-deadlift (very heavy), bench press (moderate)
Assistance exercises used as needed included partial squats, partial DL, DB bench press, dips, barbell curl (sets of 3!)
Almost every lifter used the same program with minor variation.

Here is another somewhat random forum piece talking about the first World's Strongest Man contest in 1977; Franco Columbu's accident during that event and the impact of that on the Zuver legacy at the time;

Title: **Re: World's Strongest Man 1977 - Franco's leg practically comes off**
Post by: **dutchguy** on **December 05, 2011, 01:42:24 PM**

Please post the vid, although I saw it before.....ouch!

Title: **Re: World's Strongest Man 1977 - Franco's leg practically comes off**
Post by: **wes** on **December 05, 2011, 01:43:43 PM**

:'(

Title: **Re: World's Strongest Man 1977 - Franco's leg practically comes off**
Post by: **BB** on **December 05, 2011, 02:04:53 PM**

He made something like a 1.2 million in the lawsuit that followed. That suit was also a big reason most of the WSM contests being held outside the U.S.. It was also a reason Bob Zuver of Zuver's Gym left the scene. Franco sued a ton of people after that event.

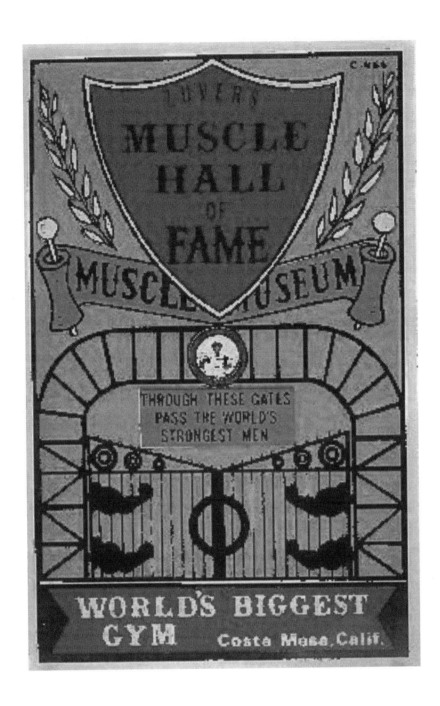

Now let's move into Dr. Ken's piece about Zuver's, for a good overview;

History of Powerlifting, Weightlifting and Strength Training - Part Twenty-Five
by Dr. Ken Leistner

Zuver's Hall of Fame Gym, Circa Late 1960'S.

Anyone who has participated in the sport of powerlifting knows that there is but one publication that represents the sport of powerlifting, and it is POWERLIFTING USA. In the past few months PLUSA, like this series on the TITAN SUPPORT SYSTEMS web site, has featured historical articles. In addition to the usual selection of fine training related materials, there is information about **the original Westside Barbell Club.** Certainly, when the modern era lifter hears "Westside," they immediately visualize Louie Simmons and his stable of incredible lifters and all of their national and world records. I would imagine that the Reverse Hyper Machine and other innovative training devices and techniques that Louie is so well known for would also quickly come to mind. **The PLUSA material is a reminder that there was an earlier, original Westside Club, one that I was lucky enough to train at a number of times. The club founded by Bill "Peanuts" West goes back further than his home garage in Culver City, California** where I was one of the fortunate lifters to walk up the street and then the driveway into a unique gathering of absolutely great powerlifters and track and field athletes. **Though I had trained at Zuver's Hall Of Fame Gym further south in Orange County's Costa Mesa, and years later traveled to California to specifically visit Bob and Jean Zuver, it was through Zuver's 165 pounder Lenny Ingro, a very underrated and under publicized champion, that I came to West's garage gym.** Ingro, who did the bulk of his training at Zuver's, did his Saturday training in West's garage and was very much a part of Peanuts' crew.

As the many writings of Louie in PLUSA, and the historical Westside article in the June issue clearly notes, there was a training system or template that Peanuts and George Frenn utilized with almost all of those who trained within the confines of the garage. At Zuver's there was also a template and it could be said that with some individual variation and the necessity to improve points of weakness, most of the Zuver's lifters trained in a similar manner. Bob Zuver had a very competent collection of lifters who influenced the "way things were done" and of course, was no doubt smart enough to inject the wisdom and ideas that came from the many luminaries who visited his unique establishment. **Zuver's was a magnet for some of the best of the day.** Dave and Laree Draper's web site has a number of articles and forum threads pertaining specifically to Zuver's Hall Of Fame Gym

Like Westside, both the original and Louie's establishment, there was a general system of training that most of the fellows pursued. 198 pounder Bill Witting and multi-time champion Tom Overholtzer set the squatting standards while many throughout a range of weight classes were recognized as excellent deadlifters. There were a few who benched big but Zuver's philosophy dictated that "the work necessary to increase the bench press by twenty-five pounds could result in a fifty pound increase in the squat or deadlift," thus, lots of effort went into those lifts. Remember though, this was Southern California in the '60's and there was still quite a bit of emphasis on exercises that intended or not, certainly resulted in large muscular physiques. If a "general program that everyone used" at Zuver's could be presented, it would look very much like the following:

Monday:

- Bench Press
- Dumbbell Bench Press
- Dip
- Squat

Wednesday:

- Incline Press
- Deadlift
- Deadlift Assistance

Friday:

- Repeat of Monday workout

Dependent upon where one's bench press was relative to a stated goal or the date of an upcoming contest, the sets and reps would vary. However, as a general rule, the warm-up would consist of a set x 6 reps and one or two sets x 3 reps. If there was "a usual" it would have been 3 sets x 5 reps or 3 sets x 3 reps with the working weight of that day and most often, a back off set x 5-8 reps. The bench press would be followed by the Dumbbell Bench Press and Reverend Bob had welded short angled racks, long enough to easily and safely hold a pair of his largest dumbbells and the gym dumbbells did go as high as 200 pounders as I recall. The small racks were angled so that one could sit at the end of a flat or incline utility bench, literally hug the heavy dumbbells to one's chest, and then roll back onto the bench with the dumbbells. This eliminated the often dangerous or energy sapping need to clean the dumbbells to the chest before attempting to lie back in place for the actual bench press movement, or finding spotters who were both strong enough and experienced in handling heavy dumbbells who then had to simultaneously hand the dumbbells off to the lifter. When the set was completed, a spotter could then help the lifter to a seated upright position by merely laying his palms onto the trainee's upper back and literally flipping him upward.

Our group of trainees never had a problem handling dumbbells in the 150 range using this procedure. Most of the powerlifters did 8 sets x 3 reps in the dumbbell bench press though some of the bodybuilders used reps in the 6 to 8 range.

Zuver's Gym had a **twelve foot long dip rack that had what resembled a small railroad flatcar, sans handles, beneath it. The cart was meant to support huge dumbbells that would be worn on a hip belt so that one could add up to a few hundred pounds over bodyweight for the dip exercise.**

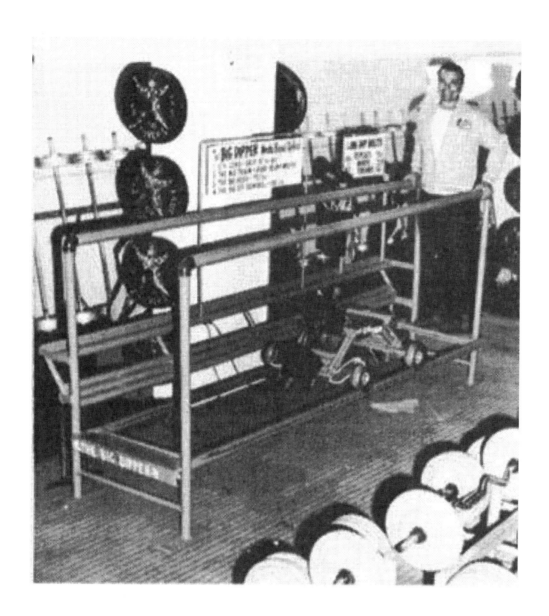

Like the dumbbell bench press, the weighted dips were also done for 8 sets x 3 reps by the powerlifters. The squats that followed the upper body work on Mondays were done in a similar manner to the bench press regarding sets and reps.

See more Zuver Gym information at:

www.davedraper.com- More Zuver's Information
www.davedraper.com- Zuver's Gym Photo Gallery
www.davedraper.com - About Zuver's
www.oldtimestrongman.com - Zuver's Hall of Fame

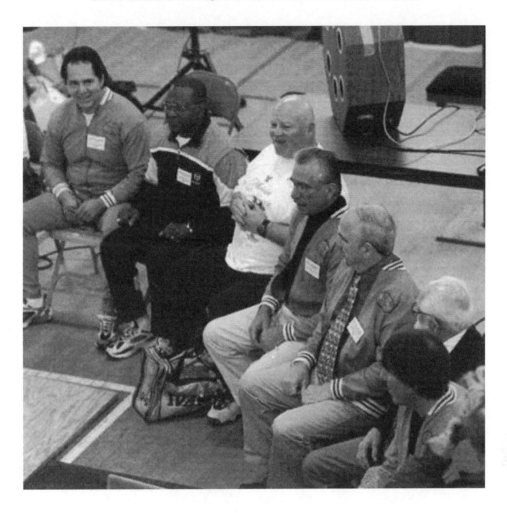

Inductees to the California Powerlifting Hall Of Fame, Class of 2005, included Zuver's Hall Of Fame Gym members, left to right: Rudy Lozano, Willie Kindred, Tom Overholtzer, Len Ingro, Bill Witting, (Jack Hughes, long time referee who no doubt red-lighted many of the attempted lifts by Zuver's team members!), and Jim Waters.

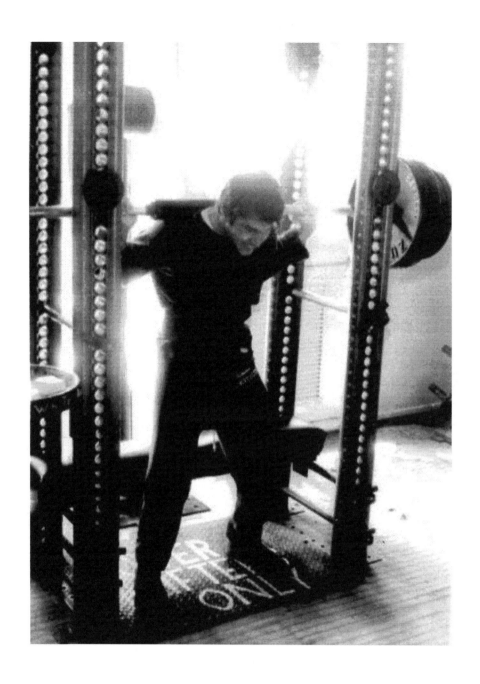

Before it was "Doctor" Ken, plain Ken often got crushed at Zuver's, this time in the bench squat within one of the unique Zuver's Gym power racks.

Was Ken trying to match Bob Zuver himself here? (see next picture)

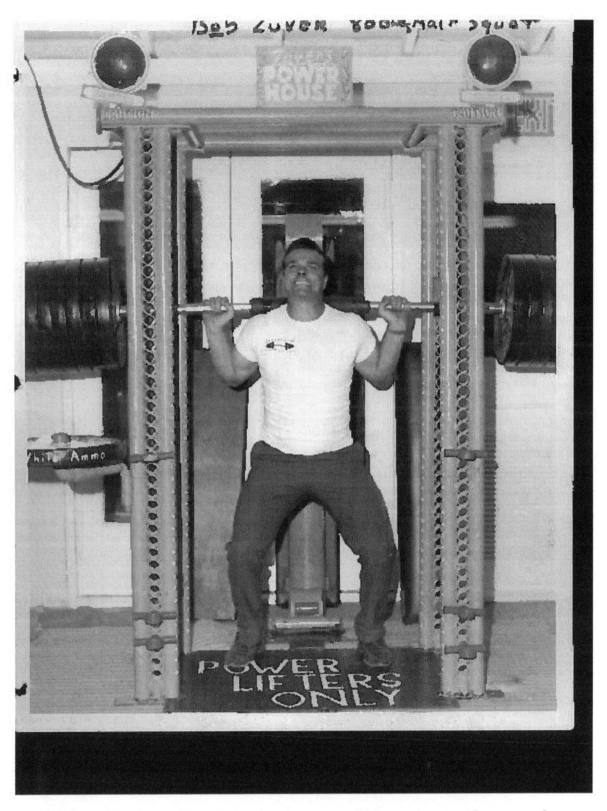

And here is the other huge power rack Zuver's was famous for;

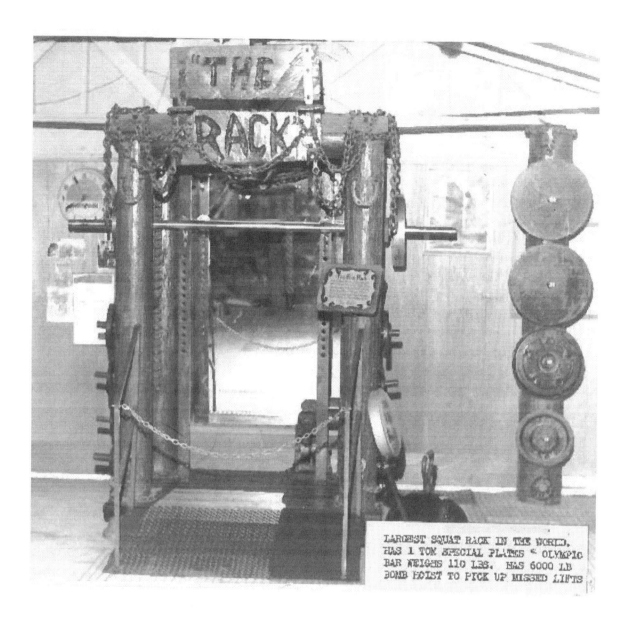

LARGEST SQUAT RACK IN THE WORLD. HAS 1 TON SPECIAL PLATES & OLYMPIC BAR WEIGHS 110 LBS. HAS 6000 LB BOMB HOIST TO PICK UP MISSED LIFTS

Friday's workout was similar with adjustments made on the bench press so that the lifter did not over train. Squats again would follow the upper body work and the load for full barbell squats would often be lowered to again, avoid overtraining although for some, this would instead be a day of partial squats. In a uniquely designed power rack, a padded bench would snap securely into place over the support pins to allow for bench squats to the desired depth. In another rack, an aircraft bomb hoist, no doubt salvaged from a World War II relic, had been refurbished into workout order and was available to lift huge weights off of pinned lifters doing heavy quarter and one-eighth level squats. On Wednesdays, incline pressing with a barbell was done by almost everyone "on the program" and the sets and reps again mimicked the bench press protocol. This would be followed by Deadlifts which would also follow the same set/rep scheme. The assistance movements done for the deadlift would follow on this day and may have consisted of pull downs, various rows, and/or shrugs.

Curls with both the fixed straight barbells and fixed EZ Curl bars that went from 20 to 200 pounds in five pound increments were done at the discretion of the trainee on any or all of the training days. When I asked Bob, "Who is going to use a 200 pound EZ Curl bar?" I was told that Paul Anderson had been by to visit just the week before our initial appearance at the gym and he in fact did curls with the 200 pound fixed EZ Curl bar. I figured I had used up my quota of stupid questions and listened rather than asked from that point onward!

In retrospect, the typical Zuver's Hall Of Fame Gym had for most, an overabundance of work that directly affected the deltoids and other pressing-involved musculature. However, we thrived on the program, enjoyed it, and most of the powerlifters at least, followed a very similar routine template. On Saturdays, Ingro as noted earlier, might lift with the Westside group while Overholtzer, Witting, Lozano, Kindred, and Jim Waters for example, might stay together as a group and do no more than the three lifts as they prepared for a contest. Like other gyms and training centers of the past and very much unlike today where cookie-cutter facilities exist, Zuver's had a great atmosphere, fueled by a group of men intent on pushing each other to improvement. The strains of Gospel music playing above the din of the clanging iron, the illuminated signs of spiritual encouragement and quoted scripture added to the unique atmosphere, one that produced many successful lifters.

Almost two decades of commitment to an ideal has benefited Orange Countians with the opportunity for a better way of life, Bob Zuver, owner and president of Zuver's Fitness Center Inc, started out in a simple garage in Costa Mesa 17 years ago with the belief that men and women have the right to enjoy life to its fullest. He dedicated himself and his business to fulfilling that right in the lives of hundreds and thousands through the years with the concept that to live right is to be fit, and that fitness is fun.

Today, over 1,000 of the highest quality items of exercise and gym equipment in the nation can be found in Zuver's Costa Mesa factory showroom.

Zuver's inspiration and motivation is sustained by the conviction that his business is not just for his own profit, but for the profit of the lives of others. Bob says, "I've seen so many men fight and scratch to get ahead in the business works, and when they make headway or approach retirement, they are two wasted to enjoy it because they didn't take the time or have the discipline to invest in their health and fitness along the way."

Beyond a doubt, the business man is a prime target for high blood pressure and heart attack. With a small investment, says Zuver, a business establishment can have the equipment necessary to build and maintain fitness and even the very life of its executives and sales representatives. In fact, all across the country more and more firms are setting up small fitness rooms for their employees. It has even shown to improve actual business performance.

Zuver's Fitness Center is totally unique in the field of weight and gym equipment manufacturing. There are the only firm in the nation to—

- Stock a complete line of highest quality equipment form light duty selectorized equipment to the country's very best free weight equipment, used by the LA Rams for over four years now);

- Custom build any piece of equipment;

- Staff experts in weight training programs and nutritional guidance;

- Offer free and complete training for individuals interested in setting up, owning and operating their own gym business.

Bob Zuver describes himself as a man of deep personal conviction who "will never compromise service or quality" for the sake of profit. "My business is to give others the best life has to offer."

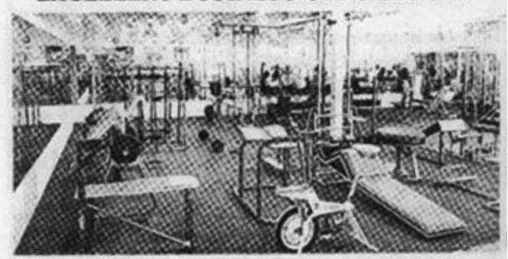

EXCELLENT BUSINESS OPPORTUNITY

OWN A TOP BODY BUILDING GYM

Duplicate one of California's world-famous body building gyms in your city. Complete package $15,000 and up. ★ Quick return on investment ★

Featuring Zuver's famous circle gym equipment. The same equipment used by all the top west coast body builders.

COMPLETE ADJUSTABLE LINE
- Flat Bench
- Incline Bench
- Decline Bench
- Calf Machine

SELECTORIZED PULLEY MACHINES
- Double Pulley Cross Overs
- Top and Bottom Pulleys
- Lat Machines
- Rowing Machines

PLUS—THE MOST COMPLETE AND SOPHISTICATED BODY BUILDING EQUIPMENT LINE.
Benches, Power Racks, Back Machines, Leg Extension Machines, Roman Chairs, Hyper Extensions, Bars, Weights, Dumbells, Etc.

Your bodybuilding gym becomes a retail store selling vitamins, supplements, T-shirts and soft goods. Many west coast gyms sell $6,000 to $8,000 a month on vitamins alone.

Start planning to open your body building gym now! Find your building and open your doors for business in 45 days or less.

Zuver's complete services provide the administrative, bookkeeping, memberships, financial planning and advertising materials for your business – Free, with your complete package.

Enclose $5.00 for complete information on how profitable the gym business can be for you.

Write to: (Please include your phone number)

Zuver's Famous Circle Gym Equipment
3320 W. McArthur Blvd., Santa Ana, CA 92707
714 • 979-9790

Featured in the CBS World's Strongest Men Show

And now, here's an article you'll enjoy: **Ken Leistner's memories of Zuver's.**

September 1988 Ironman wherein Dr. Ken's memories of Zuver's article was published. Voila!

Dr. Ken Leistner: Memories of Zuver's Hall of Fame Gym

Dr. Ken Leistner: Memories, Zuver's Hall of Fame Gym

Originally published in Ironman Magazine, September 1988
Reprinted with permission of Dr. Ken and Ironman publisher John Balik

In college during the volatile 1960s, I enjoyed playing football. Lifting weights and becoming stronger was also high on my list of things to do, and a number of college teammates at the University of Cincinnati felt the same. One of my teammates was Larry Gordon. He was easily noticed due to his outstanding physique. If he wasn't a bodybuilder, he had certainly lifted weights in a serious manner. He was a former Mr. Cincinnati winner, and quite strong in many lifts, especially the bench press. At 5'10" and 190 pounds, his All State running back status paled in comparison to his lifting accomplishments.

Larry decided to leave school, at least for a while, with the intention of traveling to California. Six months later, he returned much bigger and unbelievably stronger. He raved about a gym that sounds like it had fallen off of another planet. A gym where sirens announced the lifting of a heavy squat; where one could test ones strength against a variety of odd shaped dumbbells and globes. Here strong men strained to become stronger under the guidance of a Lutheran minister who allowed only gospel and religious music as background to the clanging of heavy iron.

Oversized fiberglass gorillas and a two-ton front door added to the atmosphere. Everyone's purpose was to become stronger, this at a time when most "serious" California gyms were dedicated to the enhancements of their members' muscular measurements.

This strength training oddity was Zuver's Hall of Fame Gym.

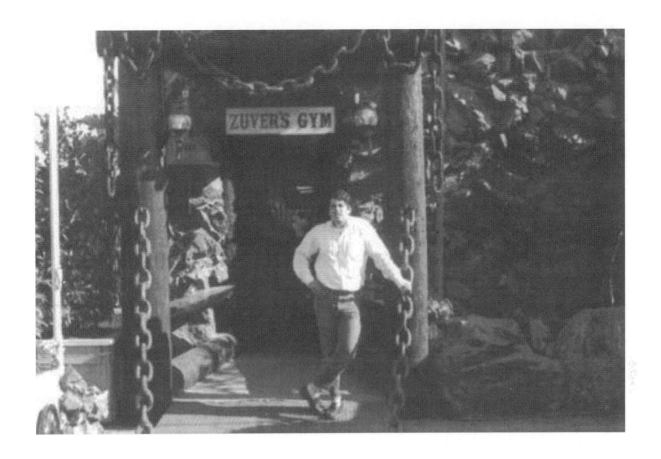

In 1968 I found myself sitting in Zuver's Gym, receiving the first of many lectures from the Reverend Robert Zuver. In time, I became quite friendly with Bob, his wife Jean and their two sons. His son Ricky "The Rhino," in fact, was forever exhorting gym members to "help Ken on his next squat." A different type of gym? Words still, after two decades, fail to describe it, and the feeling one got upon the initial visit.

The walls that supported the very high ceiling were decorated with signs exhorting one to further heights. The good Reverend included many spiritual messages, meant to augment the muscle that filled the air. Signs reminded one that "Profanity Is Not Tolerated On These Premises," nor was it. Unlike the typical gym, members policed newcomers, reminded them that respect was to be shown to all others, and the equipment, at all times.

Each of the three competitive powerlifts was given a special place. Many heavy duty benches, forerunners to today's sturdy, high tech products, lined one wall. Like other California gyms, a particular training philosophy dominated the programs of most of the members and competitive lifters. The primary auxiliary exercises were dumbbell bench presses and dips, done with very heavy weights. Special short benches would be pulled close to angled dumbbell racks, built so that one could in fact bring the 100- to 250-pound bells to ones chest without dangerously cleaning them. These benches were constructed so that a spotter could literally launch the trainee back towards the angled rack, allowing for replacement of the dumbbells, which were held close to the lifter's chest the entire time.

Few gyms have angled dipping bars, which allow for a variety of grips, and Zuver's was the only one that had a 12-foot version, allowing for more than one lifter to train simultaneously.

In order to safely allow for the use of 300-pound dumbbells, a converted railroad flatcar rode on a track beneath the dip bars. This added to the safety and convenience of moving such heavy weights from one end of the bar to the other.

While the lat pulleys were very strong, one cannot forget the day Wayne Coleman, later to gain fame as professional wrestling's Superstar Billy Graham, loaded the weight carriage to an absurd limit. Although the carriage failed to move, the solid iron lat bar handle literally curled around Coleman's upper back, ensuring this semicircle of iron would forever remind others of his legendary strength.

A refreshing pause by the water fountain was met by the clanging of fire bells. In a tribute to the firefighters who trained in his establishment, Bob had covered the fountain with a fire helmet, which, when lifted on its hinges to allow access to the drinking spout, triggered the bells.

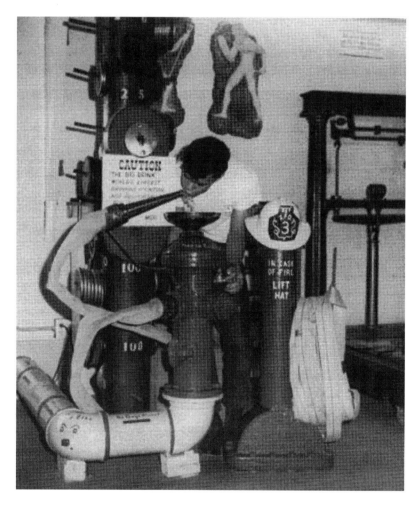

The specialized squatting racks also were never to be forgotten. One had its own 300-pound bar, indicating that only the heaviest of squats could be done within its confines.

Bob's walls were mounted with 100- and 200-pound plates for the stouthearted. An airplane bomb hoist provided a foot-operated safety spot within the rack, an innovation that protected both the lifter and his spotters.

The power rack in the back of the gym had lights and sirens, which alerted other gym members that a member of Zuver's competitive powerlifting team was about to make a personal record attempt. This, of course, allowed everyone present to cheer the lifter on, and made for enthusiastic training sessions.

Every piece of equipment was by far the most heavy-duty I had seen up to that time, anywhere. Conventional leg extension, curl and press machines were available, all handcrafted by Bob and his young sons. Bob felt that one could lift as heavily as possible only if he had the confidence that comes from the knowledge that the equipment was the best, the sturdiest and the safest available.

Bob's expertise led him to manufacture his own line of strength training equipment. These design innovations are still utilized today, although I am sure many are not aware of their origins.

He also provided all of the unique lifting apparati used in the early World's Strongest Man contests. Needless to say, "well equipped" was an understatement at Zuver's Gym.

Interestingly enough, the gym was not located on commercial property. Bob had long maintained an interest in physical fitness, and had converted his garage into a small but functional home gym. His bench, squat racks and other odd pieces were homemade, yet good looking, and well used by many youngsters in the neighborhood.

Bob's interest in Costa Mesa's youth eventually led to his garage being an unofficial meeting area and positive hangout for many formerly disruptive adolescents, youngsters who had been led into positive pursuits by the Zuver family. In time, Bob's wife insisted that he either give this up, or build a real gym. They purchased the house across the street from the one they lived in, and converted it into a gym. At the time I wandered into the gym, they had expanded it a number of times, and it provided an excellent training facility, although they would not even have showers installed until late in 1968.

Bob's collection of strength "odds and ends" was given a permanent home on a specially constructed platform in the rear of the gym. My favorite was the Big Barrel, a metal monstrosity filled with 200 or 250 pounds of constantly shifting water. I became the twelfth man to elevate the barrel overhead, a feat requiring one to first roll it up the length of his body before attempting an overhead thrust.

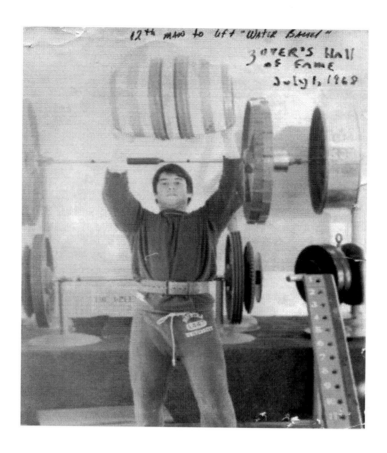

When I returned to New York, I told many tales of Zuver's Gym and the great powerlifting team they had. Len Ingro, Tom Overholtzer, Bill Whitting, Jim Waters, Willie Kindred, Rudy Lozano and others won local, state and national honors, often jostling with the more famous club from Bill West's Culver City garage.

Upon a return visit to Southern California two years later, I returned to Zuver's Gym, only to find it had again expanded and now housed a complete women's fitness area. The approach to the gym, what had in fact been the driveway to the house, featured a life-sized gorilla statue, huge iron gates shaped like a pair of muscular arms and a cascading waterfall that fell over huge boulders that formed the new front of the gym. It was a sight to see, and a sight to remember.

For those who do remember Zuver's Hall of Fame Gym, it was fondly recalled as an inspirational and colorful home of powerlifting. The wonderful workouts, unusual and enthusiastic environment, and the great lifts born of camaraderie and encouragement all come to mind when the name is mentioned.

More than a challenger for the powerlifting titles, Zuver's Gym remains one of those chapters of strength training history that make the sport what it is today. No gym has ever quite recreated the championship atmosphere fashioned by Robert Zuver.

Enthusiastic thanks for Dr. Ken for this glimpse of the special place that was Zuver's. For a photo collection and other memories of Zuver's from people there at the time, here's a choice IOL forum thread you'll get a kick out of.

To sink your teeth into the era in which Zuver's fits, start here, with **a Zuver's memory excerpt from West Coast Bodybuilding Scene.**

Our old forum friend, Bill Luttrell (RIP), offered up **his later memory of Zuver's.**

Edited September 2008: Bob Zuver died August 22, 2008 in Lake Forest, California after a battle with cancer. Rest in peace, Bob; we thank you for the great memories.

Here is some more stuff from Ken, found on the Irononline site;

From Dr. Ken Leistner;

I've written full articles in Iron Man re: my time at Zuver's. Jack and I were there when the house that the gym was located in on Hamilton Ave first opened. We were the first guys to use the showers as the tiles were put in the day before. For a while, we lived in the little trailer behind the house, urinating out the back door into the vacant lot or walking down to the gas station that was on the corner (the big street that went down towards the wealthy area/town where Nixon used to live and hang out). For $30.00 a month, it was a good deal! We helped Bob rush over to the Freeway to load a section of guard rail that was torn out in an accident. We got it before the highway crew removed it and it became an incline bench! It was a great place to get big and strong although Bob did have quite a few competitive bodybuilders on the premises. Great, supportive atmosphere with religious music blasting the entire time. Sept. 1988 Iron Man has full article I wrote.
Dr. Ken

July 1, 1968: I took about a dozen attempts on this day, a continuation of all of the times I missed lifting this 225 or 250 pound barrel that was 3/4 of the way filled with water. It continuously shifted and I had horrible "cleaning" technique. I rolled the thing up my chest and face and it was as painful as it sounds. With Jack yelling encouragement such as "forget it, you'll kill yourself" and others saying "enough already, put it down before you get hurt", I finally clean and jerked the thing. Bob and Jim Waters who I guess kept track of these things, told me I was "the twelfth man to do it" with Pat Casey completing it a few weeks before I did.

Laree mentioned this, and I am really short of time right now to add much, but I was there from 1973 until the successor Zuver's on 19th in Costa Mesa and one on El Toro road in what is now Lake Forest, closed. The move to the newer gyms from Hamilton Street (Bob's house) was sometime in around 1978. I would say the newer gyms lasted about 2 years before the whole thing closed. The photos posted are from the late 60's, but nothing on Hamilton Street changed until the end. I went by the property maybe 8 years ago and the stone door was still there on the gym building. The place was a complete dump, but man there was a bunch of iron in there and many characters using it to its fullest. By the early 70's, I recall 5 world record holding powerlifters training there. In the late 70's, it became much more of a bodybuilding gym. A very serious one. Good time

There was a thread I posted on ironage (Henrik?) not long ago on this subject that I will try to find that discussed where the equipment went.

Bill

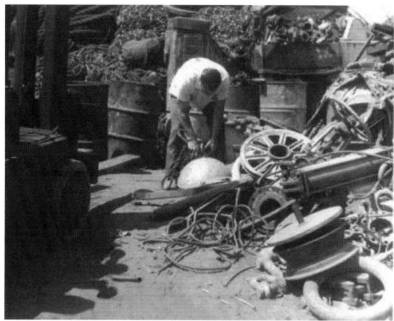
Bob finding the blob at scrap yard

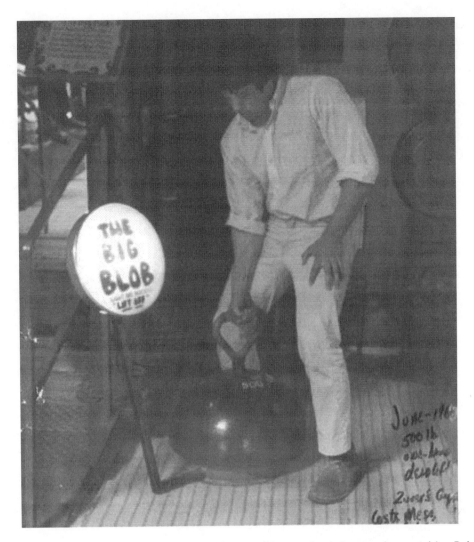

That's the big blob at Zuver's gym that I was telling Dave and Laree about. I remember watching Bob Zuver pick that up with one hand and walk around with it. This was around 1967-8. I remember it sat on a platform scale that went up to 500 hundred pounds. I never got it off the scale completely but I got the needle down to 150 lbs. or so. I love these photos of that old gym. It's a shame that place ended up dismantled. I look at those plates that Zuver had made up with his name on them and just wonder what those would cost today. Thanks for sharing these Jeff and Laree.

Here is a photo of Bob himself dueling with the mighty blob in one of the Zuver's strength shows, which it appears Dr. Ken was trying to reproduce in the picture above.

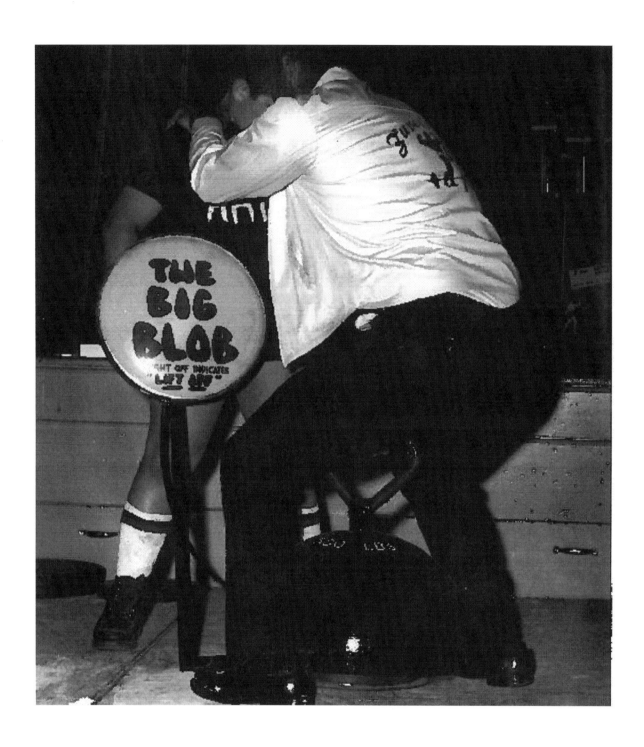

When Kathy and I opened the Iron Island Gym, we had York weights only at that time, perhaps 12,000 pounds worth. York was the standard for decades and the 45 and 35 pound plates were milled. We weighed the plates when we loaned them out to someone who was running a PL meet in pounds (we also had two full kilo sets and one bumper set for the Olympic lifters). All of the 45s that they used on the meet platform and warm-up room, perhaps twenty or so, which was a good random selection from what was on the gym floor, weighed within 2-4 oz. of the stated weight, using the same model scale that was used in the O lifting competition at the Barcelona Olympic games. They were dead-on! We wanted plates like Zuver had, because just like you, I thought they were the coolest.

Bob had a small area foundry making them and I had bought unfinished plates at Bell Foundry in LA during the weight shortage of 1974 when the EPA closed perhaps 80% of domestic foundries with the change in air pollution control laws. We decided to go to York and proposed that they make me 230 "Iron Island" 45 pound plates. They did after first making "our" mold and casting the plates. They were great and I still have a few of them in the garage that we use. It gave us distinction, similar to that of Zuver's. At the time, York did not make custom plates but after doing our's, they did a batch for the Univ of Hawaii, and then made it a policy while Vic Standish ran the foundry, to make custom plates. They closed the foundry a year ago so that's a lost opportunity. However, back then, our mold cost $1200.00 and they wanted a minimum order of 100 plates of that specific denomination. I am sure that a foundry would make the plates (perhaps not mill them as York did with our Iron Island 45s so that they too were accurate in weight) after first casting a mold for you. I would estimate the cost of the mold relative to the inflation and consumer goods increases that have occurred in the past ten years or so. I think the overall cost of the plates, when their standard Olympic plates of that time sold for $.90 per pound retail, came out to $1.42 per pound, including the cost of the mold which we included in the first batch of 180 plates (a later order of 50 plates made the total 230). I hope this gives you an idea of the cost.

Dr. Ken

More stuff from the Draper forum

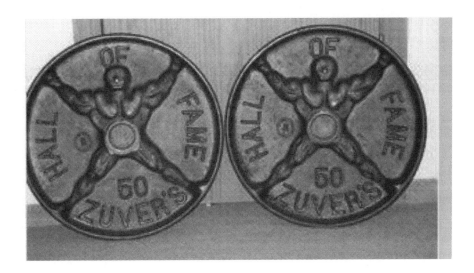

Here's a post of Bill Luttrell's I lifted from the IOL archive for those who missed it, and to get all the Zuver's material collected in one place... Laree

Here's another old (and long) story that may be of some interest. The Chet Yorton discussion, as well as Bill K's description of the Kenya gym brought this to mind. Sweet memories ... to the tune of Frank Sinatra's "It Was a Very Good Year."

The original Zuver's Gym was a large (maybe 30' X 100') rectangular building that Bob Zuver had built in the large backyard of his home on Hamilton Street in Costa Mesa. The area was zoned "commercial" only because it was with a hundred yards or so of Harbor Boulevard, a major North/South artery in Orange County that leads to Newport Beach, a couple of miles away. Everything in it was hand built by Bob: the dumbbells, the chin area, the odd but wild looking (and sometimes frighteningly dangerous - but thankfully few in number) machines, and the benches.

The front door was a foot-thick steel and stone contraption. Must have weighed at least a ton or so. A 30' gorilla stood out front on what had been the driveway. The benches were adorned underneath with cut-out and painted steel rhinos that had been welded on. Large movie-prop rocks sat in the corners. On the open-beam wood ceiling hung some of those coconut "heads" that have faces on them that make them look like pirate's heads. Right in the line of sight when you were laying on the benches. Very strange. My training partner Dave made jokes about them constantly - and usually in the middle of my toughest sets. We still laugh about that.

Little active maintenance was done by Bob or his employees, so the place was, to be kind, filthy. For example, on the floor where for years massive guys did pullovers and banged huge weights on the floor at the bottom of the reps, the carpet (?) was long gone and the concrete floor was depressed by three or four inches - exposing the aggregate rock in the concrete mixture. A jackhammer couldn't have done a better job. Concrete dust sprayed out to the sides for a foot or so around these craters. Same thing around the benches, where plates were thrown on the floor. Before being ground in with the rest of the dirt and dust, white lifter's chalk lay heavily strewn about on the floor around the benches, squat rack, and deadlift platform, as well as on all of the oly bars and larger dumbbells.

As with Dave's Dungeon at Gold's, the place had one purpose only: training to get huge. Cardio was unheard of - a foreign word. It was very much a "guy's" place. All function leading to but one end. Who cared about a little dirt? It worked, as I've never seen so many big guys in one place. As Gold's became the Mecca for bodybuilding on the west coast in the 70's, Zuver's was to powerlifting. When I first joined, five members held world records. Bill Kazmaier and other heavyweights visited. Lots of very large, very thick guys dressed in everything from cutoffs and tees or tanktops to overalls. In fact, shirts and shoes were kind of "optional." Definitely no fancy gym clothes. No lycra within miles. As with Bill's African gym, guys sometimes brought their dogs along. Quite amazing when compared to today's commercialized gyms.

However, by the late 70's the winds of change were upon us. Arnold had brought bodybuilding to the world. There was money to be made in bodybuilding. Possibly even big money. So, around late 1978, Bob closed the backyard gym and opened up a shiny new one a couple of miles closer to the beach on 19th Street in Costa Mesa. The place was to have been a "showcase" for further expansion. A "model" for future investors. Only this gym was geared to bodybuilding, not powerlifting. Gone was the deadlift platform. All the equipment was new or freshly painted. Mirrors lined all the walls. Women (gasp!) joined and trained hard after seeing what Rachel McLish had done and Cory Everson was doing. No more throwing stuff on the floor, and no chalk allowed. ;-(Real workout clothes and shoes required. A similar gleaming facility (with a separate "aerobics" area!) was opened in the affluent and fast-growing south OC location of El Toro. Bob began to gear up to make equipment in a nearby manufacturing facility.

Ostensibly, the whole thing from there was supposed to be a springboard for a proposed expansion with Joe Weider to be called "Weider/Zuver's Gyms." Always on the lookout for a buck to be made in the bodybuilding world, Joe was of course quick to notice the success of Gold's and World as they franchised their names around the world. At one point, World Gym tee shirts were the number two selling tee shirt in the world, behind only the Hard Rock Cafe megasellers. BIG bucks were being made. Joe apparently wanted some of this action, and wanted a gym with a track record and name (along with the gorilla and rhino stuff to market) to go with it. Bob saw an opportunity in terms of financial clout he otherwise lacked. The marriage seemed to have potential.

Although perhaps the thought or dream of owning a gym crosses every Musclehead's mind at some point in time, the actual reality of the business of operating a gym (much less a string of gyms) can be either lucrative or very cruel. It's no accident that most don't make it. Not surprisingly, in a year or so, and before really getting much past the starting gate, the whole merger/expansion/franchising thing fizzled and stalled.

There was something about a disagreement between the two main players.

By 1981, strapped by the expansion of the two showcase gyms, Bob sold all his equipment and closed the doors. The gym on 19th Street became a dry cleaner, then some kind of a graphic arts company. The one in El Toro became a real estate office. Sometimes, the best investments are those you don't make.

And, I still miss the old gym on Hamilton Street ... As Bill K. said, "it was all so simple then ..."

Bill (Luttrell)

The Excerpt of the Dick Tyler book that shows up on the Draper forum was originally published in a magazine article, as was pretty much everything else in the book. The book contains excerpts from Tyler's days writing for the earlier versions of Weider's publications like Muscle Builder magazine, and we actually have that article, just as laid out in the magazine. Forgive the redundancy, please, but I thought reproducing the full article here would be a nice touch.

POWER LIFTING

THE POWERLIFTING PARADISE

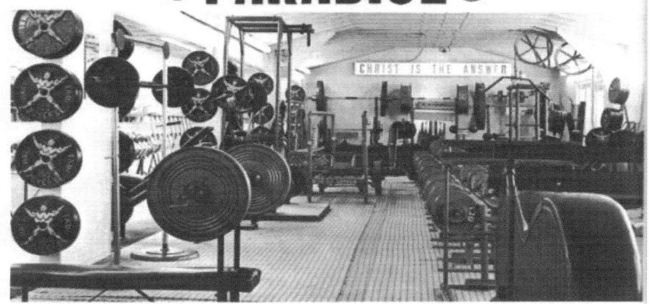

A Garden of Eden for California power lifters, Bob Zuver's Costa Mesa gym sports more weight and unusual heavy duty equipment than any training facility in the world.

BY THE SWEAT OF HIS BROW THE REV. BOB ZUVER HAS ERECTED A MONUMENT TO HIS FAITH IN HIS FELLOW MAN

By DICK TYLER
West Coast Editor and Director

THOUSANDS of years ago the Egyptians built the mighty pyramids. It took the labor of thousands of slaves and as long as twenty years to complete just one of these massive structures. In many ways the miracles wrought by ancient man seem more spectacular than some of the achievements we take pride in today. I thought achievements by the literal "hand of man" were slowly fading until one day I overheard some men talking in a gym. "You wouldn't believe it," said one of them, "it's the most incredible thing I ever saw." Hmm, that got my attention so I strained to hear more. "The place has more weight than I've ever seen in my life," he continued, "and the apparatus defies description." That did it. "What are you talking about?" I asked. "Zuver's gym." "Whose gym?" "Zuver's. It's the most incredible gym I've ever seen." He proceeded to tell me things that didn't seem real so I dismissed the whole bit to the fact that the guy was smoking something weird. I would have kept this line of reasoning if I hadn't begun to hear similar stories. Each tale seemed to get wilder than the one before.

Finally I heard tell of a wall that had been hand built from boulders averaging a *(Continued on page 52)*

32

POWERLIFTING HALL OF FAME

(Continued from page 32)

ton apiece by Bob Zuver. It sounded like the pyramids all over again. It was one boulder too many for me. The next thing I knew I was calling Zuver and arranging a story.

Try as I might I couldn't convince Art Zeller that the stories about Zuver's Gym were for real. "Look," he said as we drove along the freeway to Costa Mesa where the gym was located. "I'll take the shots for you but a gym is a gym is a gym is a gym. The only thing that really makes one different from another are the guys who train there." I looked out the window at the passing palm trees that seemed to glory in the California winter sunshine. "Guess we won't know till we get there."

Zuver's Gym is located at 443 Hamilton Street in the little southern California city of Costa Mesa which is a few miles south of Long Beach. As we pulled up I noticed a small sign that was shaped like a dumbbell. On it was printed the name of the gym. That was the last small thing either Art or I was to see while we were there. We got out of the car and walked a few paces until we reached the sign. Only then did we realize that the gym was set back off the street. Leading from the street to the front was a long promenade. On either side were potted plants and between those plants were Zuver Olympic barbell plates. What plates they were! Molded into the facing of each was a golden muscle man spread-eagled so that it appeared as if he were holding the rims apart. As you get closer to the front door the plates went from 50 lbs. to 200 lbs. a piece! That's what I said —each plate weighed as much as 200 lbs. There, finally, looming in front of us was the massive wall I had heard about. In front of that was a spectacular fountain. A draw-bridge crossed what seemed like a moat. All this was surrounded by a massive chain that entwined over an archway, that was surmounted by a loaded Olympic set. We hadn't even reached the door and I had enough for a story. "Hi," said a voice. I looked to see a good looking man with a pleasant smile. "I'm Bob Zuver." We shook hands. "I see you've been looking at the place." "That wall . . . ." I said shaking my head. "That wall," said Zuver, "weighs 65 tons. Each boulder you see weighs an average of 2,000 lbs." "That must have cost a fortune to build," I said. Zuver smiled. "Not so much when you build it yourself." "You really built that by yourself." I said in disbelief. "That's right, my sons and I would take the truck and go as far as 120 miles into the mountains to get the boulders. It took a lot of time and work but the boys in the gym helped and we all had fun building it."

By this time I was getting a little tense. Was this guy pulling my leg? Was he serious? "Now over here is the big door bell," said Zuver as he pointed to a huge bell. Then he walked over to an enormous key. "And this . . . ." "Don't tell me," I interrupted, "is the big key." "Right. Which fits into the big key hole." "Which opens the big door," I said. "Right again," said Zuver. "I guess you've noticed how I refer to everything as 'big'." "I've noticed." "That's because I want everyone who trains here to think big and to act big. However, if he's too big to be nice, he's too big for the gym. Christ, and our faith in him, is big why shouldn't our lives try to match the bigness of that faith?" I looked at him intently. His eyes were set. He believed what he was saying. That gave me a nice feeling. "Now here we have the big door handle," he continued, "which is a dumbbell that weighs 320 lbs. The big door alone weighs 4,000 lbs. and took a year to build. It's perfectly balanced and even a child can open it." With that he opened the big door. If the outside had startled me, it was like a shrug compared to the explosion of sights that greeted Art and me as the huge door opened wide to reveal what must be the greatest array of tonnage ever assembled in one area for the training of the human being.

On racks angled against the wall were dumbbells that went in five pound jumps from 10 lbs. to 300 lbs. I didn't want to meet the one who used 300-lb. dumbbells in his workout. In the center were racks that contained curling bars that went in 5-lb. jumps from 40 to 300 lbs. "Bob," I asked, "who could ever curl a 300-lb. bar?" "Paul Anderson did it," he said without hesitation. I decided not to ask anymore dumb questions.

As I looked around I saw "the big rope" which is the world's largest rope climb. I tried to figure out who would have hands big enough to hold on to it much less climb it. Bob started showing us around. "Now, here is the world's largest dipping rack," he said as we went over to a set of bars that I was told measured 12 feet long. "What are the wheels under the bars for?" asked Art. "To hold the weights when you're through," said Bob. "Now here is the big hook we use to hold the weights around the lifter's waist." With that he showed us a hook attached to a belt. "The hook alone weighs 75 lbs."

Next we came to the big lat machine whose cable had a 5 ton test. After seeing what I had so far I wondered if that was strong enough. The weight holding apparatus alone was a 100-lb. anchor. At the far end of the gym was one of the greatest assortments of odd lift weights I have ever seen. A power rack nearby had lights that would flash red when you stepped under the bar to let people know a strongman was ready to lift. A row of benches just made for bench pressing was next. And on a platform was the heaviest bench in the world weighing 652 lbs. It was complete with a seat for the spotter.

Zeller then asked for a drink, and

laughingly remarked "At the big fountain." Zuver pointed toward the world's biggest fountain. That's right—it was a fire hose. "That's the big scale there," said Bob, "and here we have the world's largest squat rack." He led us to what looked like some medieval torture device. When you stand inside its confines red lights blink. "The bar alone weighs 200 lbs. and the whole thing can be loaded to a ton." "Isn't that pretty dangerous," I asked. "I mean, who could spot you?" Zuver didn't answer. Instead he pressed a button and down came two hooks on some kind of hydraulic lift which grabbed the weight and lifted it clear of the man using it.

Bob could see the look on my face. "Look," he said with a smile, "I know this is all a little kooky but why should we take training so seriously. Let's have fun while we work out." This was all we needed to relax. I found that Bob Zuver was one of the finest and most sincere men I have ever met. He is an ordained evangelist minister who quite literally practices what he preaches. He feels that Christ is the answer and goes out to the youth with the word of God for the soul and barbells for the body. He does a great deal of work with delinquents and has marked success.

Looking around all these weights I had to ask. "Bob, who can lift all this iron?" "You mean do we have men strong enough to lift really big poundages?" I nodded. "Well, a gym member by the name of Wayne Coleman loaded so much weight on the lat machine that he couldn't lift it." "See!" I said. "So," continued Bob, "he just bent the bar around his neck." I cleared my throat. "Okay." Then I spotted a giant weight that was tagged "the blob". "What's that for and who can lift it?" "It's for one arm deadlifts, it weighs well over 500 lbs. and I can lift it." With that he took hold and proved that he was as good as his word. "Does strength run in the family?" asked Art. "Well, I personally started lifting years ago with the great Olympic lifter Pete George back in Ohio. Since that time the call of power has been a great part of my life. I've tried to imbue my two boys with the love of health and strength." "Did you succeed?" I asked. "My older boy, Bob Jr., is a fine lifter," said Bob with a flush of pride, "and the boys coach for the Powerlifting Hall of Fame. My youngest son, Ricky, is probably one of the strongest youngsters in the world. He got the nickname of the 'rhino' and with good reason." "What are some of his lifts?" "At the age of eight, Ricky was able to squat with 250 lbs. and at ten he was able to deadlift 325 lbs. while weighing 115 lbs.

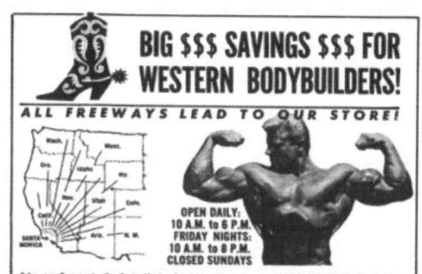

Bob's lovely wife, Jean, then asked if we would like refreshments. Art said thanks but that he had more than enough to drink from the big fountain.

At that moment a group of men smartly dressed in Zuver lifting outfits entered the gym for a training session. We were introduced to the team captain, Bill Witting, who introduced us to the rest of the crew, Rudy Lozano, Jim Waters, Willie Kindred and Chester Horvath. Not present were such power stars as the 165-lb. California champ Leonard Ingro and the 181-lb. national squat record holder Tom Overholtzer who can pound out 575 lbs in that lift. "That's quite a team," said Art. Bob nodded. "I just hope that one day very soon we'll hold the national team championship."

"You've mentioned several times about a powerlifting hall of fame. What's that all about?" We walked over and sat on a big bench. "Well, there are weightlifting halls of fame so I decided I'd start one for the power lifters. In order to gain entrance you have to be able to lift a required poundage in the selected lifts."

We walked outside again and I asked Bob about his future plans. "The next thing we have planned is an outdoor training area under a cliff-like overhang called, "the cave". Then there are the plateaus in which the men will be training on these cliffs and descend from them by fire poles." At one time, I would have thought he was kidding but after seeing what I just had, I didn't even blink.

We said goodbye and I was reluctant to leave. It had been a memorable experience. I had seen a gym that was unique in all the world but what was more important, I had been privileged to meet a fine man who was dedicating his life to the youth of his country. I thoroughly believe that if you are a strength fan you owe it to yourself to visit Zuver's Hall of Fame Gym. You'll never forget it. It's a *big* experience.

1968 IFBB JR. MR. AMERICA and ODD LIFT CONTEST

SUNDAY, JULY 28 — 2 P.M.
Mountain Park Amusement Center
Holyoke, Mass.

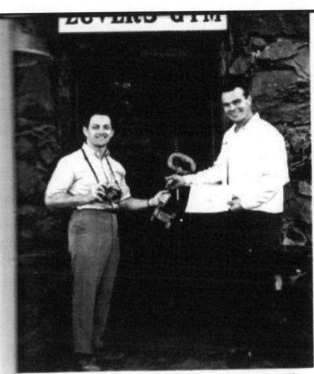

Gym designer Zuver offers key to the zany establishment to MB photographer Art Zeller. Zuver claims it's the biggest key in the world and it really works.

Outside the moat which separates gym members from lesser mortals Jim Waters, Willie Kindred, Bill Witting, Rudy Lascane and Chester Horvath (l. to r.) construct the "Big Pyramid."

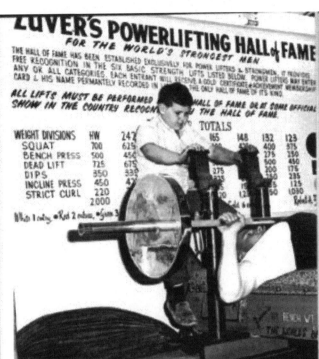

The world's heaviest proning bench weighs 652 pounds. Behind it are the standards which must be met to enter Zuver's Power Lifting Hall Of Fame. It'll take a lot of work on that super bench to get in there.

It's no simple task getting into the big gym. In fact, it takes the combined power of five strongmen to just open the door.

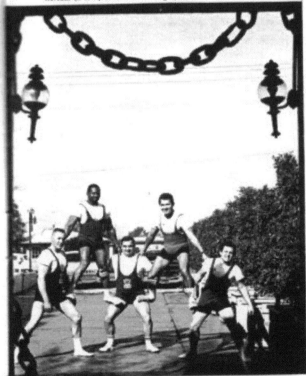

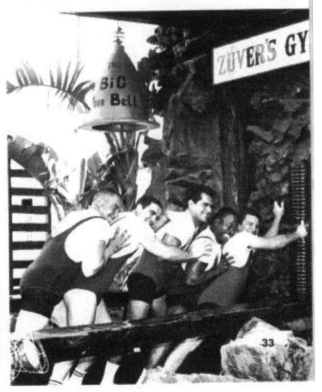

THE POWERLIFTING

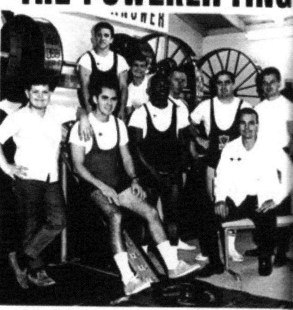

Inscription on world's biggest squat rack removes Mom-ism from any weight man. It says hydraulic apparatus will remove weight from back of pinned squatter.

A line up of Zuver's lifters pose in front of some bizarre apparatus the purpose which is still undetermined. Zuver is at right seated; his son, sturdy Ricky The Rhino is at far left.

Willie Kindred on the Big Dipper shows the Big Hook in action.

John Guarnieri works the Big Lat bar as the enormous pulleys attached to the ceiling groan under the weird-looking load.

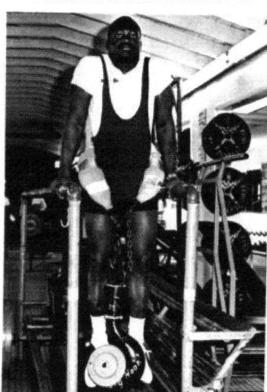

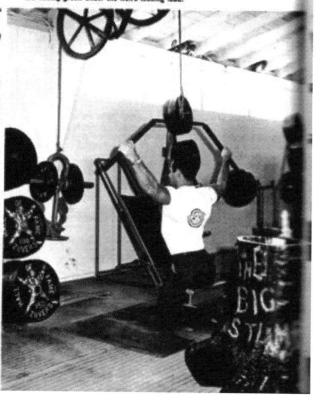

PARADISE *Continued*

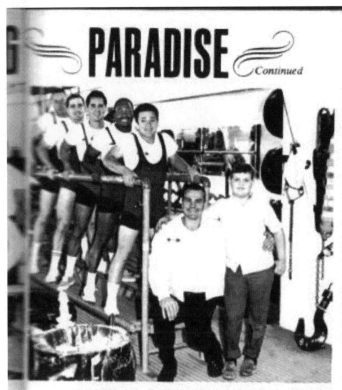

Bob and Ricky show five of their lifters on the Big Dipping Bar, world's biggest dipping rack. To the right is the Big Hook (weight: 75 lbs.) which the strong dippers use to attach dumbbells to themselves.

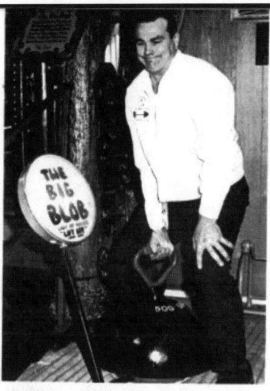

The Big Blob is a pitifully heavy 500-lb. deadweight. When lifted clear of the ground, as powerhouse Zuver is doing with one-arm, the giant bulb goes off to indicate clearance.

Bill Witting presses in the Zuver Power House as Willie Kindred and Jim Waters await their chance at tenancy.

Strongmen get thirsty and to quench their thirst Zuver has installed the world's largest drinking fountain—a fire hose and hydrant.

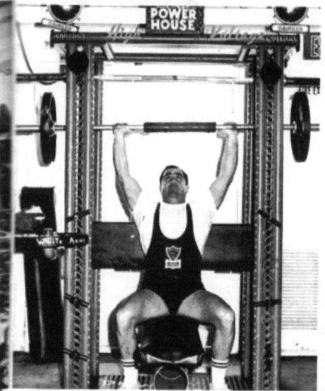

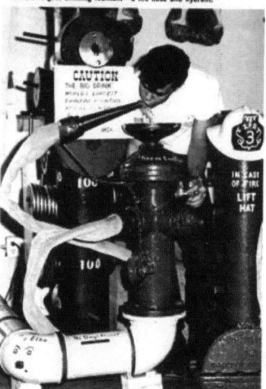

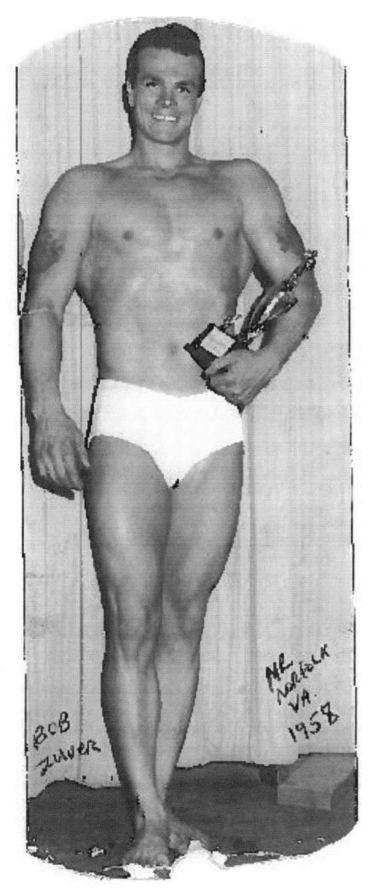

What about Bob Zuver & his family?

Former weightlifting champ, Bob Zuver, became an ordained minister after building *Zuver's Gym* and the *Muscle Hall of Fame*. What's interesting about this gym is that all of the presentations are physically large. For instance, three of the presentations are a huge fiberglass gorilla, a ten-foot tall superman and a fiberglass elephant lifting a barbell. The main entrance doors weigh two tons and the drinking fountain is a fire hydrant. When Zuver was asked why everything was made large in scale, he said, "To build fitness and strength, not only in the physical realm, but also in the mental *and the spiritual* realms." <u>Every Christian is part of the body of Christ, and the responsibility of everyone is to strengthen each other</u> and work together to build a huge, fit body of Christ.

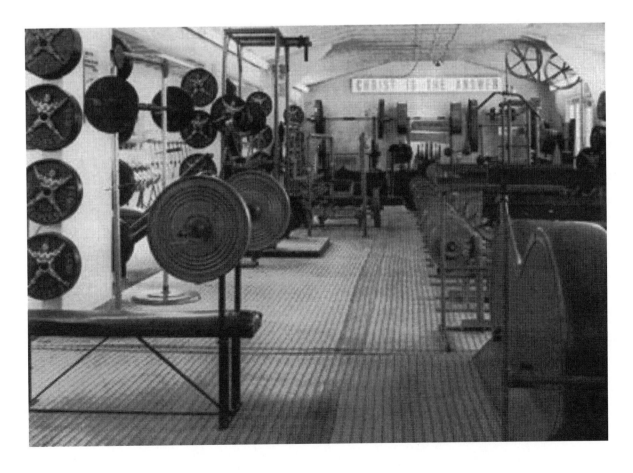

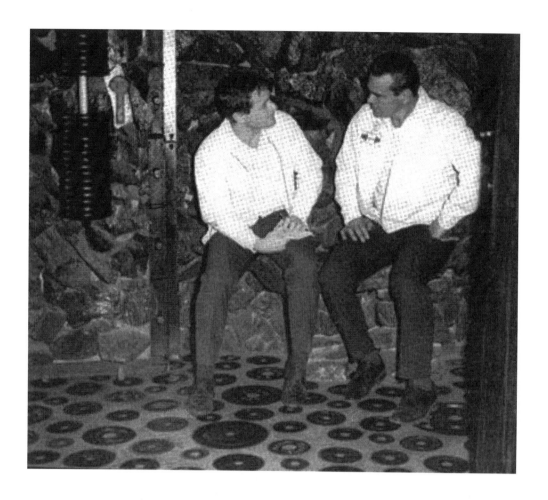

Here we see Bob talking to Dick Tyler during the interview for the magazine article

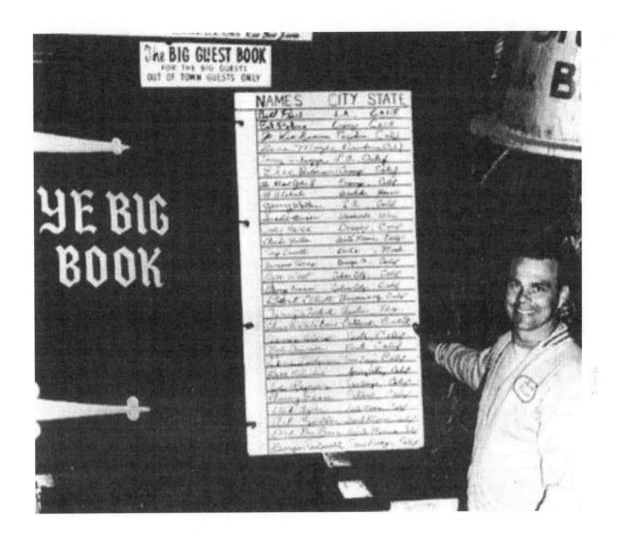

Bob posing with "The Big Guest Book". Too bad we can't read all those names!

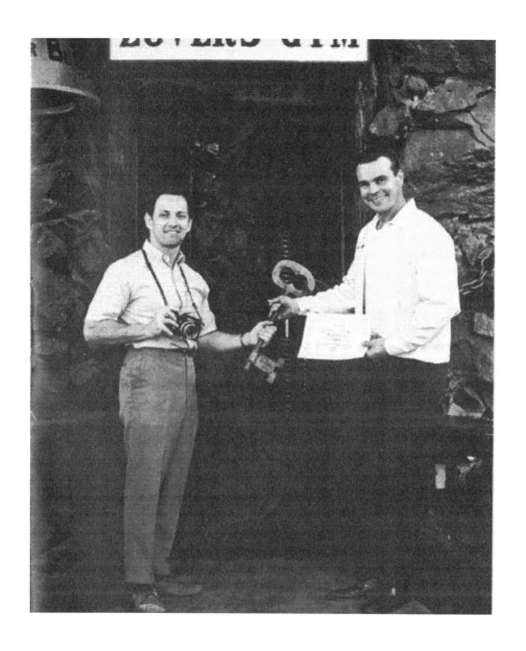

Artie Zeller gets the Big Key in a symbolic gesture. Artie took the pics for the Tyler article, and was the photographer for most of Dick's articles in the Weider magazines

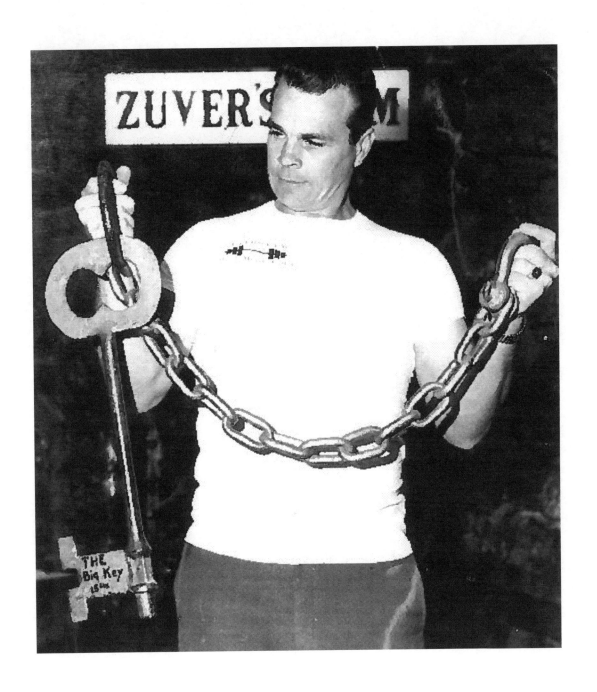

Here's a close-up of Bob with the BIG KEY

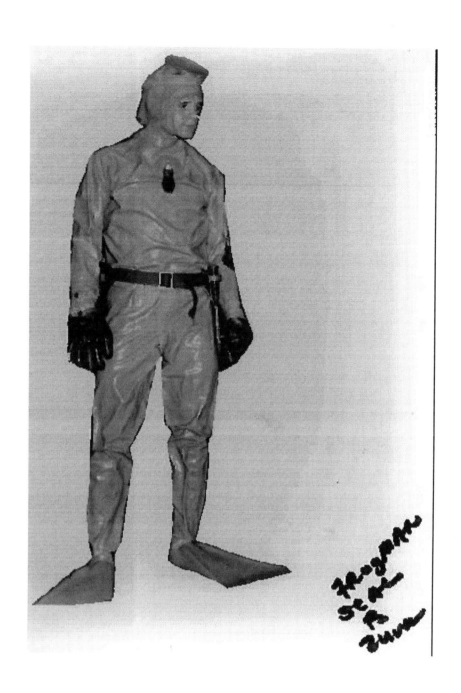

Bob was a Navy Seal in the '50s

Found this online apparently from Bob shortly before he passed;

Entry: 63855
UDT UNDERWATER DEMOLITIONS TEAMS INFO ON BUDDIES
                                                       ROBERT ZUVER SR. wrote on
January 16, 2008

City and State: LAKE FOREST CA

Unit: UDT 4

Service or Relationship: NAVY VETERAN

Comments: I am interested in making contact with any of my old UDT 4 buddies stationed in Norfolk, Va. Little creek base. During 1948 to 1953. Would like to know where they are and what they are doing now. Especially one man named Carl Zeigler. During 1949 and 1953. If you know about anyone please contact me. I now live in Lake Forest, Ca. Thanks. Bob Zuver.

Keywords: Udt 4. Little Creek , Va. Bob zuver. 48 to 53. Ed KraZEL- SHIP 136 ? NAME CARPALETTI ? Carl Ziegler .


```
Here is an article from the man himself, which will
provide a glimpse into his mind-set
```

Bob Zuver: What it Means to Be Fit

Bob Zuver
Sportscope Magazine, 1977

Over 10,000 people have come through the doors of my gym in Costa Mesa at various stages of the elusive quest for physical fitness. Now, after 17 years of being the in the business of fitness, if there is any one principle I would communicate to an individual engaged in that pursuit, it would be this: moderation and balance.

Contrary to what may seem obvious, one of the greatest hindrances to the development of physical fitness is overzealousness. It leads a person to make impossible demands on the body. One day someone much like yourself decides it is time to shape up and shape up right now. You enroll in a health club, work out vigorously five or six times a week and even go on a diet of lettuce leaves and bird seed!

What happens to our fitness zealot (and I have seen it countless numbers of times)—you burn yourself out in no time at all physically, emotionally and psychologically. Training soon becomes a drudgery and in no time at all you are back, further back, than when you started: shackled, burdened and guilty.

Forget about trimming down and shaping up on thirty days or bust. Instead of being a burden requiring strict discipline, becoming physically fit can be and should be fun.

How? By being moderate and being consistent. Consider exercising in terms of a regular and lifetime investment, not as a short term all-out blitz. Fun and enjoyment comes from seeing results and improvement and continuing that way to get the most life has to offer in good health and good shape.

Then there is balance. Without emotional and psychological harmony, a person cannot be considered to be in a state of physical fitness. For 17 years I have had the opportunity to share that concept, the importance of the spiritual aspect of life.

As a minister, it was always me desire to have a church to have a positive effect on people's lives. But instead, the Lord led me to a ministry of fitness, combining the development of the body and the spirit—development mentally, spiritually and physically, or total fitness.

When a person comes to my gym or my gym equipment center, they can experience three things: big, fun attractions, a serious program of physical development and the availability of spiritual counseling.

In keeping with my belief that total fitness is for everyone, Zuver's Fitness Center is in the business of offering the finest and most durable gym and exercise equipment available…to churches, recreation centers, schools, institutions, homes and businesses. The line ranges from the original heavy duty Circle Gym weight training equipment to the lighter exercise equipment to meet the needs of anyone and everyone.

Zuver's Fitness Center also offers complete training for anyone interested in owning and operating his own fitness and health center. We have a complete service to fully equip a gym, teach weight training, exercise and nutrition tot eh gym owner, as well as train him in the management of the new business.

It is a rewarding pursuit for me to offer this opportunity so that with a minimal investment, an individual can not only own his own business, but also be in the business of making total fitness—health and happiness—available to others.

Bob Zuver was clearly a man before his time—this was written in 1977!

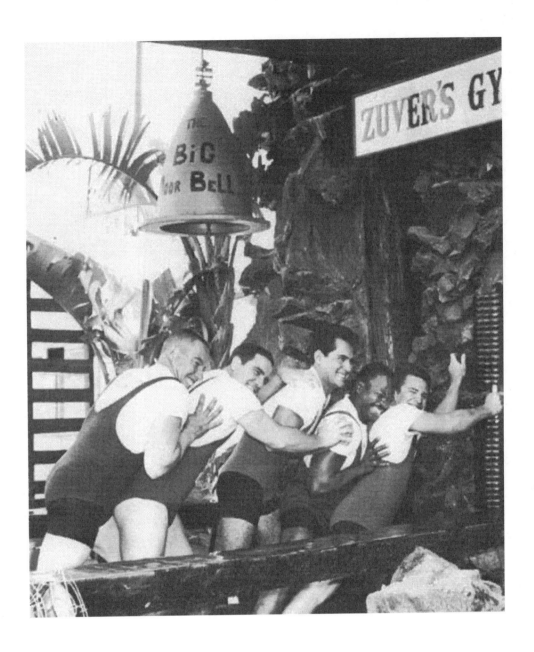

It should certainly be obvious that though Bob had a serious side, he had to have one heck of a sense of humor, and must have been a blast to hang out or train with.

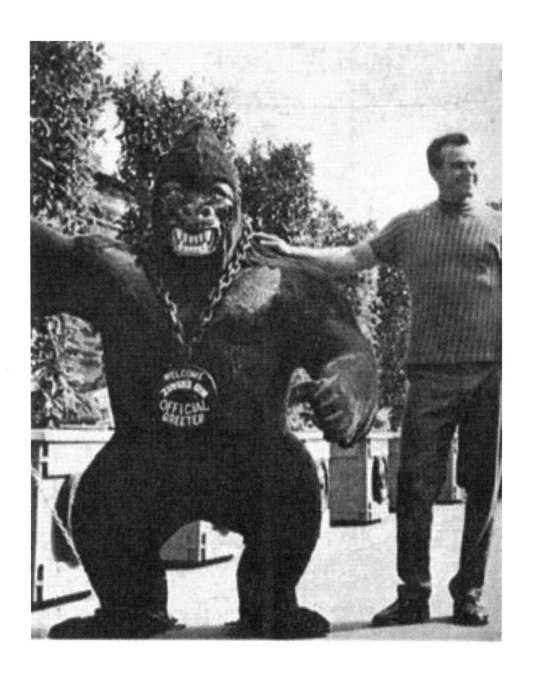

What an imagination!

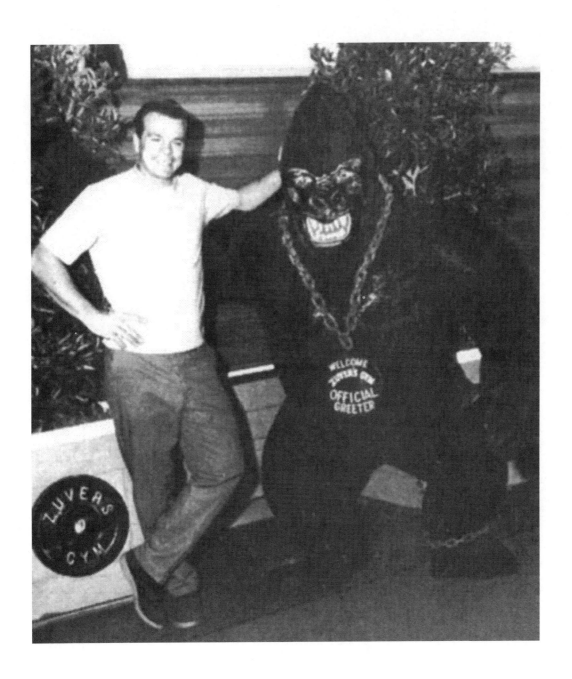

Bob was not alone in his efforts

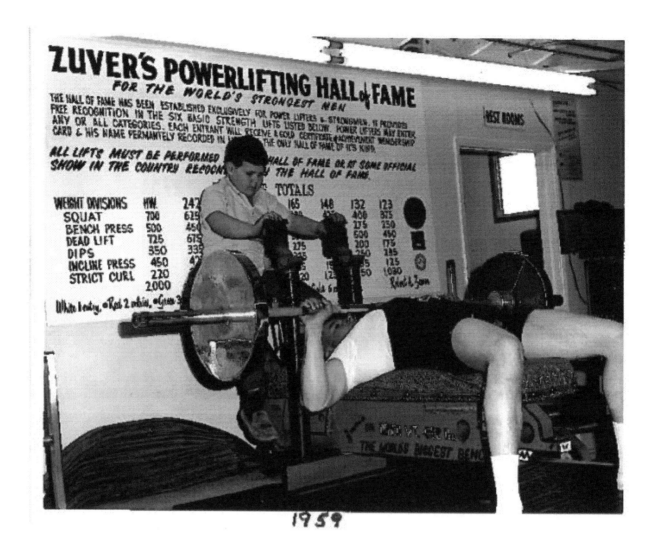

Bob's son Ricky spotting Jim Waters

The picture like this that has been circulated on the web was cutoff in the middle... this one shows almost the whole body of the lifter & a much better shot of the bench itself

A search for "Rickey the Rhino Zuver" turned this up at Draper forum

BuffBarrera
Starting to like posting

Registration Date: 01-26-08
Total Posts: 165

OFFLINE

User Options

06-29-11 08:37 PM - Post#696320

- Laree Said:

- ccrow Said:

I used the powder years ago, I don't think there is anything decent on the market now.

Worse than dirt!

So true. I used to drink liver powder I bought from Ricky the Rhino (RIP) at Zuver's Gym. Mixed it w cold water and held my nose. Drank it exclusively in our backyard, no matter the hour, in case I couldn't keep it down. Those were the days (not).

Here we see the proud papa with son hitting a big lift;

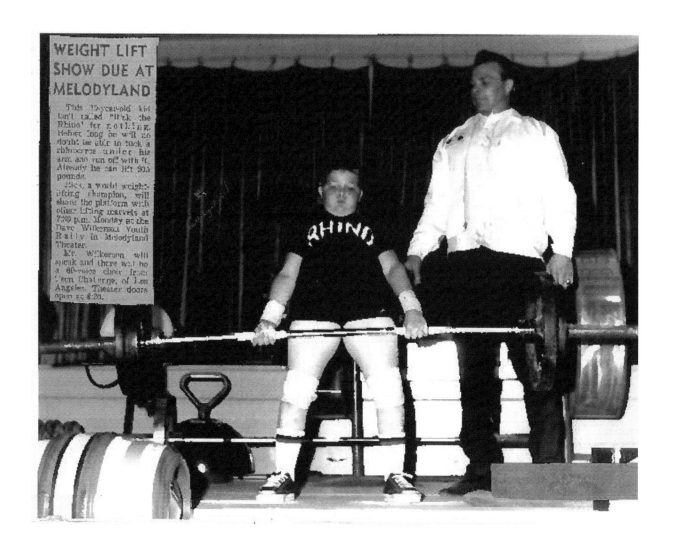

Bob Junior also was a regular at the gym

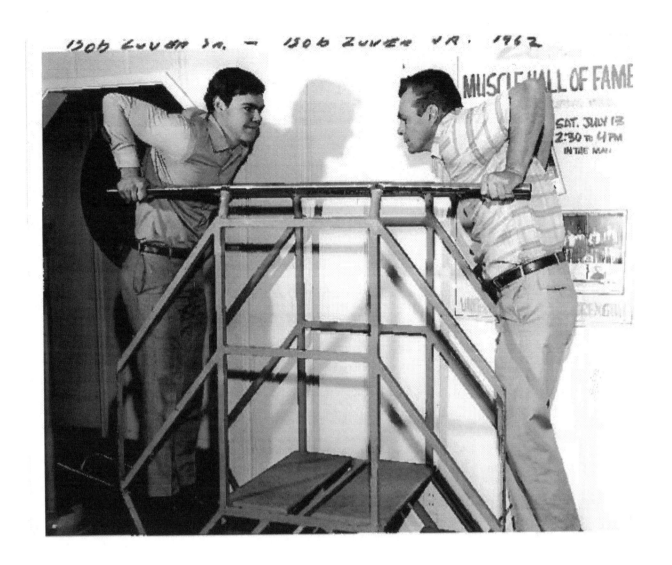

So what drove Bob & his family to create this awesome place?

The following piece will explain that;

The first page shows the publication where this article was published;

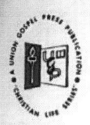

The Sunday School Times AND Gospel Herald

© Union Gospel Press, 1972

July 1, 1972
Volume LXX
Number 13

NONDENOMINATIONAL RELIGIOUS SEMIMONTHLY

STATEMENT OF FAITH

1. We believe in the Scriptures of the Old and New Testaments as verbally inspired of God and inerrant in the original writings, and that they are the Word of God and the final authority in faith and conduct.

2. We believe in one God, the Creator of all things and man; eternally existing in three Persons, in a threefold relationship, that of Father, Son, and Holy Spirit.

3. We believe that Jesus Christ was begotten by the Holy Spirit, born of the Virgin Mary, and is God incarnate, the God-Man.

4. We believe that man was created in the image of God, that he sinned, and thereby incurred not only physical death, but also the spiritual death which is separation from God, that Adam's sin is imputed to the whole race of mankind, and that all human beings are born with a sinful nature and in case of those who reach the state of moral responsibility, become sinners before God in thought, word, and deed.

5. We believe that the Lord Jesus Christ died for our sins (the sins of all men) according to the Scriptures as a substitutionary sacrifice, and that all who believe in Him are freely justified and stand before God accepted in the character and merit of Jesus Christ.

6. We believe in the bodily resurrection of Jesus Christ, in His ascension into heaven, and that in His present life He is the Head of the church, the Lord of the individual believer, the High Priest over the house of God, and the Advocate in the family of God.

7. We believe in the personal, imminent, and premillennial second coming of Christ, first to receive His own to Himself, and later, to set up His earthly kingdom and to reign over redeemed Israel and all nations of the world; that is, to bring peace and blessing to the whole world.

8. We believe that all who by faith receive the Lord Jesus Christ as Saviour are born again of the Holy Spirit, receive the Holy Spirit and a new nature, and that they also are anointed with the Spirit and by the Holy Spirit baptized into the body of Christ.

9. We believe that God is the spiritual Father only of those who trust His Son, Jesus Christ, as Saviour; that only those saved through faith in Christ are spiritual brothers.

10. We believe in the bodily resurrection of the just and the unjust, everlasting blessedness of the saved, and the everlasting punishment of the unsaved.

—Union Gospel Press

CONTENTS

GENERAL
- 4 Muscleland Ministry
- 7 One Nation, Under God
- 8 Better Leyte Than Never!
- 10 Reach Out with God's Word!

WORD OF LIFE
- 12 Sermon: Holy Spirit Conviction
- 14 Exposition: Ninth Commandment: Let's Be Honest About It!
- 15 Studies in Exodus: Ten Words for the Space Age
- 16 Bible Backgrounds: For the Survival of Galilee
- 31 Explanation: Illustration Barrel

CHRISTIANITY IN STORY FORM
- 18 Boys and Girls: There Is a Time
- 20 Youth: Play Ball!
- 24 Adults: See You in the Morning

DEPARTMENTAL
- 2 National Weakness: The Price of Unbelief
- 19 Quick Quips
- 21 What Is Worldliness?
- 22 Broken Homes Cause Broken Children
- 22 Welcome Children's Questions
- 23 Everyone Likes to Feel Special
- 27 Symbols of the New Awakening
- 28 Field Trips in Church Education
- 30 The Dawn of a New Age

FRONT COVER: Entrance to Zuver's Gym, Costa Mesa, California. This unique approach to religion is featured in "Muscleland Ministry" in this issue.

The SUNDAY SCHOOL TIMES and GOSPEL HERALD is edited and published semimonthly by UNION GOSPEL PRESS, 2000 Brookpark Rd., Cleveland, Ohio 44109. Mailing address: Box 6059, Cleveland, Ohio 44101. (Second-class postage paid at Cleveland, Ohio.) SUBSCRIPTIONS payable in advance. United States: $3.75 for one year, $6.50 for two years, $11.00 for four years. FOR POSTAGE AND HANDLING, each year add 75 cents for subscriptions to Canada. Add $1.00 each year for subscriptions to other foreign countries. PLEASE SEND CHANGE OF ADDRESS four weeks in advance for uninterrupted service. Include old address label with your new address.

Muscleland Ministry

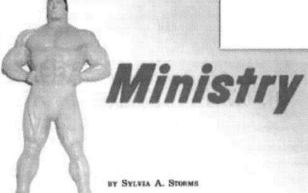

BY SYLVIA A. STORMS

THE sandy-haired youth in the jeans frowned slightly and jammed his hands into his pockets. Then with a shrug he reluctantly followed the probation officer through the black iron gate. Just inside, the young man stopped dead in his tracks and stared.

"This is a gym?" he exclaimed. "You've got to be kidding."

The officer smiled. "This is the place I've been telling you about!"

The sight before the boy was hardly that of an ordinary gym. Zuver's Gym and Muscle Hall of Fame in Costa Mesa, California, has to be one of a kind. And the same goes for

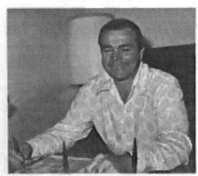

Bob Zuver in his office

its owner, Bob Zuver, an ordained minister and former weight lifter, who originated and built the gym and its equipment. He says that it's a "fun place to work out."

Inside the heavy iron gate stands a fearsome-looking fiberglass gorilla. Not far away are a ten-foot superman and a fiberglass elephant lifting a barbell with its trunk. The door leading into the main gym weighs two tons!

Everything inside is big. There are a one thousand-pound lift, a five hundred-pound "blob," and several unique racks. Bells ring and lights flash when they're lifted. There is also the world's biggest drinking fountain, made from a fire hydrant!

How has God chosen to use the gym and its fantastic equipment to win souls to Christ? Let the Zuvers tell it.

"You need something unusual to interest the kids and the others who come in regularly to keep in shape," said Bob.

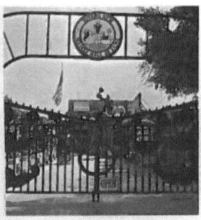

Iron gate entrance to grounds

"The main purpose of the gym," added Jean, his dark-haired wife, "is to build fitness and strength, not only in the physical realm, but also in the mental and the spiritual realms."

Zuver's Gym has an amazing outreach. Six hundred members work out regularly and thousands of others—men, women, and children—have visited the gym on tours and have heard of Jesus Christ. Housewives, former drug addicts, ex-convicts, and, yes, even musclemen belong to the club. And the ministry doesn't stop there. Bob is available for counseling, and he works closely with police and probation authorities. Additional gyms have been set up at the juvenile hall, at Joplin Ranch, and at other youth and prison farms.

Zuver's name is a household word to "muscleheads" and weight lifters throughout the world. Not only is the name synonymous with the zany gym, but it also stands for equipment made by the Zuvers in their own factory and sold to gyms throughout the country.

Some of the world's biggest names in weight lifting have visited Zuver's Gym to set records. An all-Orange County lineup of lifters Bob coached won the 1968 United States Senior National Powerlifting Championship team award. The gym has more unusual heavy-duty equipment than any other training facility in the world. Because of this, many of the country's strong men have heard of Christ.

"Weight lifters need Christ, too!" declared Bob. "That's why God literally built this gym!"

It all began in a small garage in 1960. After a whirlwind conversion at the age of thirty, Bob Zuver attended a Bible college and became a nondenominational minister. During this preparation, he taught Sunday school. One Lord's Day after class, two boys came to him and asked whether he would teach them a few things about weight lifting. Bob agreed to help out with a few pieces of equipment he had in his garage.

The word spread. Within a month one hundred boys were meeting there. Within three months the garage was bursting at the seams with boys, and Bob realized that he'd need to find a bigger place quickly.

"We started out with a makeshift bench and one set of weights," he explained. "Gradually we added to it and expanded. Every time we reached a point where we needed money, the Lord provided. When we were ready to pour the foundation for the new place, the Lord sent a Christian, who owned a cement company and who *happened* to hear of our need, with several thousand dollars' worth of cement. We stepped out in faith, and the Lord met each step."

Asked for past history, Bob and Jean emphasized, "We're interested in what God is doing now and is going to do in the future. This is His ministry, and we're just working for Him."

Bob had been a contractor and a Navy frogman before his conversion, and Jean had been a professional dancer. Both were interested in drama, and they met in an acting class. They were married later, while Bob was stationed in Virginia with the Navy. After his discharge they came to California.

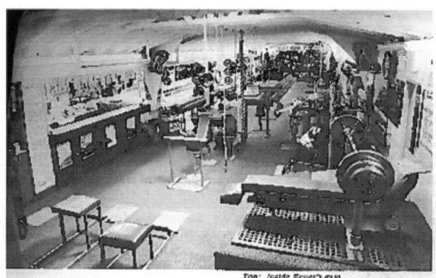
Top: Inside Bower's gym

Bob was at loose ends, and his nerves were very bad. He was searching for peace of mind.

"For some reason I was on my way to China to find it. I thought, How many problems can you have just walking around in a bunch of rice paddies?" he said seriously.

But the Zuvers never got to China. One evening not long before they were to sail from California, Bob was on his way to a gym. He passed a little Assembly of God church and decided to go in. The Lord saved him that night. Within a short time, his entire family of fifteen (two brothers, their wives, and their children) were brought to Christ through his witness. One brother became a minister and a missionary to Mexico. The other is a Christian businessman. In each case, God has used the background of the individual to fulfill His purpose.

Bob and Jean both had been trained for the physical fitness and beauty contest business. God was to use them in this special field.

"We have prayed over every piece of equipment in the gym and for every person who walks through the door," Jean said. "The Lord has shown us that if you claim big things for Him, you'll get them. That's the reason for the 'God Is Big' sign on the wall. God isn't limited in His thinking. We shouldn't be either. Everything we have in the gym is

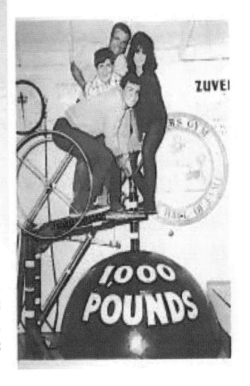

big. It's a means of bringing people in to hear the gospel—a conversation piece and a fun place, as well."

The Zuvers don't push religion down the throats of their members. If the Lord leads, He'll open the way to speak His Word, they believe. Many people come into the gym out of curiosity.

One curious man saw the "Christ Is the Answer" sign, which is located at the end of the room. (It is twelve feet long!) He saw the "Gospel Barrel" which holds tracts and devotional material. Bob spoke to him briefly about the Lord. But it was a year and a half later when that man came knocking on the Zuvers' door at home.

"I remember the things you told me," he said to Bob, "and I'm ready now to accept the Lord."

The same sign has been instrumental in other decisions for Christ. One man who came to the Zuvers' door early on Sunday evening asked to see the gym. He didn't see much more of the gym than the sign, though.

"I've been running from God," he told Bob, "and I believe that He sent me here to talk to you."

The Zuvers work most frequently with youngsters. The police and probation officers send many kids to the gym. As a result, many of these have found Jesus Christ, including several gang members in Costa Mesa. Others come from Calvary Chapel, Melody Christian Center, and other churches located throughout the county that work with young people for physical rehabilitation. Bob helps rebuild their bodies, which many times have been wasted from drug addiction. And he encourages young converts to grow in grace at the same time.

Jean works with the ladies on Tuesdays and Thursdays in weight reduction and fitness programs. Many have confided in her their special problems, and she has often been able to point them to the one answer, God's Son.

"A lady came in one day with a load of troubles," she recalled. "She'd been coming in quite regularly, but I was waiting on the Lord before I approached her. When everyone else left, I was able to lead her to Christ. Now He is carrying her burdens."

Zuver's Gym has a young man named Mike who works out with the men on Monday, Wednesday, Friday, and a half-day on Saturday. He told me that he had barely made it through high school. He had done time in jail for three counts of burglary, and he had taken drugs. God dealt with him through Campus Crusade, and at the age of twenty-one, he accepted the Saviour at a Billy Graham crusade in Anaheim. When he first visited the gym, he was a longhaired new Christian.

"I was probably the first longhair Bob ever allowed in the gym," he said with a smile, as he pointed to a posted list of gym rules. "He's pretty strict with the rules, but he bent them a bit that day! Finally I learned to cut my hair and clean up!"

Mike felt the Lord leading him into the gym business, but he had his doubts. "How can you have a ministry in a gym, I thought, with all those 'muscleheads' running around?"

But he went to Bible college in preparation, and Bob gave him a job.

"I had a lot to learn about God's ways," Mike declared. "He's so big and powerful that we can't box Him in. The gym is not just a physical thing. We're here to win souls. Nobody in the gym business has ever sprung forth in this way for God, to my knowledge."

It's the prayer of the Zuvers that other Christians interested in the business will catch the spirit and open Christ-oriented gyms throughout the country.

"We'd like to see a Christian gym in every major city," they said fervently. "We believe that Christ is the answer for everyone, and we're willing to help any church or Christian couple by teaching them how to run a gym and by setting up the gym at near cost. Something is needed to replace the non-Christian health clubs, and this is a fantastic means of winning people to the Lord!"

And this brings us right back to Bob's statement earlier that "weight lifters need Christ, too!" And it's a wide-open ministry! ★

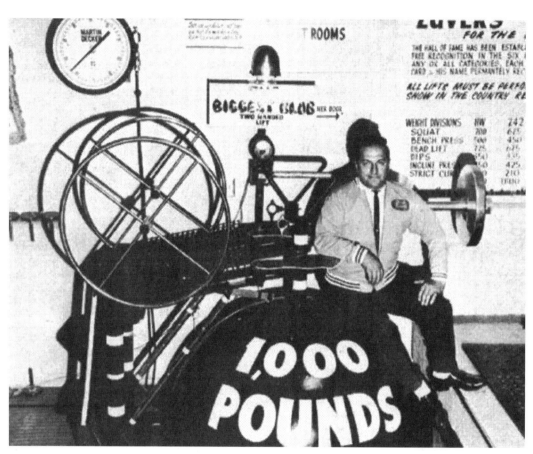

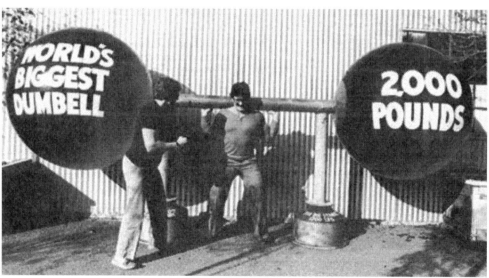

http://www.davedraper.com/fusionbb/showtopic.php?tid/204/post/1666/hl/

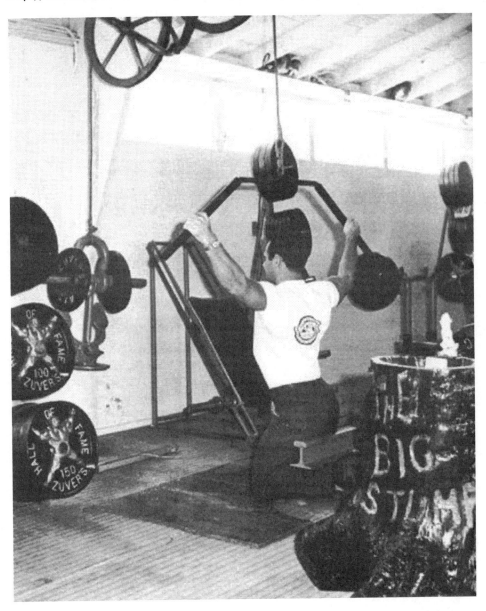

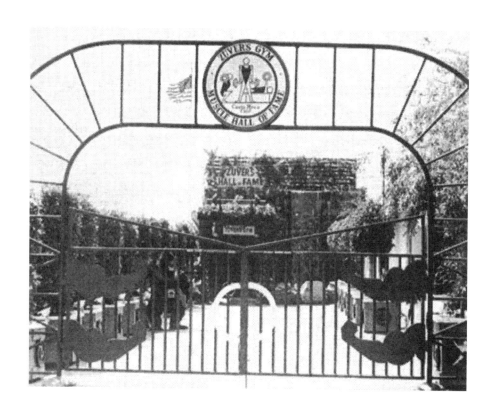

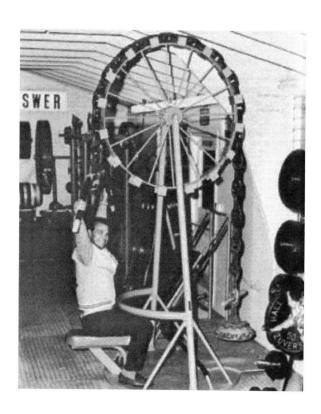

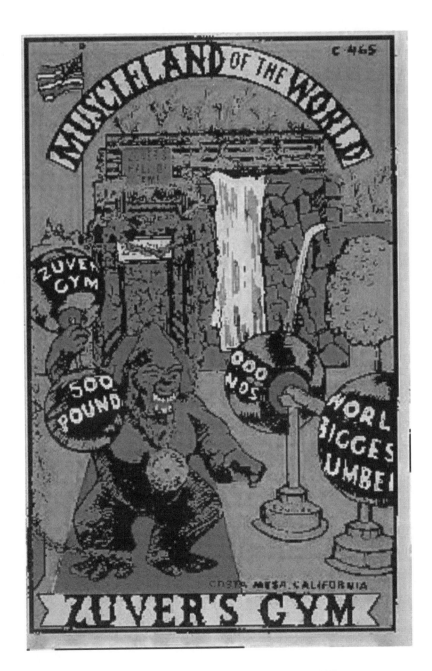

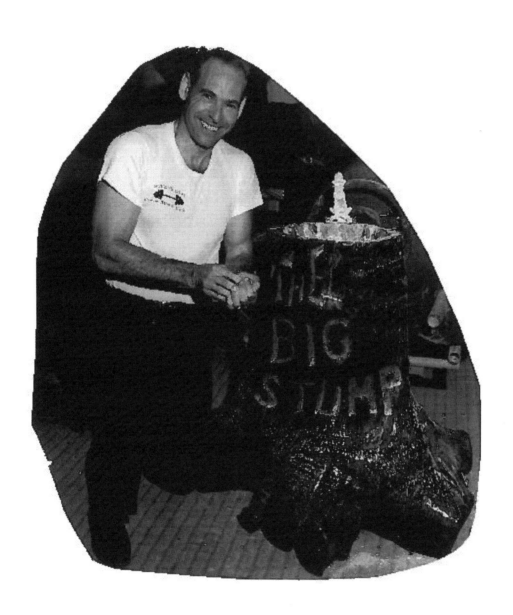

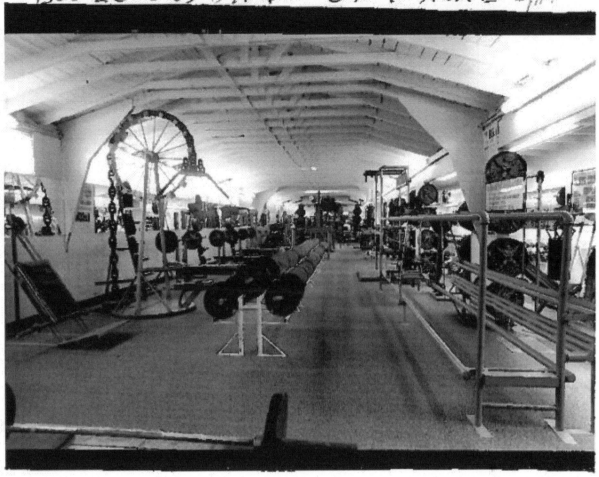
Bob Zuvers Hall of Fame Gym.

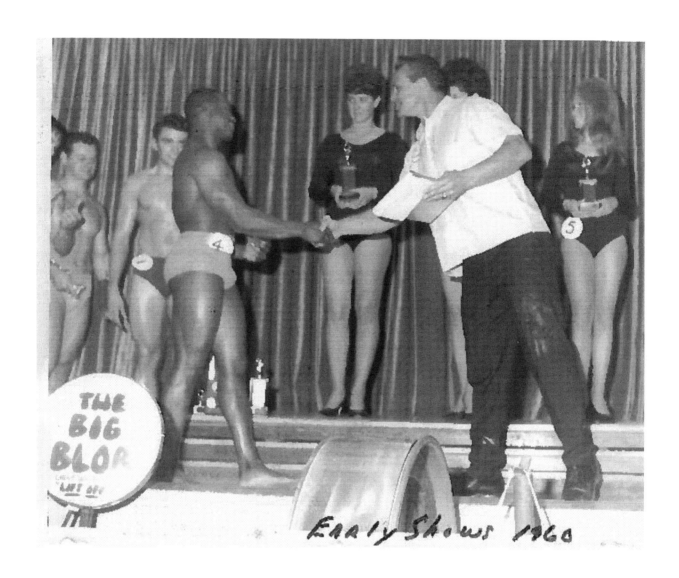
Early Shows 1960

Mecca of Power

By John | Published: October 11, 2010

I was in Fairfield, CT last month for a certification and Zach Even-Esh took a drive up from New Jersey to say hello. Zach and I have been emailing for over a year and finally got the chance to meet up. He loaned me a collection of old PL'ing articles for light reading on the plane ride home. I was reading an old article from Joe Weider in 1969 by Dick Tyler entitled "Weighty Happenings in the West". The article talked about the powerlifting scene on the West Coast. In the article he talks in great length about a Mecca for powerlifting in Costa Mesa called Zuver's Hall of Fame Gym. The gym reportedly had some of the biggest most exotic equipment in the land. A 300 lbs door handle and a collection of "unliftables". I did some research and found the gym was located on Hamilton Street a few miles from my gym. On my way to work the next day, I decided to get a coffee and explore Hamilton Street in Costa Mesa. The street is only 5 blocks long and straddles Harbor Blvd, a main artery in the OC. I drove up and down the street hoping to catch a glimpse of the 60-ton back wall of the gym that was hand built with boulders harvested from Big Bear. I got out of the car and invested the WWII era homes and to my disappointment nothing remains of Zuver's spot. I had hoped my impromptu treasure hunt would bring back some cool relic but I came up empty handed. It did however get me thinking about what makes a "temple of power".

It just so happened I had a question sitting in my inbox when i got back to the office asking, "what should I look for in a gym?"

Seems ironic since I just been on a hunt of an old strength, I own and operate a gym, travel the world teach people how to lift weights and training as a pro athlete for a decade. My perspective of what makes a good gym goes far beyond the palaces I have trained in recent years. Check out the pictures of the NovaCare Center in Philadelphia for reference. It goes back to my beginnings…a garage packed with weights, a high school weight room or some local place like Zuver's Hall of Fame. Places where you keep your rep count in the chalk dust on the floor.

What makes a good gym goes deeper then than just the superficial stuff like good equipment, good scenery and amenities. But since this is a major component let's start there. I know walking into a gym there are a few things that instantly make me feel at home or want to turn and run. A strong man once said, "I have never seen a bad gym with a platform". Just for clarification, a platform is raised wooden structure where Olympic weightlifting, deadlifting and squatting take place. One sheet of plywood lying on concrete does not constitute a platform, regardless of what someone might tell you. Heavy dumbbells are a dead give away. If you see dumbbells ranging up to a 100 lbs you know are safe, if those dumbbells are in the 150+ range you know strong people are lurking. Chains, bands and chalk are another indicator this could be a safe haven. But in today's world of gimmicks and bullshit those could be smoke screens used as accessories to confuse you…so proceed with caution. The final two beacons of hope are a squat rack and iron plates. If you walk into a gym and they have more leg extension machines than squat racks, run.

This too can be deceiving, as many gyms that work with Olympic lifters use squat pillars or Vulcan racks, so I would tell you to refer back to the first part of this paragraph. And finally…iron plates. I am not talking about metal plates coated in plastic or rubber, but old iron plates that are heavy, dense and full of inertia. The kind of iron that get sweaty with the slightest humidity and has a thin coat of dirt, rust and dust. The kind of plates that make a comforting jingle on rep 10…11…12…and so on.

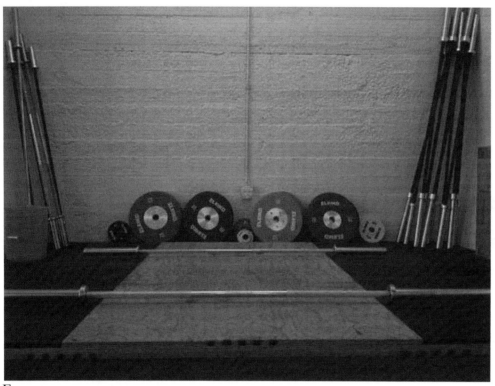

Energy.

Energy is the single most important factor in making or breaking a gym. If you are not a little nervous pulling up in the parking lot then you might as well keep driving and find a better place. I remember the first time I was invited to Zangas' garage to lift weights and walking in to see 585 lbs on the squat bar. I thought strange place to store the weights. Then I saw a massive dude with a knee wraps, a thick belt and thicker neck step underneath and pull it off the rack like it was nothing. I got flooded with a feeling of nausea and curiosity at the same time. I got the same nervous feeling walking into the Cal weight room in 1993.

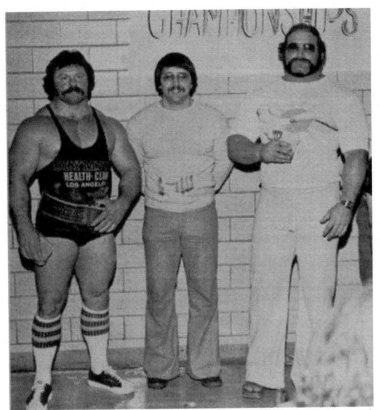

Earlier this year I headed to Columbus, Ohio for a CrossFit Football certification at Rogue Fitness. I had grown up hearing the legends of the original Westside Barbell Club in Culver City and had followed many of the WSB protocols in recent years. I decided I would stop by and meet Louie Simmons and visit his gym, Westside Barbell. For more than a few decades WSB has housed some of the strongest men on the planet and Louie has been an innovator in anything strong. His gym did not disappoint. Pulling up I could hear the blaring sounds of gangster rap from the car. The gym was packed with everything from mono lifts to reverse hypers and a bunch of shit I couldn't describe. The place had an energy that was unmistakable and a feeling like some crazy shit goes down on a regular basis. Sign me up.

At the end of 09, I took a trip to visit Mark Rippetoe in Wichita Falls, Texas. Rip's gym, Wichita Falls Barbell Club was another one of these locations. Filled with iron plates, home-made squat racks, platforms and dust it would make anyone worth their salt smile. I have never visited or trained there but Dave Tate's place in Ohio at Elite FTS and Metroflex in Arlington, TX are a few more.

Between the ages of 24-28, I had some of my best training days. I was the strongest in that window of my football career. During the season I trained with Mike Wolf and Tom Kanavy in a converted storage room the Philadelphia Eagles called their weight room. It had no windows, no ventilation and no mirrors. Just weights, loud music and anger. Some of my best workouts came on Friday afternoons in that shit hole we called a weight room. In the off-season, I trained with a group of NFL players in Tampa with Raphael Ruiz of 1441 S&C. We trained in a warehouse with no A/C and big skylights in the middle of summer in Tampa. The place was packed with free weights, a few huge gymnastics tumbling mats and pissed off competitive individuals.

Attitude.

I have always felt if the gym was too nice, too shiny and packed with too many smiles the result were less than optimal. I always looked to the Rocky movies for direction. In Rocky III, Rocky got his ass beat by Clubber Lange in the first fight. Rocky was training in a hotel ballroom…Clubber a basement. After he lost he moved to South Central to train "hard", he came back and crushed Clubber. In Rocky IV, Rocky skipped the glamor and heads straight to Siberia to train in a barn in the cold and snow. Drago trains in a modern facility but his training montage is pretty inspiring as well. The result is a great fight sequence.

The gym becomes an extension of the attitude and mindset of the people that train there, regardless of the equipment or location. If you walk into a Curves Gym do not expect to find dumbbells up to 100 lbs or chalk. If you show up at WSB and the first thing out of your mouth is "Squats?! Those will destroy my knees" you might need to run. If you walk into Metroflex and see Ronnie Coleman with 800 lbs on the bar don't ask him when the spin class starts.

In the end, what makes a mecca of power? Energy and attitude.

If you have energy and attitude in your training the volume gets turned down on all rest of the bullshit.

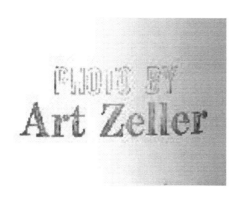

ZUVER'S HALL OF FAME
POWERLIFTERS

443 Hamilton Street
Costa Mesa, California
646-5184

The Hall of Fame has been established exclusively for power-lifters and strong men. It provides free recognition in the six basic strength lifts listed below. Power-lifters may enter any, or all of the categories. Each entrant will receive a gold certificate of achievement, membership card and his name permanently recorded in lights in the only Hall of Fame of its kind. Please be sure to notify the Hall of Fame before your planned visit.

Rev. Robert A. Zuver

All lifts must be performed at the Hall of Fame, or at some official show in the country recognized by the Hall of Fame.

ENTRANCE TOTALS

Weight Divisions - Hvy.	242	198	181	165	148	132	123
SQUAT............700	625	550	520	500	425	400	375
BENCH PRESS........500	450	435	400	350	325	275	250
DEAD LIFT..........725	675	625	610	590	535	500	450
DIPS..............350	335	325	300	275	250	200	175
INCLINE PRESS......450	425	400	375	325	275	250	235
STRICT CURLS.......220	210	200	180	165	150	135	125

White - 1 Entry; Red - 2 Entries; Green - 3 Entries; Blue - 4 Entries; Silver 5 Entries; Gold - 6 Entries

For information concerning power-lifting, contact Jim Waters, Records Chairman c/o The Hall of Fame.

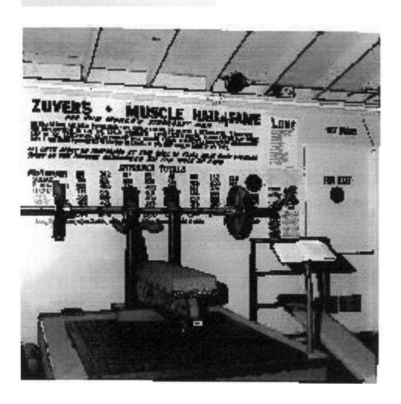

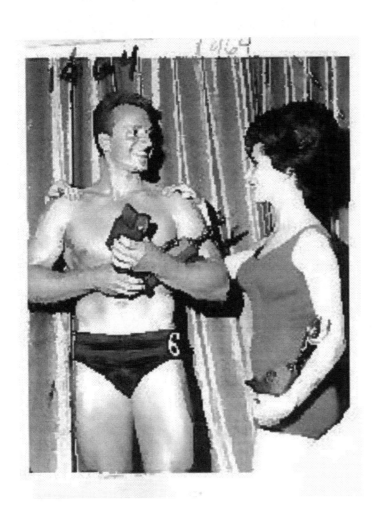

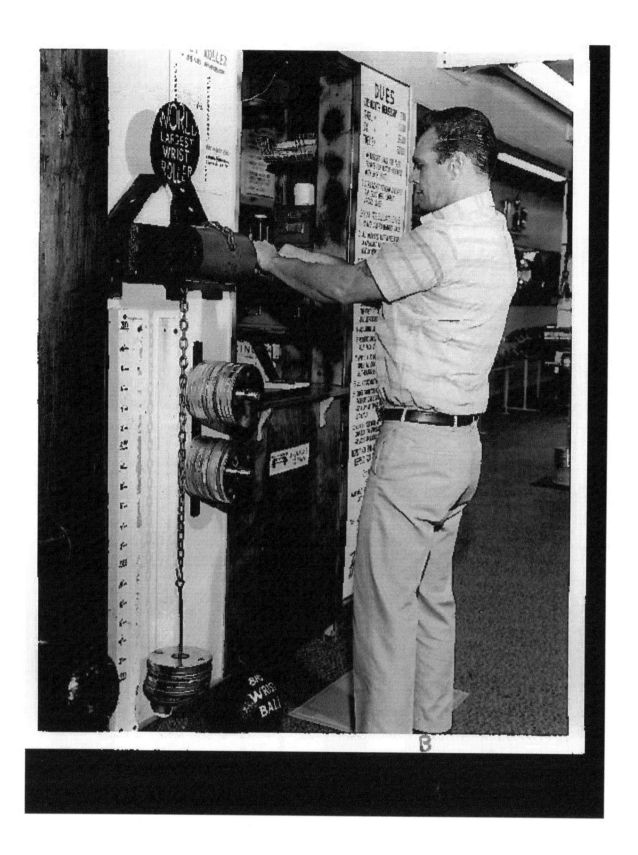

The Big Meara Bench

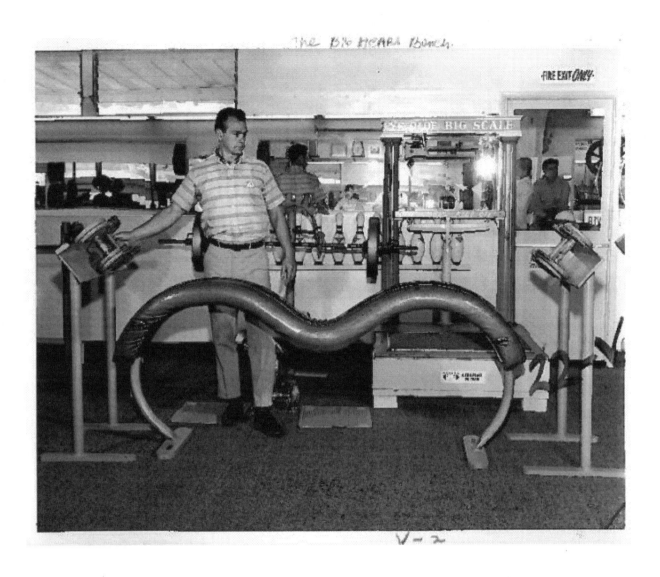

V-2

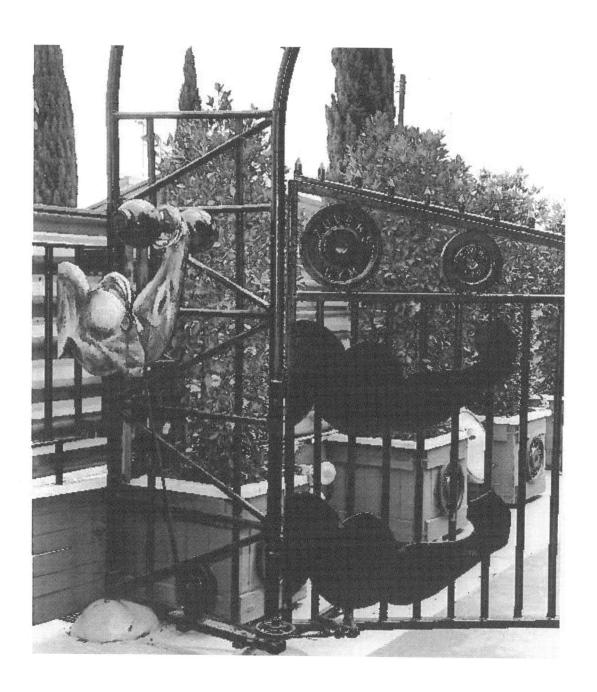

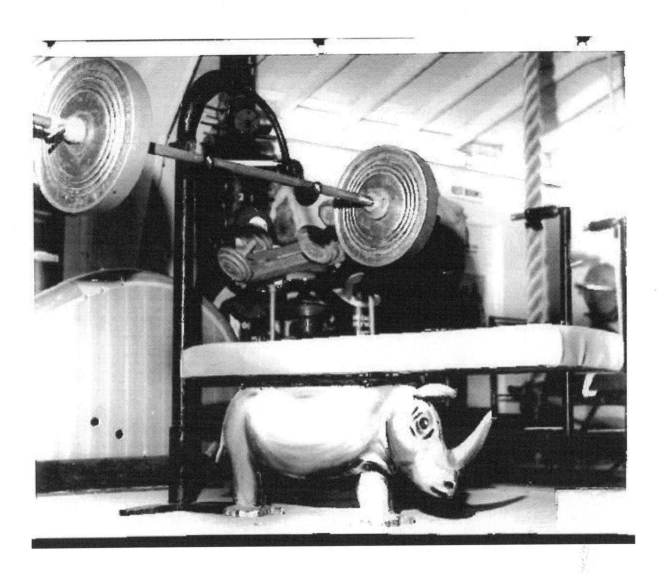

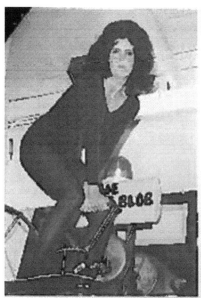

Joan tries to ride the "big bike."

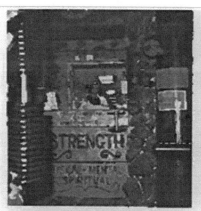

Ron talking on the big phone in doorway to gym. The gym features physical, mental and spiritual strength.

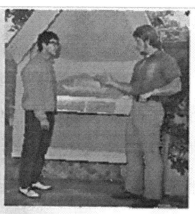

Mike counsels a youth at the little chapel on the patio. Note the open Bible. Tract literature is inside the two drawers.

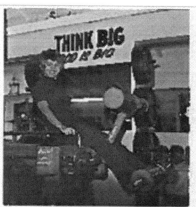

Girls also work out at Zony's.

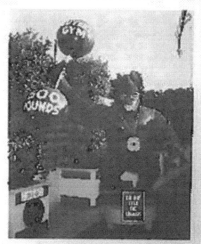

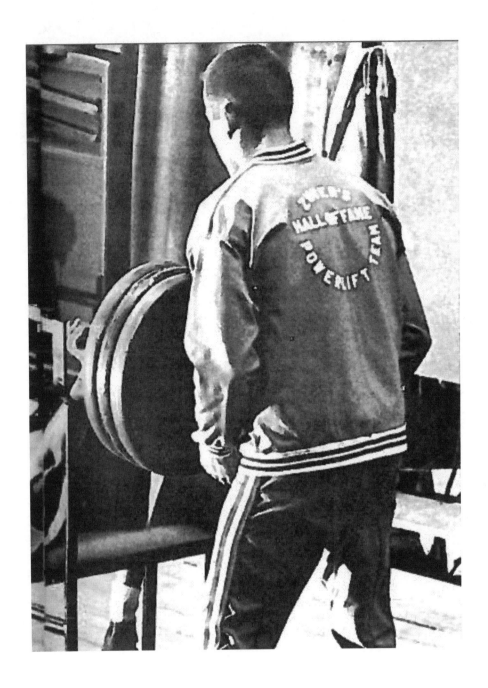

The Muscle Builder & Power issue from May of '69, with the great cover shot of Arny that was posted back in the Culver City section, contained this powerlifting report in which the Zuver's team is featured;

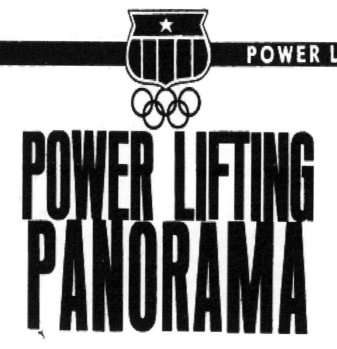

POWER LIFTING PANORAMA

AT the time of this writing, only two contests have been held and they were at opposite ends of the country. The New England AAU Open Power Lift was held at the Boston YMCA November 16, 1968 and some impressive lifts were made. Robert Garrow, 132-pounder, recorded a 290-pound Bench Press in good style. The lift was a New England record but was 29½ pounds shy of the American record held by Rudy Hernandez. Bill Loiacano, 148-pounder, made a 510-pound Deadlift which turned out to be the only lift which was close to any American record in this class. In the 165-pound class, Steve Crandall of Arizona Bench Pressed 370 pounds only 6 pounds short of the 376-pound American record held by Robert Burnett. On a fourth attempt, Steve made 380 pounds, which is fantastic but it will not count for a record. In the same class, Robert Crampton proved that he was no slouch by making a 360-pound Bench Press. The other two lifts in this class were under par. The Bench Press stole the show again in the 181-pound class as 2 men exceeded the 400-pound mark. Tom Familiari made 430 pounds and Jim Leland Proned 400 pounds. Both are excellent lifts.

On the other side of the country, in San Diego, on December 8, 1968 the San Diego Open and Novice were held. Most of the lifting was of inferior quality with the top lift of the meet being a 605 deadlift by Harold Love who won the 198-pound class and the Outstanding Lifter Award. Zuver's Hall of Fame won the team trophy. Tom Overholtzer, who recently moved up in class to the 198's took a sur- *(Continued on page 69)*

POWER LIFTER OF THE MONTH

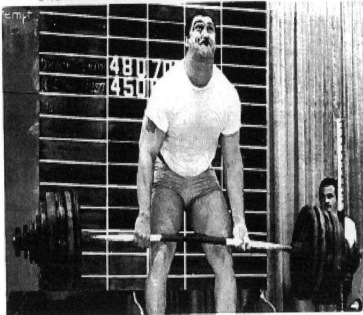

WE CONGRATULATE George 'Ernie' Pickett on his selection as the Power Lifter of the Month. Ernie is the only man that we know of who has demonstrated his ability as an Olympic lifter, having represented the U.S.A. at Mexico City in the heavyweight class, and as a power lifter of note having placed 2nd twice in 1967 and 1968 behind Don Cundy. Ernie was also one time World Record holder for the Military Press. Ernie is shown here making an easy 750-pound Deadlift. He also has Squatted with over 600 pounds and has Bench Pressed 450 pounds. With little doubt, we feel that if Ernie could devote a bit more time to his Power Lifting he would erase the heavyweight Deadlift record and the Total record. Best of luck Ernie. We wish you the very best in both forms of lifting.

AMERICAN POWERLIFT RECORDS
(some pending)

123-LB. CLASS
- Bench Press.......... 272 — E. Hernandez
- Squat.......... 456½ — D. Meyer
- Deadlift.......... 480 — N. Cross
- Total.......... 1160 — D. Meyer

132-LB. CLASS
- Bench Press.......... 319½ — E. Hernandez
- Squat.......... 476 — D. Meyer
- Deadlift.......... 543 — A. Lord
- Total.......... 1215 — A. Lord

148-LB. CLASS
- Bench Press.......... 355½ — B. Thurber
- Squat.......... 457 — B. Thurber
- Deadlift.......... 563 — D. Blue
- Total.......... 1300 — B. Thurber

165-LB. CLASS
- Bench Press.......... 376 — R. Burnett
- Squat.......... 535½ — L. Ingro
- Deadlift.......... 663 — R. Burnett
- Total.......... 1550 — R. Burnett

181-LB. CLASS
- Bench Press.......... 450½ — R. Ray
- Squat.......... 676½ — J. Barnes
- Deadlift.......... 650½ — P. O'Brien
- Total.......... 1605 — J. Barnes

198-LB. CLASS
- Bench Press.......... 468½ — R. Ray
- Squat.......... 628 — B. Wirling
- Deadlift.......... 688½ — J. Ozurenko
- Total.......... 1670 — R. Ray

242-LB. CLASS
- Bench Press.......... 527½ — R. Myers
- Squat.......... 750 — J. Cole
- Deadlift.......... 770½ — B. Young
- Total.......... 1975 — J. Cole

HEAVYWEIGHT CLASS
- Bench Press.......... 617½ — P. Casey
- Squat.......... 800 — P. Casey
- Deadlift.......... 784 — D. Cundy
- Total.......... 2040 — R. Weaver

POWERLIFTING

INTERNATIONAL POWER LIFTING SCENE

By OSCAR STATE, Secretary International Weightlifting Federation

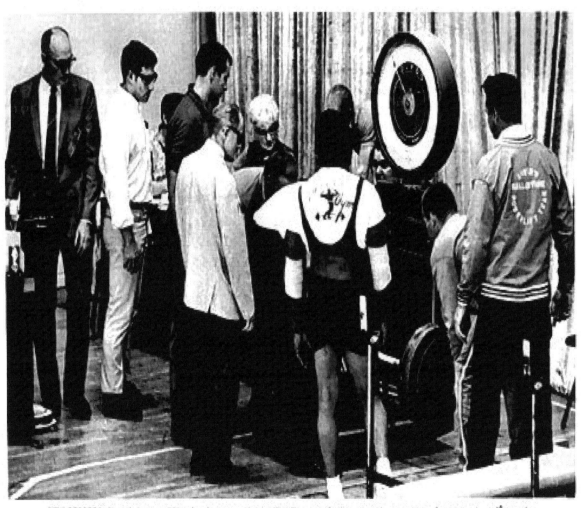

NEW RECORDS: Now that power lifting has become an internationally recognized sport, and news will be developing fast all over the world, we have commissioned our International Editor, Oscar State, Secretary-Treasurer of the F.I.H.C., to handle this new department. Here you will find the latest records, new developments, and news items as they develop in different parts of the world—outside, and, at times, inside the U.S.A.

Here is another Muscle Builder piece featuring Zuver's guys;

POWER SCENE

By GEORGE FRENN

ONCE again, the records for the 198-pound class in powerlifting have been rewritten. This time by Tom Overholtzer, who represented Zuver's Hall of Fame. The competition was held in Bakersfield on March 29, 1969. Tom started with a 435 Bench Press on his third attempt, enroute to a new Squat record of 674 pounds and a mediocre Deadlift of 560 pounds. These lifts totaled a remarkable 1675 pounds which wipes out the record set by Ronnie Ray, the 198-pound champion. The Squat record was formerly held by Bill Witting at 630 pounds. The face value of the Squat was 680 pounds. The plates weighed light. Rudy Lozano and Willie Kindred, who also represented Zuver's showed that they have been steadily improving since their showing in Los Angeles. At the same Bakersfield competition, Rudy, as a 148-pounder, Benched *(Continued on page 87)*

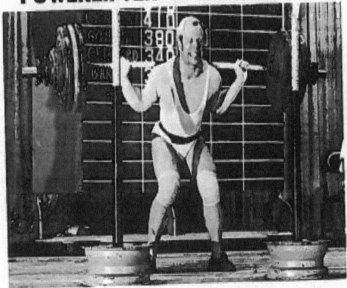

POWERLIFTER OF THE MONTH

JERRY JONES is a powerlifter of exceptional talent. Not heard of until he competed in the National Powerlifting Championships in Los Angeles, he was most impressive there with his powerful squatting—as seen in this photo of Jerry completing a 590-pound full Squat.

Jerry placed third in the Nationals with a 1560-pound Total, behind Jack Barnes, the champion, and Tom Overholtzer, the runner-up. He gave them a run for their money when he Bench Pressed 330 pounds, Squatted 590, and Deadlifted 640 for a new meet record. We wish Jerry every success in his bid to win the 1969 National Championships—and we know he's going to be a tough guy to beat.

NEW AMERICAN POWERLIFTING RECORDS
(some pending)

123-LB. CLASS
- Bench Press ..... 272 ..... E. Hernandez
- Squat ..... 456¼ ..... D. Moyer
- Deadlift ..... 480 ..... M. Cross
- Total ..... 1160 ..... D. Moyer

132-LB. CLASS
- Bench Press ..... 319½ ..... E. Hernandez
- Squat ..... 476 ..... D. Moyer
- Deadlift ..... 543 ..... A. Lord
- Total ..... 1175 ..... A. Lord

148-LB. CLASS
- Bench Press ..... 355½ ..... B. Thurber
- Squat ..... 457 ..... B. Thurber
- Deadlift ..... 563 ..... D. Blau
- Total ..... 1300 ..... B. Thurber

165-LB. CLASS
- Bench Press ..... 376 ..... R. Burnett
- Squat ..... 536½ ..... L. Ingro
- Deadlift ..... 668 ..... R. Burnett
- Total ..... 1550 ..... R. Burnett

181-LB. CLASS
- Bench Press ..... 450¼ ..... R. Ray
- Squat ..... 676½ ..... J. Barnes
- Deadlift ..... 660½ ..... P. O'Brien
- Total ..... 1595 ..... J. Barnes

198-LB. CLASS
- Bench Press ..... 486½ ..... R. Ray
- Squat ..... 674 ..... T. Overholtzer
- Deadlift ..... 688½ ..... J. Dzurenko
- Total ..... 1675 ..... T. Overholtzer

242-LB. CLASS
- Bench Press ..... 527¼ ..... R. Myers
- Squat ..... 751½ ..... J. Cole
- Deadlift ..... 770½ ..... G. Young
- Total ..... 1975 ..... J. Cole

HEAVYWEIGHT CLASS
- Bench Press ..... 617¼ ..... P. Casey
- Squat ..... 800 ..... P. Casey
- Deadlift ..... 784 ..... D. Cundy
- Total ..... 2045 ..... R. Weaver

290 pounds, Squatted 410 pounds, and Deadlifted 510 pounds for a 1210 Total. Willie made a 365-pound Bench Press, Squatted 465 pounds, and almost made 480 pounds, and then he Deadlifted 565 pounds for a 1395 Total.

You will remember that it was our prediction that the 198-pound class Squat would soon be upped to the 700-pound area. However, we thought that it would come much later in the year. We feel that the 198-pound record for squatting should level off at 710 to 715 pounds with the total record somewhere around 1725 pounds.

Jack Barnes, the 181-pound champion, has not competed since he set the 181-pound Squat record at 676½ pounds. Jack recently Squatted 700 pounds in training and he expects to do this poundage in his next competition.

John Kanter has moved out of the 242-pound class up to the heavyweight class. He now weighs 265 pounds enroute to a new high of 275 pounds bodyweight. We don't agree with this move because he has not turned in his best performance at any of the three bodyweight classes that he has lifted in. John has had bad luck in his competitions and has moved up in bodyweight class in order to get a new start. We would like to see him stay at the 242-pound class and perfect his technique at this bodyweight.

Jon Cole, the 242 pound champion and record holder, has not been doing heavy power training since his record breaking competition in November, 1968. Jon has been concentrating on his Olympic lifting, as he hopes to make the Olympic team as an Olympic lifter. He said that he still maintains a 450-pound Bench Press, a 700-pound Squat, and a 700-pound Deadlift.

Bill West, one of the early pioneers of the Powerlifting Game, has gone to Indio, California on location for a new movie in which he will play the part of a cavalry sergeant in a stockade. Bill plans to continue his power training, however, because he took his entire gym and all of his heavy iron with him. He built a lifting platform and had it shipped down to the desert along with 800 pounds of iron, bench press bench and squat racks.

George Frenn, the ex-242 pound champion, has been training hard for the hammer throw, as he plans to beat the Russians when they come to Los Angeles in July, 1969. He has been doing heavy squats and deadlifts and occasionally a bench press or two, some cleaning and snatching. Frenn's squat and deadlift have been going out of sight and this has pushed his Olympic lifts up. In recent training sessions at Gold's Gym in Venice, California, George Squatted 785 pounds and just barely missed 820 pounds. The 785-pound Squat was judged to be very deep. Three weeks before this George Deadlifted 805 pounds in perfect style. He did this with very little assistance from Bill West, his main training partner. At the same workout in which the 785-pound Squat was made, Bill West made 655 pounds. The idea was that George was to remain 100 pounds ahead of West as a bet. Some of Frenn's other lifts include a 285-pound Snatch for 2 reps and 300 for 1 recently, a 285 Military Press, and a 325 Power Clean. The Snatch is particularly good as Frenn weighs 236 pounds and the Snatch record for the 242-pound class is held by Bob Bednarski at 332 pounds. New faces at Gold's Gym include Don Tollefson, a 255 pound discus thrower from Oregon. Don has thrown 193 feet 8 inches. At 6 feet 3 inches tall, he has Benched 350 pounds, Squatted 525 pounds and Deadlifted 655 pounds. He will make a 700-pound Deadlift soon.

Gary Young, from Portland, Oregon lifted 1905 in his last contest. Apparently the 800 pound deadlift, which he was so confident of making, has eluded him like a thief in the night. The most that he has made since his setting the record of 770½ pounds is 755 pounds. Gary has squatted 725 pounds recently in a contest along with bench pressing 435 pound.

Leonard Ingro has announced that he quit powerlifting for good. He feels that he won everything that he could—including the Nationals. Leonard still holds the Nationals Squat record of 541½ pounds for the 165 pound class. Robert Burnett probably had something to do with Ingro's retirement from the game. Burnett holds the total record at 1550 pounds. Ingro's best total was 1420 pounds.

Ronnie Ray jumped bodyweight classes long enough to Bench Press 500 pounds at 219 pounds. He also Squatted 585 pounds and Deadlifted 630 pounds. In our opinion, Ronnie could Bench Press 500 pounds at 198 pounds and total 1700 pounds at this same bodyweight. It sure would be a good contest to see Tom Overholtzer and Ronnie Ray square off for a meet. Even though Overholtzer is the record holder, we feel sure that Ray would win because of the fact that Ray has never been pushed in any competition that he has been in. Another good contest would be one with Gary Young, John Kantar, George Frenn, and Jon Cole. This would have to be the contest of the century. The real battle would be between Cole and Frenn. Both lifters have never been pushed and each are capable of much more than they have done.

A new face has cropped up at Joe Gold's Gym and this man could be the one to break Pat Casey's Bench Press record. This giant is Wayne Coleman, a 300 pounder who looks more like a physique contestant. His nickname is 'Abs.' Wayne made a 550 Bench Press last week with only 5 weeks of heavy bench pressing behind him. Frenn said that he had a chance at the record if he continued to keep the heavy training going. Wayne also Squatted 650 pounds and Deadlifted 650 pounds. His arms measure 21 inches cold. Man, what a man!!!

As we look over the results of the different powerlifting competitions, we are finding more and more new names and seeing less and less of the greats of yesteryear. One oldtimer who decided to make a comeback just to prove that he could still make a 550 pound Squat is Louis Paul. Louis is better known for his Deadlift of 640 pounds at 198 pound bodyweight. Louis made 505 pounds in the Squat last week after 3 weeks of training and said that when he gets to 550 pounds, in about 4 weeks, he plans to quit and continue his running.

Pat Casey told George Frenn that he would return to powerlifting this year. Pat said that he now can Bench 475 pounds, Squat 675 pounds and Deadlift 675 pounds. Pat's bodyweight is 258 pounds. The big Irishman is a policeman in Seal Beach for that city. He undoubtedly will go up to about 280 pounds in an attempt to win the Nationals. We feel that he could because there are no more good heavyweights after Don Cundy, the present champion.

Mel Hennessey is back lifting after that bout with high blood pressure which he had at the Los Angeles Nationals. Mel wants to win at least 1 title before he hangs it up. Mel said at the Nationals that he though he would break all powerlift records that night because he at the time was making a 750-pound Squat and Deadlift.

Acknowledgements

I would like to thank my friend Jean Zuver for providing original pictures for the chapter you just read; some of which have been previously posted on the internet, some you have not seen until now, I suspect. I would also like to acknowledge Dave & Laree Draper, and thank them for the awesome content on their website & forum. I suggest you check out Dave's books & other offerings available at the Irononline site; I am a big fan.

http://www.davedraper.com/index.html

Dave is a revered icon of the Golden Age, and a heck of a nice guy according to anyone who has ever had the pleasure of rubbing elbows with him. I am also indebted to one of the denizens of the Irononline forum, a guy that goes by the name "Neander", and who hosts one of the great Old-School treasure troves on the internet known as the Ditillo blog.

http://ditillo2.blogspot.com/

Dr. Ken Leistner also has a great website with lots of Old-School resources that I have borrowed from here & elsewhere;

http://www.titanstrengthandpower.com/powerlifting_articles.html

My new friend Sam Calhoun provided many pictures and some documents from his personal collection, and was right there in the thick of things at Tanny's & Muscle Beach in their boom times. Thanks, Sam! My friend Joe DiMarco, an original Culver City Westside crew member, continues to be an inspiration & is still training & building equipment in his 80s.

This site has also been an Old-School detectives dream and an invaluable resource that I suggest you take advantage of;

http://musclememory.com/

Joe Roark and his "Iron game History" has also been a tremendous help;

http://www.ironhistory.com/

http://www.la84foundation.org/5va/iron_frmst.htm

This website is yet another great resource that I have frequented and enjoyed;

_____ Iron Age Home

Thanks also to all the other websites & blogs I have referenced & used excerpts from along the way.

Please check out my website; http://www.christianiron.com/Pages/default.aspx

Check out the rest of my books there;

http://www.christianiron.com/Pages/VaultofSecrets.aspx

Stop in and visit my Old-School based Facebook page;

http://www.facebook.com/pages/Forgotten-Strength-Secrets

Thanks for reading the book, and I hope you have enjoyed it!

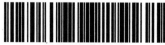

Made in the USA
Lexington, KY
22 March 2014